Level 3

How to get through

NVQ3

for

Veterinary

Nurses

Alison Lomas
BVetMed MRCVS

Annaliese H. Magee
VN AVN Dip (Surgical)

Lorraine Allan
BVSc MRCVS PGCE, D32/33/34
Veterinary Nursing Lecturer, Myerscough College

Margaret Blezard
VNCertEd TDLB, D32/33/34/35
Veterinary Nursing Lecturer, Myerscough College

Edited by
Susan L. Roberts
BVMS Cert VC MRCVS

© 2004 PASTEST Ltd
Egerton Court
Parkgate Estate
Knutsford
Cheshire
WA16 8DX

Telephone: 01565 752000

First published 2004
Reprinted 2005

ISBN: 1 901198 79 0

A catalogue record for this book is available from the British Library.

The information contained within this book was obtained by the authors from reliable sources. However, while every effort has been made to ensure its accuracy, no responsibility for loss, damage or injury occasioned to any person acting or refraining from action as a result of information contained herein can be accepted by the publishers or authors.

PasTest Revision Books and Intensive Courses

PasTest has been established in the field of postgraduate medical education since 1972, providing revision books and intensive study courses for doctors preparing for their professional examinations. Books and courses are available for the following specialties:

MRCGP, MRCP Part 1 and 2, MRCPCH Part 1 and 2, MRCPsych, MRCS, MRCOG, DRCOG, DCH, FRCA, PLAB.

For further details contact:

PasTest, Freepost, Knutsford, Cheshire WA16 7BR
Tel: 01565 752000 Fax: 01565 650264
www.pastest.co.uk enquiries@pastest.co.uk

Cover design by Andrew Shoolbred
Text prepared by Vision Typesetting Ltd, Manchester
Printed in Europe by the Alden Group, Oxford

Level 3

Contents

Unit 6: Medical nursing 131

Level 3

Foreword

In my capacity as principal and senior lecturer of a VN Training college, I was delighted when *How to Get Through NVQ2 for Veterinary Nurses* was produced. Many of my students found it extremely helpful, and referred to it throughout their studies.

Now the sister volume has been written for NVQ3 candidates and this promises to be equally successful at helping candidates prepare for the NVQ exams and appreciate the key points of their coursework.

The format of the book follows the objective syllabus exactly with each section numbered in the same way as the units in the syllabus. This is very useful for the student nurse revising for his or her exams, as it allows the candidate to check they have covered all the relevant information to the appropriate depth.

Each subject is clearly laid out with a bullet point outline of the section given first. The information is then explained clearly and concisely, and with technical accuracy. There are good diagrams, tables and plates used throughout the book to illustrate key points.

At the end of each unit, there is a self-test section of multiple choice questions. This allows candidates the opportunity to check their knowledge and understanding, and the answers and explanations are given at the end of the book.

Overall I feel this would be a very valuable addition to a student or practice library, as it is an excellent study aid for any nurse working towards their level 3 qualification. I also have no doubt that not only will this be useful for students, but also invaluable for qualified staff or those involved in nurse training.

Julie Ouston
MA, VetMB, MRCVS, PGCE, D32/33/34
Principal: MYF Training, Aldershot

About the authors

Alison Lomas qualified from the Royal Veterinary College in London. She is currently working in small animal practice at Hird & Partners in West Yorkshire.

Annaliese H. Magee qualified from Edinburgh's Telford College in 1997. She has worked in small animal and mixed practices. She gained the assessor examination in 2000 and the surgical diploma in 2003. She is now Head Nurse at Hird & Partners, Halifax, West Yorkshire.

Susan L. Roberts is a Glasgow graduate and was a clinician in small animal and mixed practice for 30 years. She now runs a peripatetic cardiology referral service in the north of England. Susan is also editor of *Veterinary Practice Nurse*.

About the contributors

Lorraine Allan is a Veterinary Nursing course tutor and lecturer at Myerscough College, Preston.

Margaret E Blezard is a Veterinary Nursing lecturer and Level 2 course tutor for Veterinary Nursing at Myerscough College.

Special thanks to Myerscough College; the staff, students and animals and especially to Mark Rosbotham for his invaluable photographic assistance.

Also to AxiomVetLab (www.axiomvetlab.com) for supplying the colour photos of blood cells. AxionVetLab retain copyright of these photos.

Level 3

Introduction

This book is written for veterinary nurses who are revising for their NVQ3 exam. Written and reviewed by experts who have had to sit the exam themselves, it is the only book that reflects the structure of the syllabus so that you follow each element by element. *How to get through NVQ3* is designed to be used for constant reference. You can either read the book from cover to cover or dip into the areas which you find particularly difficult.

How to get through NVQ3 explains the exam and gives you top tips on how to prepare for it. There are multiple choice questions at the end of each unit and the answers are thorough so that you can understand why A,B,C,D or E is the correct answer to question 1, etc.

Each element is broken down into What you need to learn sections to help you pass your exam. You can then tick off what you have learnt so far and plan the rest of your revision.

There are useful bullet points for you to remember rather than long-winded paragraphs and the text is also broken up by invaluable diagrams and photographs to help you visualise the points being made.

There is also a useful colour plate section of blood cells so you can identify what you would see under a microscope.

Finally, there is a comprehensive index that will help you find more specific areas.

How to prepare for your NVQ3

The National Vocational Qualification (NVQ) 3 exam is held every July and December. The awarding body is the Royal College of Surgeons.

The NVQ (and SVQ, the Scottish equivalent) are vocational qualifications that are based on agreed national standards of competence. Veterinary nurses train in a veterinary practice so that their skills can be assessed both at work and in an exam.

The NVQ exam consists of two written multiple choice question papers of 90 minutes each. Veterinary nurses are also expected to complete a portfolio at NVQ3. There is also a practical oral exam on:

- Diagnostic nursing
- Surgical nursing
- Radiography
- Medical nursing.

Multiple choice questions (MCQs)

MCQs are the most consistent, reproducible and internally reliable method we have of testing how much a person can remember. They also test reasoning ability and an understanding of basic facts, principles and concepts that can be assessed.

The best way of passing your exam is to know the answers to all of the questions, but you need to be able to transfer this knowledge accurately onto the answer sheet. All too often, people suffer because they haven't given themselves enough time, they haven't read the instructions carefully or they have failed to read and understand the questions.

First of all, make sure you have time to answer all the questions. If you're stuck on one MCQ leave it and go on to the next one, making a note that you need to return to that question later. The exam lasts for 90 minutes. Try and save some time to go over your answers and complete any that you may have missed.

You must read the question carefully. You should be clear that you know what you are being asked to do. Once you are sure, mark your answer boldly, correctly and clearly.

The best way to get a good mark is to have as wide a knowledge as possible of the topics being tested in the exam, rather than focusing on particular areas, hoping they will come up. Use this book to help test yourself and your colleagues. Go back over the areas which seem weak. Use the index to help you.

Last but not least, get a good night's sleep before the exam – you'll be more mentally alert to get through your NVQ3.

Portfolio tips

Modules 6 to 11, consisting of 52 case logs including expanded case reports in all. A daunting prospect? But think back to your first case log at Level 2, you were probably just as overawed. Now you are in the swing of things the Level 3 portfolio should not unnerve you at all, if you actually think of the 52 as case studies rather than in isolation. In fact it should be quite exciting for you to demonstrate and reflect on whole cases that you have seen through.

Cross-referencing will be vitally important for Level 3 for two main reasons:

1   fewer cases will need to be chosen by you and your assessor. However they should still be chosen with care to include a broad spectrum of cases covering major body systems and as many aspects of the occupational standards as possible. But also so that:
2   you will be able to use this opportunity to demonstrate the major contribution that you have played in the total veterinary care of the patient.

As a student veterinary nurse you are an extremely versatile member of the veterinary team. You help to provide the diagnostic tool by being involved with laboratory investigation and diagnostic imaging. You then contribute to the medical and surgical treatment, often have the immense responsibility of anaesthetist, actually pre and post operatively nurse the patient and then advise and counsel the client.

All of these logs could be cross-referenced demonstrating the total veterinary care of just **one** patient.

There is an opportunity to discuss your contribution to the smooth running of your training practice, by demonstrating your involvement with maintenance and availability of equipment and supplies. As health and safety legislation becomes even more vital for us all, you can apply your underpinning knowledge to the important risk assessments and maybe even suggest ideas for improvement. Health and safety, just like your portfolio, is an ongoing and progressive mission!

Knowledge and demonstration of exotic care plays a large part in both the Level 3 syllabus and portfolio. These cases provide an exciting challenge from the norm. Remember that these cases can still usually be cross referenced and that the term *exotic* does not have to be anything other than a *small furry*.

When choosing your case remember that there does not have to always be a successful outcome. Many cases are very rewarding but equally some may be extremely sad. There is always a bright side and this will give you plenty of opportunity for your reflective student comment! A typical entry in the student comments box is: 'I really enjoyed working on this case.' This is meaningless! It is important that you actually reflect on your involvement and show how you have learnt from it.

General portfolio guideline tips

- **Portfolio guidelines** for each module and relevant **occupational standards** should be constantly referred to by both you and your assessor. This is vital to ensure that all of the scope and all of the performance criteria are included in the whole of the module. Remember that it is unlikely that one log can provide all of the evidence. This could be included in later logs or your assessor can include questions and answers to prove that you have all of the underpinning knowledge, even if you have not been involved in a relevant case.
- **Simulated cases** are not permitted in Level 3. All case logs should be completed relevant to an actual case. Remember that when your IV makes a routine visit to your practice they will actually cross check your logs with client records to verify your involvement. In the unlikely event that your practice does not have certain equipment or never perform certain tasks, such as ultrasound or the administration of blood or colloids, then your IV must be informed **early** in your portfolio progression. Provided that your VNAC has plenty of notice of the situation they may be able to arrange an authentic case for you or a short secondment to another practice.
- **RCVS Annexes.** Make new photocopies of all annexes and start to fill them in at the beginning of Level 3. They must be continually updated amended by you and your assessor.
- Back up computer work and keep up to date photocopies of everything.
- Correction fluid is NOT allowed. To obliterate confidential client details a black marker pen should be used and then the back of the sheet should also be obliterated.
- Bullet points are clear and concise. Extra detail can be included in expanded case reports.
- Enter all case log boxes.
- Spelling and correct use of English language and veterinary terminology is vital for Level 3. Exceptions will only be permitted if indicated on the log by your assessor. However progression will still be accounted for.
- Abbreviations and all clinical parameters should initially be accompanied by a full explanation of the norm. Recognise that even if certain points were explained fully at Level 2, these details will not be included with your Level 3 portfolio and your assessor and IV may have changed.
- **Case identification** should be kept as clear and unambiguous as possible. It is advisable not to use a computer reference as your main log identification, however this should still be listed for everyone's reference.

eg of log identification for Module 9c Surgical nursing – general
SN 3(Computer 13966)

- It is vital that the main ID is easy to follow, particularly when cross referencing. For example:

LOGSHEET 7b – Fluid Management

> 3.   **Major presenting problems and history:**
> - 8% dehydration due to vomiting and anorexia for 5 days
> - severe abdominal pain exhibited by patient often lying in 'praying dog' position
> - admit for X-rays, general anaesthetic and laparotomy to investigate and remove possible intestinal foreign body
>   **CR** – RAD 5 (Computer 13966)
>   – SN 3 (Computer 13966)
>   – AN 2 (Computer 13966)

- **Generic drug names** must be used throughout but also include
- (brackets are useful) the retail drug name.
- **Calculations**
  It is not always necessary to include calculations for dispensed and administered medicines as this will have been demonstrated at Level 2, however it is vital that complete calculations are included in fluid therapy and anaesthetics.
  Dose rate calculations for anaesthetics should clearly show the working in milligrams (mg) as well as mls.
  All calculations should clearly state the units involved. For example in Fluid management calculations each step should clearly state – the fluid deficit in ml, the total volume required in ml per hour, ml per minute and the drip rate as drops per minute and drops per second.
  - **Anaesthetic monitoring records** should also include all agents and medication in mg and ml where necessary.
    Even though there is no requirement to include whether the ET tube was cuffed or not, this information should be added, especially in the case of cat anaesthesia studies. Also include this piece of vital information on the log sheet.
- **Hospitalisation records** should always be included where indicated by the portfolio guidelines, particularly in the case of the expanded case reports. Photocopies are authentic evidence provided that they have been dated and signed by your assessor, and they must show where you actually nursed the patient. False entries on a photocopied sheet are easy for an IV to detect that a student was not actually involved in a case. This is a common unacceptable falsification.

- You should highlight your involvement with the case, particularly if more than one nurse also had input.
- **Radiography** log sheets should only demonstrate one projection on each log, even though you probably actually exposed 2 views on the one film. The other view could however be mentioned on the log.
- **Appendices** as with Level 2 should be used to show extra evidence and save some time for yourself. Suitable appendices would be biological parameters (including exotics), exotic care, radiography processing, details of anaesthetic machine and circuits, preoperative preparation of patient etc. etc.
- Ensure that all appendices are clearly signed and dated by yourself and the assessor and include your RCVS enrolment number. All this information must be included on ANY other extra evidence.
- Make certain that all appendices are clearly cross referenced between case logs and include them **all together** either at the very front of all of the logs or at the very back It is confusing for your IV if appendices are interspersed throughout your portfolio.

Sixty per cent of the portfolio must be completed by the time you actually APPLY to sit the Level 3 external examination. In fact your Practice principal must sign a declaration on your examination form to that effect. The 15th April and 1st October are the final dates for the receipt of examination applications at the RCVS. The RCVS will not accept ANY late entries, for whatever reason, so this does mean that you and your assessor should set an absolute target for the end of March or the middle of September. (There is a 2 month *window* for application entries, so there really is no room for excuses here.)

The remaining 40% should be completed as soon as possible. It is very tempting to put completion on hold until after the final examination, but it will be even harder to pick up again afterwards. A gap of only a few months may mean that the evidence you have already provided would no longer be current and therefore may not be accepted by your IV.

Always check with your IV/ VNAC if you have any worries or problems that cannot be resolved by discussion with your assessor.

Remember that even though you will have striven for a successful outcome in the external (RCVS) examination you cannot achieve unit certification for Level 3 and be listed as a VN until your portfolio has been successfully verified.

Good luck!

Margaret E. Blezard
VNCertEd TDLB, D32/33/34/35

Level 3: Unit 5

Laboratory diagnostic aids

3.5.01   Laboratory health and safety

What you need to learn

* You need to be able to describe the important points of legislative Acts and Regulations that affect laboratory work:
  * Health & Safety at Work Act (1974)
  * Control of Substances Hazardous to Health (COSHH) Regulations 1988
  * Control of Pollution (special waste) Regulations (1988)
  * Collection & Disposal of Waste Regulations (1988)
  * Environmental Protection Act (1990)
  * Reporting of Injuries, Diseases and Dangerous Occurrences Regulations (RIDDOR) (1995)
  * First Aid at Work.
* Identify common hazards in the laboratory and the relevant warning/hazard signs:
  * chemical
  * biological
  * toxic fumes
  * eye contamination
  * cuts
  * other injuries.
* Identify the correct disposal of laboratory waste:
  * normal
  * clinical
  * special
  * glass.
* Describe the action that should be taken in the event of an accident or emergency in the laboratory:
  * spillage of chemicals
  * spillage of biological fluids/substances
  * toxic fumes
  * eye contaminations
  * cuts and other injuries to personnel
  * zoonoses.

There are many potential hazards in the veterinary laboratory and it is very important to be aware of the risks so that accidents can be avoided. There are a number of laws and regulations designed to protect people who work in laboratories. These include:

- **The Health and Safety Act (1974):** This act is designed to maintain and improve health and safety standards at work. It provides protection against risks in the workplace and controls the storage and use of dangerous substances. It explains the duties of an employer to protect his/her employees. It also ensures that the activities of workers do not endanger anybody.
- **The Control of Substances Hazardous to Health (COSHH) Regulations (1999):** This is the main legislation covering the control of risks to staff from exposure to harmful substances at work. The aim of the regulations is to reduce occupational illness. Substances harmful to health include cleaning materials, waste products, disease-causing organisms and numerous other items. The COSHH regulations include risk assessment; monitoring and controlling exposure to harmful substances; and training, information and supervision for the handling of hazardous substances.
- **The Control of Pollution (Special Waste) Regulations (1998), Collection and Disposal of Waste Regulations (1998) and Environmental Protection Act (1990):** These acts describe the safe handling and disposal of products including clinical waste and chemicals. They cover the correct disposal of such materials so that damage to the environment is minimised.
- **Reporting of Injuries, Diseases and Dangerous Occurrences Regulations (RIDDOR) (1995):** These regulations describe the procedures which must take place if death, serious injury, or work-related disease occur in the workplace. The supervising staff must report to the Health and Safety Executive (HSE) if:
  - an injury occurs which necessitates more than three days off work for the affected person;
  - a reportable, work-related disease is diagnosed. In veterinary work this could include leptospirosis, aspergillosis, anthrax, tetanus, or tuberculosis;
  - there is a dangerous occurrence. This can include explosions, chemical leaks, collapse of the building or of equipment and many other things.
- **First Aid at Work:** Standard first-aid procedures should be available in the veterinary laboratory. It is important that first-aid equipment, such as eye wash, is easily available and in working condition.

Common hazards in the laboratory include:

- chemicals – detergents, chemical stains, reagents, acids and alkalis
- biological agents – bacterial swabs and cultures, viruses, parasites
- toxic fumes – any agent which can be inhaled including gases, aerosols and spores
- eye contaminants – any kind of liquid or dust particle which can be splashed in the eye (in the case of contamination the eyes should be rinsed immediately with an eye wash)
- sharp objects – including needles, vials, glass slides, etc; these can cause cuts or scratches, and can provide a route of infection for zoonotic diseases.

To avoid injury certain precautions should be taken in the laboratory:

- There should be no food or drink in the laboratory at any time.
- Protective coats, gloves, and if necessary eye glasses, should be worn when handling hazardous material.
- Long hair should always be tied back.
- The laboratory should always be kept clean and free of clutter.
- No unauthorised personnel should be allowed to use the laboratory without supervision. This includes work-experience students.
- Waste should be disposed of safely. This means that items such as needles and glass should be placed in a sharps bin; and biological material, such as body fluids, tissue samples and contaminated equipment, should be placed in the clinical-waste bin. (NB Samples containing infectious agents such as culture plates should be sterilised before being placed in clinical-waste bags.)
- Special waste – this includes veterinary clinical waste such as body fluids, tissues and cadavers.
- A normal waste bin should be provided for uncontaminated material such as paper.
- Hands should be washed when leaving the laboratory using an appropriate antibacterial soap.
- A number of hazard symbols are used to warn the handler of the potential risks.

Figure 5.1 Hazard symbols.

In the event of an accident in the veterinary laboratory:

- The safety of personnel is the most important issue.
- First-aid and resuscitation techniques must be administered where necessary. Medical attention should be sought where necessary.
- If there are serious injuries an ambulance should be called.
- Medical attention should also be sought if:
  - toxic fumes may have been inhaled
  - any chemical or biological substance has been splashed in the eyes
  - the accident has involved contamination with a potentially zoonotic disease.
- Any spills should be contained and disposed of safely. This may include neutralising acid or alkaline spills.
- If an infectious agent is involved, thorough disinfection or sterilisation may be necessary.
- The incident should be recorded in the practice accident book.
- If the accident is of a serious nature it should be reported according to the RIDDOR regulations.

(See NVQ Level 2, 2.1.06 First aid in the workplace).

3.5.02 Laboratory apparatus

What you need to learn

☙ You need to be able to describe the care and cleaning of routine laboratory apparatus:
  - ❧ glassware
  - ❧ microscope
  - ❧ centrifuge.
☙ Describe the special care and maintenance of electronic analysers:
  - ❧ biochemistry
  - ❧ haematology.
☙ Describe systems for monitoring the regular quality control checks of in-house equipment.

The apparatus within the veterinary laboratory is expensive and very sensitive to damage. Careful maintenance is vital to ensure that the apparatus remains fully functional and that the results provided by the precision instruments are accurate.

Equipment present in most laboratories includes:

- various glassware including pipettes, bottles, blood tubes and slides
- a microscope
- a centrifuge
- biochemistry, haematology and electrolyte analysers.

Cleaning and care of laboratory equipment

- Glassware is often disposable, and should be placed in suitable clinical-waste containers after use.
- Reusable glassware should be soaked in disinfectant before cleaning.
- Any visible material should be carefully removed using disposable gloves and a soft brush or cloth.
- The glassware should then be soaked in disinfectant. Some practices use ultrasonic cleaning baths at this stage.
- The glassware should then be rinsed, drained and left to dry.
- According to health and safety regulations, all electrical equipment should be checked regularly for safety.
- The microscope should be switched off and covered when not in use to avoid contamination from spills and dust.
- The microscope should be stored away from vibrating objects (such as the centrifuge) or liquids (eg stains, etc) to avoid damage.
- The eyepieces and lenses should be cleaned regularly using special lens paper which is designed not to scratch the glass.
- The oil immersion lens should be cleaned after every use to prevent build-up of oil.
- The centrifuge should be regularly cleaned and serviced to ensure reliability.
- When the centrifuge is to be used care should be taken to fasten the safety plate over the samples before the lid is replaced. This ensures that the tubes are held safely in place. Failure to do this usually results in the tubes breaking, which is potentially hazardous.
- Any spillage in the centrifuge should be cleaned carefully while wearing disposable gloves.
- Electronic analysers should be switched off and covered when not in use to avoid contamination from spills and dust.
- Electronic analysers should be stored away from vibrating objects (such as the centrifuge) or liquids (eg stains, etc) to avoid damage.
- Analysers should be serviced regularly and should always be used in accordance with the instruction manual.
- Quality control tests should be performed regularly to ensure that the results received from the analysers are accurate.
- Quality control tests usually involve running samples which have a known result (usually a low sample, normal sample and high sample are tested) and checking the results against the known results.
- Quality control can also be tested by sending samples to an independent laboratory and checking the results against the

in-house results for the same sample. These are known as external quality control tests.

3.5.03 The microscope

What you need to learn

🐾 You need to be able to describe the care and cleaning of routine laboratory apparatus. Parts include:
  🐾 foot
  🐾 limb
  🐾 body
  🐾 stage
  🐾 mechanical stage
  🐾 substage condenser
  🐾 iris diaphragm
  🐾 light source
  🐾 coarse adjustment
  🐾 fine adjustment
  🐾 nose piece
  🐾 eye piece
  🐾 Vernier scales
  🐾 eye lenses.
🐾 Describe the functions of the parts of a microscope.
🐾 Describe the correct method of using a microscope.
🐾 Describe how to examine a specimen on a microscope slide. The methods are:
  🐾 low power
  🐾 high power
  🐾 oil immersion.
🐾 Explain the use of the Vernier scale to plot the position of specimens.

The microscope is an essential tool in the veterinary laboratory. It is used for examining biological samples such as blood smears, urine samples, hair plucks, skin scrapes, fine-needle aspirates and impression smears.

The microscope used in the practice laboratory will be a light, or compound, microscope.

Other types of microscope are:

• Scanning electron microscope – used for viewing objects at 50,000 up to 100,000 times magnification.
• Transmission electron microscope – used for viewing objects at a magnification of up to 500,000 times.

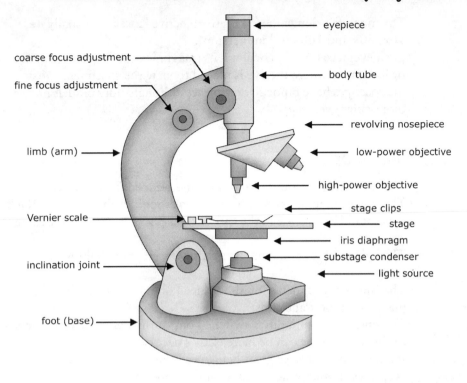

eyepiece

coarse focus adjustment

fine focus adjustment

body tube

revolving nosepiece

low-power objective

limb (arm)

high-power objective

stage clips

Vernier scale

stage

iris diaphragm

substage condenser

inclination joint

light source

foot (base)

Figure 5.2 Basic light microscope.

- The **foot** of the microscope is the base which supports the microscope.
- The **limb,** or arm, attaches the eyepiece and body to the foot.
- The **body** is the tube which supports the eyepiece.
- The **stage** is the platform on which the specimen slide is placed. The **stage clips** hold the slide in place.
- The **substage condenser** focuses light onto the slide.
- The **iris diaphragm** is an adjustable opening beneath the stage. It can be used to vary the amount of light on the stage.
- The **light source** directs light upwards onto the stage. The amount of light produced at the light source can be varied.
- The **coarse adjustment** is a knob which allows large adjustments in focus to be made.
- The **fine adjustment** is a smaller knob which allows smaller adjustments in focus to be made.
- The **nosepiece** is a revolving disc which holds the objective lenses. It is possible to rotate the nose piece so that a particular objective lens is selected.
- The **objective lenses** allow the specimen to be viewed at different magnifications. There are usually three or four objective lenses. Often one of the objective lenses can be used with immersion oil.

The magnification values of these objective lenses are usually 4×, 10×, 40× and 100× (oil immersion).

- Each **eyepiece** holds an **ocular lens** (magnification is usually 4×, 6×, or 8×) and is where the eye is placed to view the specimen. Most microscopes have binocular eyepieces although older models have a monocular eyepiece.

Using the microscope

- The microscope should be checked and cleaned if necessary.
- The lowest magnification objective lens should be in place and the lens should be as close to the specimen as possible without touching it.
- The light source should be turned down so that the light is at a dim setting.
- The slide or specimen should be placed on the stage and held in place using the stage clips.
- The microscope should be switched on. At this stage the brightness of the light source can be increased as necessary.
- If a binocular microscope is being used the distance between the eyepieces should be adjusted to suit the operator.
- The specimen should be brought into the field of view by adjusting the mechanical stage, and by using the coarse, and then fine, focus knobs. Focus adjustment knobs must always be used to move the objective lens away from the specimen. This prevents damage to the specimen or slide by the end of the objective lens.
- The condenser and light diaphragm can be adjusted until the specimen is clearly illuminated.
- Once the specimen has been examined thoroughly under low power (using the mechanical stage to move across the sample area) areas of particular interest may be viewed at higher magnification by rotating the nosepiece and selecting an appropriate objective lens.
- Oil immersion can be used to view the specimen at higher magnification. A drop of immersion oil is placed on the coverslip or directly onto the slide. The end of the oil immersion lens is lowered into the drop of oil using the fine focus knob. Care must be taken not to touch the specimen with the lens.
- To calculate the total magnification used the following equation is used:

Magnification = magnification of × magnification of
objective lens   eyepiece lens.

3.5.04   The centrifuge

What you need to learn

- You need to be able to describe common types of centrifuge:
  - electric
  - microhaematocrit.
- Describe the working parts and the function of both types of centrifuge. Terms include:
  - safety plate
  - bucket
  - rubber cushion
  - guard bowl.
- State the precautions which should be taken when using a centrifuge.

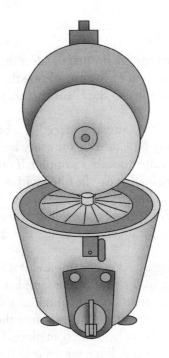

Figure 5.3   Centrifuge microhaematocrit.

There are two types of centrifuge which are commonly encountered in veterinary practices:

- the electric centrifuge
- the microhaematocrit centrifuge.

The **electric centrifuge** is a device which spins samples of liquids at high speed so that more dense particles or liquids sink to the bottom of the sample while lighter particles or fluids float to the top. The deposit left at the bottom of the sample after centrifugation is called the **sediment**. The liquid on top of the sediment is called the **supernatant**. The electric centrifuge can therefore be used to:

- separate cells from liquid in a sample
- concentrate a sediment (eg crystals in a urine sample).

The **microhaematocrit centrifuge** is used to separate blood samples which are placed in special capillary tubes.

- The microhaematocrit centrifuge allows accurate measurement of the packed cell volume of a blood sample.
- Many haematology analysers use a microhaematocrit centrifuge to separate the layers of white blood cells so that cell counts can be made.

Using the centrifuge

- The rotors of the centrifuge are housed inside a thick metal **guard bowl**. This protects the operator by preventing the rotors from bursting out of the centrifuge in the event that they become detached.
- In an electric centrifuge the sample is placed in a **bucket**. The buckets should be evenly balanced (ie for every bucket used the opposite bucket should also contain a sample). If only one sample is to be spun the opposing bucket can be filled with a water sample to provide balance.
- In a microhaematocrit centrifuge the **capillary tubes** are placed horizontally in slots. As for an electric centrifuge the samples should be balanced.
- At the base of each sample bucket or sample slot is a **rubber cushion** which prevents damage to the base of the sample tube.
- When using the microhaematocrit centrifuge care should be taken to fasten the **safety plate** over the samples before the lid is replaced. This ensures that the tubes are held safely in place. Failure to do this usually results in the tubes breaking, which is potentially hazardous.

3.5.05   Laboratory analyses

What you need to learn

- ❧ You need to be able to describe common types of laboratory analysers:
  - ❧ biochemistry wet/dry chemistry
  - ❧ haematology

☙ hormones
☙ electrolytes.
❧ Outline their uses in veterinary practice.

Analysers which are encountered frequently in veterinary practice include:

• biochemistry analysers
• haematology analysers
• electrolyte analysers
• hormone analysers.

Biochemistry machines

Biochemistry machines are used to measure levels of substances in the blood such as:

• blood urea nitrogen (BUN)
• creatinine
• albumin
• globulin
• total protein
• amylase
• calcium
• glucose
• cholesterol
• bilirubin
• alkaline phosphatase (ALKP)
• alanine aminotransferase (ALT).

Most of the commonly used biochemistry analysers are **dry chemistry** systems. These place a small amount of the sample onto a series of slides. A colour change occurs on each slide which reflects the amount of whichever substance is being measured. The machine reads the colour change and interprets it automatically, providing a value for the level of substance in the sample.

Some chemistry analysers use **wet chemistry** systems. In these systems the colour change occurs in a small well of fluid rather than on a slide. The colour change is read and interpreted automatically by the machine.

The results are compared with the normal reference range for each parameter measured. The information provided by measuring levels of these substances in a blood sample allows the veterinary surgeon to:

• diagnose disease
• monitor the progression of the disease by testing serial samples

- monitor recovery from disease
- check the health of an animal prior to sedation or anaesthesia.

Haematology machines

Haematology machines are used to measure automatically the numbers of the cells which make up whole blood. These include:

- lymphocytes
- monocytes
- neutrophils
- eosinophils
- basophils
- platelets
- erythrocytes
- reticulocytes (immature erythrocytes).

The proportion of the blood sample which is made up of erythrocytes (red blood cells) is expressed as the haematocrit or packed cell volume (PCV).

- Haematology machines are very useful for assessing whether an animals is anaemic, and for characterising the type of anaemia (regenerative, non-regenerative, etc).
- They are also used to assess disorders or changes in the white blood cells such as inflammatory change or neoplastic change (such as leukaemia).
- An assessment of platelet numbers can be useful in the diagnosis of some clotting disorders.

Electrolyte analysers

Electrolyte analysers are used to measure plasma electrolyte levels from a blood sample. Parameters measured include:

- sodium ions
- potassium ions
- chloride ions
- carbon dioxide (bicarbonate ions)
- calcium ions
- inorganic phosphate ions.

Electrolyte measurement can be of great importance in:

- diagnosing diseases such as Addison's disease (hypoadrenocorticism)
- monitoring the acid-base balance of animals which may be suffering from acidosis or alkalosis, including animals with

diarrhoea and vomiting
• measuring changes caused by dehydration

Calcium and phosphate levels are useful in animals with conditions such as hyperparathyroidism, hypocalcaemia (eg postpartum), neoplasia and ethylene glycol toxicity.

Hormone analysers

Hormone analysers are used to measure levels of hormones from blood samples. The hormones that are regularly measured include:

• thyroxine (T_4)
• cortisol
• insulin
• reproductive hormones.

Thyroxine is the only one of these which is regularly measured using an in-house analyser. Most of the others are measured at an external laboratory.

Hormone measurement is important for the diagnosis of conditions such as hyper- and hypothyroidism, diabetes mellitus or the presence of an insulinoma (insulin-producing tumour), hyper- and hypoadrenocorticism (Cushing's disease and Addison's disease respectively). It is also used to assess the stage of the reproductive cycle in breeding animals, and to diagnose reproductive disorders.

3.5.06   Test kits

What you need to learn
❧ You need to be able to describe the principles of use for commercial test kits:
❧ FeLV (ELISA)
❧ FIV
❧ canine parvovirus
❧ Premate®
❧ allergies
❧ assessment of clotting.

A number of in-house test kits are available which are used to:

• diagnose diseases caused by viruses such as canine parvovirus, feline immunodeficiency virus (FIV) and feline leukaemia virus (FeLV)
• check hormone levels in breeding animals

• check for allergies
• check blood clotting. (Simplate II measures buccal mucosal bleeding time.)

The **ELISA** (enzyme linked immunosorbent assay) test is used to test for diseases such as FeLV and FIV in cats or parvovirus in dogs. There are also ELISA tests available which detect whether an animal is suffering from allergy (eg detects antibodies to fleas, pollen and house-dust mites).

The **FeLV ELISA** test detects viral **antigens** in the blood. The test well is impregnated with antibodies to FeLV. Any viral antigens in the blood sample bind with these antibodies and activate a dye. This produces the coloured line or spot seen in a positive result.

The **FIV ELISA** test detects **antibodies** to FIV in the blood. The test well is impregnated with FIV antigens. Any antibodies in the blood sample bind with these antigens and activate the dye.

The canine **parvovirus ELISA** test detects viral **antigens** from a faeces sample. It works in the same way as the tests described. Care must be taken when interpreting the results as animals which have been vaccinated with a live parvovirus vaccine may shed viral antigens in the faeces for 5 to 12 days afterwards, giving a false-positive test result.

The **Premate®** test is an ELISA test which measures progesterone levels in serum or plasma. It is used to detect the rise in progesterone levels which occurs when a bitch ovulates so that the breeder can choose the optimum time to mate the bitch. It works in the same way as the tests described. Blood samples are taken every 24–48 h from the bitch. Before the bitch ovulates the progesterone levels are low (>2 ng/ml) and the test shows a dark pink colour. When the bitch ovulates progesterone levels rise and the test becomes lighter pink in colour. Breeders often choose to mate the bitch when levels reach >10 ng/ml.

The **Allercept®** e-screen test is an ELISA test which detects immunoglobulin E (IgE). It is used to determine whether an animal is suffering from an allergy. A serum or plasma sample is used. The test works in the same way as the tests described. The presence of IgE in the sample causes a colour change in the sample well. This test suggests that allergy is likely and further samples can be sent to an external laboratory to determine exactly to what the animal is allergic.

3.5.07　Blood

What you need to learn

- You need to be able to describe terms related to blood:
  - plasma
  - serum
  - anticoagulant
  - haemolysis
  - lipaemia.
- Describe the measurement of red cell parameters:
  - Mean Corpuscular Volume (MCV)
  - Mean Corpuscular Haemoglobin Concentration (MCHC)
  - PCV
  - RBC
  - Hb.
- Describe common sites that are suitable for the collection of samples and list the veins involved in these species:
  - dogs
  - cats
  - other companion animals eg birds, rodents, lagomorphs, reptiles.
- Identify the equipment needed for the collection of blood:
  - syringe
  - needle
  - Vacutainer etc.
- Describe the principles of venipuncture in these species:
  - dogs
  - cats
  - other companion animals.
- Describe suitable techniques for handling/restraining animals during the collection of blood samples:
  - cats
  - dogs
  - other companion animals
  - manual
  - chemical.
- Describe the tests which are carried out on whole blood, serum and plasma:
  - haematological
  - biochemistry.
- Describe haemolysis and outline the precautions which should be taken to prevent blood samples haemolysing:
  - serum
  - plasma samples
  - sampling technique

* lipaemia
* patient preparation
* storage
* transport
* smear preparation.

🐾 Describe the different anticoagulants used to obtain whole blood samples:

* ethylene diamine tetra-acetic acid (EDTA)
* heparin
* ammonium and potassium oxalate mixture
* sodium fluoride and potassium oxalate mixture
* disodium hydrogen citrate.

🐾 Describe the system of colour coding commercial blood containers/vacutainers.

🐾 Describe how to store and preserve samples if testing is delayed:

* whole blood
* plasma
* serum.

🐾 Describe principles of using electronic analysers to calculate total blood cell counts.

🐾 Describe the principles of obtaining a white/red blood cell count electronically.

Blood makes up approximately 8–10% of body mass. It is made up of various cells suspended in a liquid (**plasma**).

Plasma

Plasma is the liquid in which the cells are suspended. It contains:

* plasma proteins (mainly albumin and globulin)
* clotting proteins (such as fibrinogen)
* hormones
* metabolic substrates and products (lipids, carbohydrates such as glucose, vitamins, amino acids, etc)
* water.

When blood has clotted the clotting proteins have all been used up. The liquid remaining is called **serum**. (Serum therefore contains all the same things as plasma except clotting proteins.)

Blood sampling is performed regularly in veterinary practice.

Blood can be processed in a number of ways depending on what tests are to be performed.

* For haematology evaluation it is important that the blood sample does not clot. **Anti-coagulants** are used to prevent blood clotting.

Usually the blood sample tube is impregnated with the anti-coagulant agent. The commonly used anti-coagulants are heparin and EDTA (ethylene diamine tetra-acetic acid). Occasionally oxalate fluoride or citrate are used as the anti-coagulant.

- For biochemistry evaluation serum is usually used, so a plain tube is used for collection of the blood sample.

Haemolysis is the loss of haemoglobin from red blood cells caused by damage to the cell membrane.

- The plasma/serum of a haemolysed sample is pink to red in colour.
- It can be caused by some diseases but is more often caused during sampling and handling of the blood sample. Freezing, excessive suction when sampling, shaking of the blood tube, or centrifugation can all cause haemolysis.
- Haemolysis can interfere with many test results.

Lipaemia is the increased turbidity (milky appearance) of the plasma/serum in fresh samples. It is caused by the presence of fat (triglycerides and chylomicrons in particular) in the blood sample.

- Lipaemia is often seen when a blood sample is obtained shortly after a meal.
- Lipaemia can interfere with many test results.

Red cell parameters

The **packed cell volume (PCV)** [also called the **haematocrit (Hct)**] is the proportion of the blood made up by red blood cells (ie not including white blood cells or platelets).

- It is often expressed as a percentage.
- Normal ranges are: cat, 30–45%; dog, 37–55%.
- PCV is often increased in athletic animals, particularly following exercise (following splenic contraction).
- Generally a low PCV indicates anaemia, while a high value suggests dehydration.

The **red blood cell (RBC) count** is the number of red blood cells per litre of blood.

- Generally a low RBC count indicates anaemia, while a high value suggests dehydration.

The **haemoglobin concentration (Hb)** is the amount of haemoglobin in a volume of blood.

- It is usually expressed as grams per litre or decilitre (g/l or g/dl).
- Generally a low Hb indicates anaemia, while a high value suggests

dehydration.

The **mean corpuscular volume (MCV)** is a measure of the size of individual red blood cells.

- RBCs of normal size are called **normocytic.**
- An increase in MCV suggests that RBC are larger than usual (**macrocytic**). This can occur in regenerative anaemia (immature RBC are larger than mature ones).
- A decrease in MCV suggests abnormally small cells (**microcytic**). This can occur in iron-deficiency anaemia.

The **mean corpuscular haemoglobin concentration (MCHC)** is a measure of the amount of haemoglobin in an individual red blood cell.

- RBC with a normal MCHC are called **normochromic.**
- An increase in MCHC is usually an error in results as a cell cannot hold more haemoglobin.
- A decrease in MCHC suggests a low haemoglobin content (**hypochromic**). Some immature RBC (such as reticulocytes) are hypochromic. RBC in iron-deficiency anaemia are often hypochromic.

Blood sampling

Before taking a blood sample the correct equipment must be assembled.

- The syringe used should be of a suitable volume. It is best to use the smallest volume possible so that the RBCs are exposed to as little pressure as possible (For example, if 1 ml of blood is required a 2 ml syringe will suffice and a 5 ml or 10 ml syringe should be avoided.)
- The correct gauge of needle should be selected. The needle should be as large a gauge as possible to allow the sample to be taken swiftly, and to prevent damage to blood cells. A 22-gauge 5/8-inch or 1-inch needle is suitable for dogs and cats. Smaller gauge needles are necessary in smaller species or young animals.
- Blood can also be collected directly into a tube known as a **vacutainer**. These are usually made of glass and are sealed at one end with a rubber bung. There is a vacuum within the tube. One end of a double-ended needle is placed into the vein, the other end is then used to pierce the bung. The blood flows into the tube to fill the vacuum. When enough blood has been withdrawn the needle is withdrawn from the vein. The inside of the vacutainer is often coated with anti-coagulants such as heparin or EDTA.

The insertion of a needle or catheter into a vein is known as **venipuncture.**

- The largest accessible vein should be used for venipuncture.
- The most commonly used veins are the cephalic vein in the foreleg, the jugular vein in the neck and, occasionally, the saphenous vein in the hindlimb (Table 5.1).
- The injection site should be clipped and prepared aseptically.
- An assistant restrains the patient and occludes the proximal part of the vein. This causes the vein to fill with blood and appear more prominent.
- The needle is inserted at a shallow angle.
- The plunger is pulled back slowly, taking care not to collapse the vein with excessive suction.
- Once the required volume has been obtained the needle is withdrawn.
- The assistant puts pressure on the injection site to prevent bleeding from the punctured vein. After a minute or two a clot will form over the puncture site within the vein so the pressure can be released.
- The blood sample should quickly be transferred into the sample tube. The needle should be detached from the syringe before expelling the sample from the syringe. This prevents damage to the red blood cells.
- The collection tube should be filled to the line indicated to ensure that the anti-coagulant is diluted correctly.
- The sample tube should be rolled or inverted to mix the contents. Shaking the tube can cause damage to the red blood cells.

Table 5.1 Sites for blood sampling in various species

Species	Site for blood sampling
Rabbits	As for dogs and cats but also marginal ear vein
Small rodents	Usually jugular; may require anaesthesia
Birds	Jugular vein, ulnar vein (medial elbow), saphenous vein, tarsal vein (larger birds); may require anaesthesia
Reptiles	Jugular vein, coccygeal vein (underside of tail), intracardiac (not tortoises)

Handling/restraint for venipuncture varies with the species involved.

- Manual restraint is normally sufficient for restraining cats and dogs for blood sampling.
- Aggressive or fractious animals should be muzzled and, if necessary, sedated.
- It is usually possible to obtain a blood sample from a rabbit without sedation. The use of topical local anaesthetic at the venepuncture site can facilitate the procedure.
- Sedation or general anaesthesia is usually necessary for blood sampling from exotic species.

• It is usually safer and less stressful to anaesthetise most birds for blood sampling. An exception is large birds such as swans and geese, as blood can be taken from the tarsal vein with minimal stress.

Blood tests

To obtain information from the sample a number of tests are performed.

Serum biochemistry is used to measure levels of substances in the blood such as:

• blood urea nitrogen (BUN)
• creatinine
• albumin
• globulin
• total protein
• amylase
• calcium
• glucose
• cholesterol
• bilirubin
• alkaline phosphatase (ALKP)
• alanine aminotransferase (ALT).

Biochemistry measurements are taken from serum or plasma samples, and are not concerned with the cells contained within the blood.

Haematology is concerned with the cells which are suspended in the plasma. For this reason haematology evaluation is performed on whole blood which has been prevented from clotting.

Haematology machines are used to measure automatically numbers of the cells which make up whole blood. These include:

• lymphocytes
• monocytes
• neutrophils
• eosinophils
• basophils
• platelets
• reticulocytes (immature erythrocytes).

Haematology analysers also measure and calculate the haematological values such as PCV, RBC, MCV, MCHC.

For a full haematology evaluation it is vital that the morphology (shape and size) of the blood cells is examined from a fresh blood smear.

The morphology of blood cells can provide information about the progress of a disease (whether changes are acute or chronic; regenerative or non-regenerative) and can aid in diagnosis of blood-borne diseases such as *Leishmaniasis* and *Haemobartonella* infections.

A smear should therefore be produced and examined for every haematology sample, to confirm the results provided by the analyser.

Other tests

Many hundreds of tests can be performed on blood samples. Those commonly used in veterinary practice include:

- hormone tests (thyroid hormones, adrenal hormones, insulin, reproductive hormones, etc)
- organ function tests (bile acid stimulation test, TLI (trypsin-like immunoreactivity), folate and cobalamin measurements, etc)
- levels of drugs in the blood (phenobarbitone, thyroxine, potassium bromide)
- levels of other substances in the blood (heavy metals such as lead, zinc, etc)
- serology for infectious diseases (FeLV, FIV, toxoplasmosis, coronavirus, etc)
- electrolytes.

Haemolysis

Haemolysis is the loss of haemoglobin from red blood cells caused by damage to the cell membrane.

- The plasma/serum of a haemolysed sample is pink to red in colour.
- It can be caused by some diseases but is more often caused during sampling and handling of the blood sample. Freezing or overheating, or excessive suction when sampling, shaking of the blood tube, or centrifugation, can all cause haemolysis.
- Haemolysis can interfere with many test results.

To avoid haemolysis:

- Excessive suction should be avoided when obtaining the sample.
- The blood should only pass through the needle once (ie the needle should be removed before transferring the sample into the sample tube).
- The sample tube should be inverted or rolled rather than shaken.
- The sample should be stored at a cool but not freezing temperature

and direct sunlight should be avoided.
- The sample should be evaluated or posted to the laboratory as soon as possible.
- The sample should be properly packaged to protect against temperature variations and careless handling.
- Clean dry equipment should always be used.
- Samples should normally be taken when the patient has been starved (unless a post-prandial (post-meal) sample is required for the test, as is the case in a bile acid stimulation test) to avoid lipaemia.
- Fresh smears can be made when a blood sample is taken for haematology evaluation. This allows examination of the cell morphology and can be used to provide cell counts if the whole blood sample is damaged after sampling.

Anti-coagulants

Various anti-coagulants are available for use with blood samples. They are listed in Table 5.2 with their characteristics and uses.

Table 5.2 Anti-coagulants

Anti-coagulant	Uses	Tube colour	Vacutainer colour
No anti-coagulant (plain)	Biochemistry and serology	Brown or clear	Red
EDTA	Haematology	Pink/red	Purple
Heparin	Biochemistry, trace elements	Orange	Green or yellow
Ammonia/potassium oxalate	Glucose	Yellow	Grey
Sodium fluoride/ potassium oxalate	Glucose	Yellow	Grey
Sodium citrate	Coagulation profiles	Lilac	Dark blue

Storage of samples

Ideally samples should be processed immediately after they are obtained. This is because many results change as the sample degrades over time.

If this is not possible the sample should be stored in a manner which minimises degradation.

- If the delay is for a few hours the sample can be stored at 4°C in a refrigerator.
- If the delay is prolonged (more than a few hours) the serum or

plasma can be decanted from the centrifuged sample and frozen at −20°C.

Freezing damages the cells within blood and so cannot be used as a method of storage for whole blood. A fresh smear should be made which can then be stored at room temperature.

Counting the samples

Cell counts can be measured electronically or can be determined manually.

An automated haematology analyser known as a QBC (quantitative buffy coat) machine can be used to assess the red and white blood cells in a blood sample electronically.

• When using an electronic haematology machine a special pipette is used to draw a sample of whole blood into a microhaematocrit tube.
• A special float is then placed in the same tube.
• The microhaematocrit centrifuge is used to separate blood samples.
• The white blood cells and platelets sit on top of the red blood cells in a layer called the buffy coat.
• The buffy coat is separated into its constituent cell layers by the float, so that values for each type of white blood cell can be measured.
• The centrifuged sample is placed in a special reading machine which analyses the layers within the tube.

The manual determination of cell counts in a blood sample uses a microscope.

• A specially marked slide called a **haemocytometer** is used.
• The blood sample is diluted and placed onto the slide.
• Different areas of the grid are used to count red blood cells, white blood cells and platelets.
• Calculations are then used to estimate cell numbers for the sample.

If a haemocytometer is not available an estimation of cell numbers can be obtained as follows:

• A fresh blood film is prepared.
• An experienced technician then counts 100 white blood cells under the high-power objective of the microscope and calculates the proportion of white blood cells which are neutrophils, lymphocytes, etc.
• This can be repeated a few times to get an average value.

What you need to learn

☙ You need to be able to describe the meaning of packed cell volume (PCV), buffy coat haematocrit and microhaematocrit:
  ☙ dogs
  ☙ cats.

☙ State the normal range of PCV:
  ☙ dogs
  ☙ cats.

☙ Describe how to estimate PCV using microhaematocrit tubes:
  ☙ plain
  ☙ heparinised.

☙ Outline conditions which may commonly result in increased or decreased PCV:
  ☙ haemorrhage
  ☙ anaemia
  ☙ dehydration.

The packed cell volume (PCV) is also sometimes called the haematocrit (Hct).

The PCV is the proportion of the blood made up by red blood cells (not including white blood cells or platelets).

It is often expressed as a percentage. Normal ranges are:

• cat 30–45%
• dog 37–55%.

PCV is often increased in athletic animals, particularly following exercise (following splenic contraction). A fit greyhound can have a normal PCV of up to 65%.

Measurement of PCV

To measure the PCV of a blood sample the blood is drawn up into a capillary tube known as a microhaematocrit tube.

• If the blood sample is fresh it should be drawn into a heparinised microhaematocrit tube to prevent clotting.
• If the sample has been collected into a heparin tube prior to testing it is not necessary to use a heparinised microhaematocrit tube and a plain one will suffice.

One end of the microhaematocrit tube is sealed using a special clay seal.

The tube is then placed in a microhaematocrit centrifuge. It is important that the sealed end of the tube rests on the rubber cushion.

The centrifuge must be balanced so usually at least two samples are spun at the same time at opposite sides of the centrifuge.

When the sample has been spun it is placed on a haematocrit reader. The base of the blood column (just on top of the seal) is placed on the zero mark while the meniscus at the top of the sample is placed on the 100 mark. The position of the top of the column of red blood cells is noted and read against the scale to provide the PCV result.

The colour of the plasma should be noted when the sample has been centrifuged.

• normal plasma is pale yellow
• pink plasma indicates haemolysis
• milky plasma indicates lipaemia
• darker yellow plasma indicates jaundice (icterus).

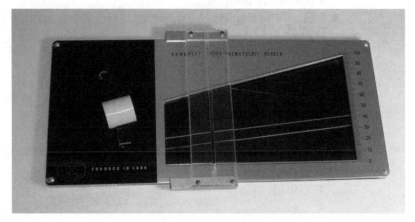

Figure 5.4 Haematocrit reader.

Causes of a change in the PCV are listed in Table 5.3.

Table 5.3 Causes of a change in PCV

Conditions causing an increase in PCV	Conditions causing a decrease in PCV
Dehydration	Anaemia
Splenic contraction (caused by fear, excitement, shock, strenuous activity)	Late pregnancy
	Sedation and anaesthesia
Anabolic steroids	Haemolysis during or after sampling
High altitudes	
Polycythaemia (rare)	
Hyperthyroidism in cats	
Errors causing an increase in PCV	**Errors causing an decrease in PCV**
Evaporation from sample	Excess EDTA
Prolonged contact with EDTA (causes cellular swelling)	Dilution (eg after excessive iv fluids)
	Coagulation of the sample

3.5.09 Blood smear

What you need to learn

- You need to be able to describe how to prepare a blood smear and how to stain it for haematological examination. The stains are:
  - Leishman's
  - Giemsa
  - Diff-Quik®.
- Describe common faults in blood smears and their causes:
  - incorrect thickness
  - unequal distribution
  - thick and thin bands
  - crenation
  - streaks and spots
  - incorrect staining.
- Describe principles of examining a blood smear and identify cell types:
  - mature and immature neutrophils
  - eosinophils
  - basophils
  - lymphocytes
  - monocytes
  - mature and immature erythrocytes.
- Explain abnormalities seen on blood smears:
  - reticulocyte
  - polychromasia
  - crenation
  - Howell Jolly bodies
  - rouleaux.
- Describe the common causes of abnormal cell counts:
  - leucocytosis
  - leucopaenia
  - lymphopaenia
  - lymphocytosis
  - neurophilia
  - neutropaenia
  - eosinophilia
  - eosinopaenia
  - monocytosis.
- Describe the principles of obtaining a differential cell count, manually and automatically.
- State the normal parameters of leucocytes:
  - dogs
  - cats.

A fresh blood smear should be prepared for every haematology sample. This should be used to check results provided by an automatic haematology analyser.

To prepare a smear:

- A small sample of fresh or EDTA-treated blood is drawn into a capillary tube and transferred onto a clean slide.
- A slide spreader (a slide with a corner removed) is placed on the sample slide at an angle of approximately 30° to the horizontal.
- The spreader is moved backwards towards the blood drop until the blood spreads along the edge of the spreader.
- The spreader is pushed smoothly and swiftly along the sample slide, taking the line of blood with it.
- A smear with a feathered edge will have been produced. This should be air-dried.
- The smear may need to be fixed prior to staining.

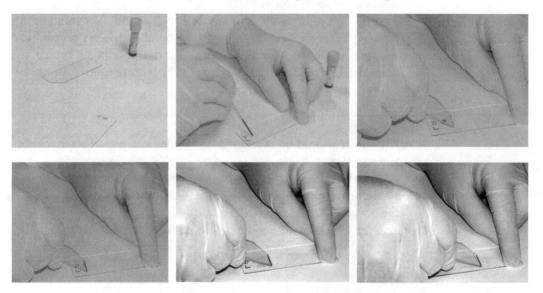

Figure 5.5 Technique of preparing a blood smear.

Stains are used to highlight parts of the different cells allowing examination under a light microscope. A number of different stains can be used:

- Rapid stains, such as Diff-Quik® or Rapi-Diff®, are commonly used in practices. These stains are usually adequate for in-clinic purposes but show little nuclear detail and so more sensitive stains are usually used in commercial laboratories.
- Romanowsky stains, such as Giemsa and Leishman's, are used in most laboratories as they show excellent detail.

• Other stains are available and are used in laboratories to highlight specific parts of the cells, or specific organisms. These include new methylene blue and haematoxylin & eosin (H & E).

Common faults in blood smears include:

• If the smear is too thick the drop of blood was too large. The smear should be one cell thick. If too much blood is used the smear will cover the whole slide and a feathered edge will not be produced.
• If the smear is too thin the drop of blood was too small.
• An unequal distribution of cells is usually caused by poor technique when advancing the spreader.
• Thick and thin bands of cells are usually caused by hesitation when advancing the spreader.
• Crenation of cells is cellular shrinking caused by water leaving the cells. Crenation happens when slides have been dried too slowly. Crenated cells have an irregular spiky outline.
• Streaks and spots can appear.
• Incorrect staining results in a smear which cannot be examined properly because the cells are poorly defined. Improper staining can be caused by leaving the slide for too short or too long a time in the staining solutions; use of the stains in the incorrect order or use of stains at the wrong concentration.

When examining a blood smear:

• The smear should be examined first under low power to check for quality.
• The feathered edge of the smear should be examined to assess platelet clumping and to look for white blood cells or any abnormally large cells.
• An area which is one cell thick should be selected so that the morphology of the blood cells can be examined and if required a differential cell count can be performed under oil immersion.

Cell types seen on a blood smear

See colour plate section in the middle of this book for photographs of mature neutrophils, immature neutrophils, eosinophils, basophils, lymphocytes, monocytes and mature erythrocytes.

Mature neutrophils are a type of polymorphonuclear leucocyte. They have a multi-lobed nucleus that stains dark purple. As the neutrophil matures the number of lobes in the nucleus increases so that mature neutrophils often have four or more lobes. (Plate 4.)

Immature neutrophils are released when there is an increase in demand for neutrophils. This happens during infection and inflammation. Immature neutrophils have fewer lobes in the nucleus and are often termed band cells. (Plate 5.)

Eosinophils are also a type of polymorphonuclear leukocyte. Eosinophils also have a multi-lobed nucleus. The cytoplasm stains pink and contains characteristic orange/pink-staining granules. (Plate 6.)

Basophils are also a type of polymorphonuclear leukocyte. Basophils are rarely seen in normal blood smears. The nucleus is bi-lobed or shaped like a kidney bean. The cytoplasm contains many granules of histamine which stain dark blue. (Plate 7.)

Lymphocytes have a large, darkly staining nucleus, surrounded by a small amount of cytoplasm. (Plate 8.)

Monocytes have a bi-lobed, darkly staining nucleus. They have pale pink cytoplasm which contains granules. (Plate 9.)

Mature erythrocytes do not possess a nucleus and have a biconcave shape. They appear red/pink with most stains. (Plate 11.)

Immature erythrocytes are frequently seen where there is an increase in demand for erythrocytes (such as with regenerative anaemia or following haemorrhage). Erythrocytes are released from the bone marrow before they have finished maturing. They often have nuclear remnants in the cytoplasm. The most immature form released is the **nucleated red blood cell,** followed by the next stage, which is a polychromatic (darkly staining) cell called a **reticulocyte.**

Platelets are small cellular fragments which are involved in blood clotting. They are smaller than red blood cells and are usually pale pink when stained. They are often irregular in shape.

Abnormalities seen on blood smears

Crenation

Crenation is cellular shrinking caused by water leaving the cells. Crenation happens when slides have been dried too slowly. Crenated cells have an irregular spiky outline.

Reticulocytes, polychromasia and Howell–Jolly bodies

Reticulocytes are polychromatic (darkly staining) cells which are slightly larger than mature erythrocytes and are darker in colour when stained.

Polychromasia means darkly staining cells (reticulocytes).

Nuclear remnants seen in immature red blood cells appear as tiny, darkly staining granules within the cytoplasm. These are known as Howell–Jolly bodies.

Rouleaux formation

This term describes the stacking on top of one another of red blood cells which occasionally occurs. It is most commonly seen when there is an excess of certain factors in the blood such as fibrinogen or globulin. Rouleaux formation is normal in the horse.

Supervital staining

Supervital stains (or supravital stains) are used to detect inclusions in the blood cells. Organisms which may be detected using supervital stains include blood-borne parasites such as *Babesia*, *Leishmania* and *Haemobartonella*.

Abnormal cell counts

The reasons for abnormal cell counts are listed in Table 5.4.

Table 5.4 Abnormal cell counts

Cell type	Increase in numbers caused by	Decrease in numbers caused by
Leucocytes	**Leucocytosis** caused by: bacterial infection, inflammation, tissue necrosis, steroid treatment, lymphoid diseases (lymphosarcoma, leukaemia), FIP, pregnancy and parturition, hyperthyroidism (feline).	**Leucopenia** caused by: viral infection, anaphylactic shock, toxicity, bone marrow disease (tumours and myeloproliferative disorders), severe bacterial infection.
Lymphocytes	**Lymphocytosis** caused by: youth/fear/stress/excitement, lymphocytic leukaemia and lymphosarcoma, FIV, hypersensitivity, autoimmunity, hypoadrenocorticism, drug treatment.	**Lymphopenia** caused by: steroid treatment, stress, acute infections, loss of lymph and lymph node damage, immunosuppressive drugs, generalised demodicosis, chronic renal failure.
Neutrophils	**Neutrophilia** caused by: fear/stress/excitement, steroid treatment, hyperadrenocorticism (Cushing's disease), hyperthyroidism (feline), infections, some types of anaemia, pregnancy (canine).	**Neutropenia** caused by: viral infection, overwhelming bacterial infection, autoimmune disorders, toxicity, radiation, anaphylactic shock, some testicular tumours, uraemia.
Eosinophils	**Eosinophilia** caused by: tissue damage from allergic reactions, parasitism, hypoadrenocorticism (Addison's disease), oestrus (canine), drug treatment.	**Eosinopenia** caused by: stress, hyperadrenocorticism, steroid treatment, acute infection/inflammation.
Monocytes	**Monocytosis** caused by: steroid treatment, stress, infections, immune-mediated disease, old age.	**Monocytopenia:** difficult to recognise as monocyte numbers are normally low.

Obtaining a differential cell count

Cell counts can be measured electronically or can be determined manually. See page 23.

Normal parameters for leucocytes

The normal white blood cell parameters in the dog and the cat are given in Tables 5.5 and 5.6, respectively.

Table 5.5 Normal white blood cell parameters in the dog

Blood cell type	Percentage %	Number (×10⁹/l)
Mature neutrophils	60–77	3–11.5
Immature (band) neutrophils	0–3	0–0.3
Eosinophils	2–10	0.1–1.35
Basophils	Rare	Rare
Lymphocytes	12–30	1–4.8
Monocytes	3–10	0.15–1.35

Table 5.6 Normal white blood cell parameters in the cat

Blood cell type	Percentage %	Number (×10⁹/l)
Mature neutrophils	35–75	2.5–12.5
Immature (band) neutrophils	0–3	0–0.3
Eosinophils	2–12	0.1–1.5
Basophils	Rare	Rare
Lymphocytes	20–55	1.5–7
Monocytes	1–4	0.1–0.85

3.5.10 Haemoglobin

What you need to learn

- What you need to learn
- You need to be able to describe the methods used to estimate haemoglobin and state the normal value:
  - dogs
  - cats
  - biochemical analyser.

Haemoglobin estimation is performed using an automated haematology analyser such as the QBC machine described earlier. The normal levels for haemoglobin in dogs and cats are given in Table 5.7.

Further values, such as the mean corpuscular volume (MCV) and mean corpuscular haemoglobin concentration (MCHC) are calculated from the values obtained.

Table 5.7 Normal haemoglobin, MCV and MCHC values in dogs and cats

Species	Haemoglobin (g/l)	MCV (fl)†	MCHC (g/dl)
Dog*	120–180	60–77	32–36
Cat	80–150	39–55	30–36

*This value is true for most breeds but values are higher (170-230) for very athletic breeds, including greyhounds, whippets, borzois and lurchers.
† fl = femtolitres; 1 femtolitre = 10^{-15} litres.

3.5.11 Blood biochemistry – blood urea/blood urea nitrogen

What you need to learn

☙ You need to be able to describe the techniques to perform BUN/Blood urea nitrogen:
  ☙ dipstick method
  ☙ biochemistry analyser.
☙ Outline the clinical conditions which can cause a high BUN:
  ☙ pre-renal
  ☙ renal
  ☙ post-renal.

Urea is an ammonia-containing waste product formed in the liver by the metabolism of proteins in the liver.

Proteins which are old or damaged are **deaminated** (amino groups are removed and ammonia is produced). The amino groups are used to provide energy for tissue respiration. The ammonia is toxic and is converted to the less toxic **urea**.

Urea is filtered out of the blood at the kidney and is excreted in the urine.

The amount of urea in the blood can be expressed in two ways:

• Plasma urea (normal ranges: dog 2.5–7 mmol/l; cat 5–11 mmol/l)
• Blood Urea Nitrogen (BUN) (normal ranges: dog 7–20 mg/dl; cat 14–32 mg/dl).

The BUN measures how much nitrogen is being carried within urea molecules in the blood. BUN, rather than plasma urea, is the value that is usually measured.

BUN and plasma urea are usually measured on automated biochemistry analysers. Dipsticks are available which measure these values in the blood but they are not very precise and are usually only useful to detect significant increases in blood values of BUN or urea. An increase in the BUN can occur for three reasons:

• **pre-renal** – increased breakdown of proteins (therefore increased

production of urea) or decreased renal perfusion (such as during shock, severe haemorrhage, dehydration and heart failure)
- **renal** – primary renal failure
- **post-renal** – obstruction to the flow of urine.

An increase in nitrogenous waste (BUN and creatinine) in the blood is known as **azotaemia.**

A decrease in the BUN can occur with a low-protein diet, liver failure, portosystemic shunt and treatment with anabolic steroids.

3.5.12   Blood biochemistry – blood glucose

What you need to learn

- You need to be able to describe methods available for the estimation of blood glucose levels:
  - reagent strips
  - biochemistry analysers
  - glucometer.
- State the normal levels of blood glucose and give examples of conditions associated with an increase or decrease of blood glucose.

Glucose is the energy source required by all cells in the body. The level of glucose in the blood is controlled mainly by two pancreatic hormones, insulin and glucagon.

Within the pancreas there are islands of endocrine tissue called the **Islets of Langerhans.** These areas contain three types of cells: alpha (α), beta (β) and delta (δ) cells.

Beta cells secrete **insulin.** Insulin is secreted when blood glucose levels rise, for example after a meal to lower blood glucose. It performs two functions:

- Insulin stimulates the synthesis of **glycogen,** which is a polymer of glucose. Glycogen can be stored in the liver and in skeletal muscle cells.
- Insulin aids the transport of glucose **from** the blood **into** respiring cells.

Alpha cells secrete **glucagon.** Glucagon is secreted when blood glucose levels decrease. It has the opposite effect to insulin. It stimulates the conversion of glycogen back to glucose, thereby raising blood glucose levels.

Plasma or serum glucose can be measured in a number of ways.

- An automated biochemistry analyser can be used following the manufacturer's instructions.

- Reagent strips can be used. A drop of blood is placed at the sample site. After a measured period of time the colour change at the sample site is compared with a reference scale so the blood glucose value can be determined.
- A glucometer follows the same principle as the dipstick but is a handheld machine that reads the colour change at the sample site on the dipstick rather than relying on human judgement.

Normal serum/plasma glucose reference ranges for dogs and cats are:

- dog 3.5–7.0 mmol/l
- cat 3.5–7.5 mmol/l.

An increase in serum/plasma glucose can be caused by one of the following:

- increased glucose production/release
- fear, excitement or stress (commonly seen in cats)
- following a meal
- traumas
- seizures
- exercise
- some sedative/anaesthetic drugs (eg xylazine, morphine, ketamine, alphaxolone/alphadolone in cats)
- acute pancreatitis (effect is rare and transient)
- decreased glucose usage:
  - diabetes mellitus
  - other hormonal conditions (eg hyperadrenocorticism, acromegaly, hyperthyroidism)
  - treatment with steroids
  - obesity
  - dioestrus in the bitch.

A decrease in serum/plasma glucose can be caused by one of the following:

- increase in insulin (either from overdose or from an insulin-producing tumour (insulinoma)
- hypoadrenocorticism
- liver disorders (portosystemic shunts, glycogen storage diseases)
- neoplasia
- sepsis
- starvation
- chronic malabsorption
- status epilepticus.

3.5.13 Blood biochemistry – other biochemical estimations

What you need to learn

❧ You need to be able to outline the common blood biochemistry estimations:
   ❧ total serum
   ❧ protein
   ❧ total cholesterol
   ❧ creatinine
   ❧ ALT (SGPT)
   ❧ SAP
   ❧ AST (SGOT), total bilirubin, calcium, albumin, amylase
   ❧ TSH
   ❧ ACTH
   ❧ Low/high-dose dexamethasone
   ❧ bile acids
   ❧ T_4.
❧ Outline factors which may affect the levels of these substances.
❧ Describe the laboratory equipment used to carry out these estimations:
   ❧ biochemistry analysers.

Many other parameters can be measured from blood samples to aid in the diagnosis of disease and to monitor the progress of medical conditions. Several of the most common parameters are outlined.

Most of the parameters can be measured in-house on an automated biochemistry analyser, although hormone assays are usually sent to commercial laboratories for tests such as radio-immunoassays.

It should be noted that this list is not exhaustive.

Enzymes

Alanine aminotransferase (ALT)

ALT used to be known as serum glutamic–pyruvic transaminase (SGPT).

The normal reference range depends on the method used by laboratory or analyser (see ranges provided by manufacturer/laboratory).

ALT is almost completely liver specific in the cat and dog. A rise in ALT levels in the blood indicates that liver cells have been damaged. The rise is proportional to the number of cells damaged.

Increased ALT activity is caused by hepatocellular damage through

- hepatitis (toxic, chronic or infectious)
- trauma
- acute pancreatitis
- neoplasia
- hepatic lipidosis (cats)
- hypoxia caused by shock
- myocarditis.

Decreased ALT activity is thought to have no significance.

NB ALT measurement does not provide information about the function of the liver.

Aspartate aminotransferase (AST)

AST used to be known as serum glutamic-oxaloacetic transaminase (SGOT).

The normal reference range depends on the method used by the laboratory or analyser (see ranges provided by manufacturer/laboratory).

AST occurs in many tissues but is present at the highest concentrations in muscle and in the liver. This lack of specificity means that AST is less useful than ALT in diagnosing liver disorders but is useful in diagnosing muscular disorders.

Increased plasma AST activity is caused by:

- liver damage
- skeletal or cardiac muscle damage
- over-exercise.

Decreased AST activity is thought to have no significance.

NB AST measurement does not provide information about the function of the liver.

Alkaline phosphatase (ALKP)

ALKP used to be known as serum alkaline phosphatase (SAP).

The normal reference range of ALKP depends on the method used by the laboratory or analyser (see ranges provided by manufacturer/laboratory).

ALKP is present in many body tissues. Increases in plasma ALKP are mainly the result of release of ALKP from the liver and bile duct; and from the bones. A form of ALKP can also be induced by steroid treatment in dogs.

Increased plasma ALKP activity is caused by

- obstruction to the flow of bile
- liver damage
- steroid treatment
- hyperadrenocorticism
- youth (growing animals release ALKP from bones)
- bone disease
- neoplasia
- starvation
- septicaemia.

Decreased ALKP activity is not though to be of clinical significance.

NB ALKP measurement does not provide information about the function of the liver.

Amylase

Amylase is also known as alpha amylase (α amylase).

The normal reference range depends on the method used by the laboratory or analyser (see ranges provided by manufacturer/laboratory).

Amylase is a digestive enzyme which comes mainly from the pancreas, liver and small intestine. It is therefore not a specific marker for pancreatic disorders but acute pancreatic inflammation can cause a marked rise in amylase.

Increases in plasma amylase activity are seen in:

- acute pancreatitis
- kidney failure in the dog (reduced kidney excretion of amylase)
- small intestinal obstruction.

Nutrients and metabolites

Plasma urea / BUN

See notes in 3.5.11.

Plasma glucose

See notes in 3.5.12.

Plasma creatinine

The normal reference range for creatinine in both the dog and cat is between 40 and 130 µmol/l.

Creatinine in plasma comes from the breakdown of creatine from muscles. It is excreted freely by the kidneys.

Increased plasma creatinine can be caused by:

- pre-renal, renal, or post-renal failure (from reduced filtering at the kidneys)
- severe exercise (from increased breakdown in the muscles).

Decreased plasma creatinine is occasionally seen in:

- muscle wasting diseases
- reduced muscle mass (eg starvation).

NB An increase in nitrogenous waste (BUN and creatinine) in the blood is known as **azotaemia**.

Total protein

The normal reference ranges are 57–77 g/l in dogs and 58–80 g/l in cats.

Total protein consists of albumin and globulins. It is normally measured in the plasma and so includes clotting proteins such as fibrinogen. Total protein measured in the serum does not contain fibrinogen and so values are slightly lower.

All proteins except for immunoglobulins are synthesised by the liver. Immunoglobulins are produced by the cells of the immune system.

An increase in total protein (**hyperproteinaemia**) is caused by:

- dehydration
- increased globulin levels
- anabolic steroids
- increased fibrinogen levels (rare).

A decrease in total protein (**hypoproteinaemia**) can be caused by

- youth
- decreased protein synthesis (starvation, malabsorption, liver disease and congestive heart failure)
- increased protein loss (protein-losing enteropathy or nephropathy, burns, haemorrhage and sepsis).

Albumin

The normal reference range in both dogs and cats is 25–40 g/l.

Albumin is synthesised from amino acids in the liver. It is a storage protein and provides amino acids for the tissues. Albumin is mainly responsible for osmotic pressure in the blood. Many substances bind to albumin including calcium, fatty acids and some hormones.

Increased plasma albumin levels (**hyperalbuminaemia**) can be caused by dehydration. This increase is relative and is caused by the reduced water content in the blood. Absolute increases in plasma albumin are not thought to occur.

Decreased plasma albumin levels (**hypoalbuminaemia**) are caused by:

- decreased protein synthesis (starvation, liver disorders, congestive heart failure)
- increased protein loss (protein-losing enteropathy or nephropathy, burns, haemorrhage and sepsis).

Globulin

The normal reference ranges are 25–45 g/l in dogs and 28–55 g/l in cats.

Fibrinogen and some globulins are produced in the liver. Immunoglobulins are produced by the cells of the immune system including plasma cells and B lymphocytes.

Increased globulin levels can be caused by:

- inflammation and infection
- neoplasia
- liver disease
- autoimmune disorders.

Decreased globulin levels can be caused by:

- decreased globulin synthesis
- increased globulin loss, as for albumin.

Total bilirubin

The normal reference ranges are 1.7–10 μmol/l for dogs and 2–5 μmol/l for cats.

Bilirubin is a yellow pigment which is mainly derived from the breakdown of erythrocytes. It is either recycled through the gut and liver, or passes out of the body in the faeces. A small amount is excreted through the kidneys.

An increase in the plasma bilirubin level eventually results in yellow discoloration of the skin and mucous membranes. This is known as **icterus (jaundice)**.

Increased plasma bilirubin levels (**hyperbilirubinaemia**) are caused by:

- increased breakdown of erythrocytes (haemolysis, haemorrhage, or transfusion)

- hepatocellular damage
- obstruction of bile flow (tumour, abscess, bile duct obstruction, right-sided heart failure, inflamed biliary tract).

Decreased plasma bilirubin levels (**hypobilirubinaemia**) can be caused by:

- reduced erythrocyte numbers from non-regenerative anaemias (malignant neoplasia, end-stage kidney failure and chronic infection/inflammation).

Bile acids

Bile acids are a measure of the **function** of the liver.

Normally a **bile acid stimulation test** is performed. This involves taking a **pre-prandial** (fasting) blood sample, then providing the patient with a fatty meal. A **post-prandial** blood sample is taken two hours after the meal. The bile acids are then measured in the two samples to assess the response of the liver to the fatty meal.

The reference ranges for biles acids in dogs and cats are given in

Table 5.8 Reference ranges for bile acids

Species	Pre-prandial bile acids (μmol/l)	Post-prandial bile acids (μmol/l)
Dog	<30	<50
Cat	<25	<30

Table 5.8.

Bile acids are synthesised in the liver and function as emulsifying agents during fat digestion. Most bile acids are recycled through the gut and liver. The plasma bile acid levels normally increase slightly following a meal, although most of the bile acids are extracted through the liver. Where liver function is impaired more bile acids leak into the blood.

Increased bile acid levels can be caused by:

- impaired liver function
- biliary obstruction
- portosystemic shunt.

Decreased bile acid levels can be caused by:

- intestinal obstruction
- severe malabsorption.

Electrolytes

Calcium

Calcium (Ca^{2+}) is a very important ion. It is involved in muscle contraction, blood clotting and nerve conduction as well as providing the structure of teeth and bones. Calcium levels are very tightly controlled by parathyroid hormone (PTH).

The main actions of parathyroid hormone are:

- increasing the absorption of Ca^{2+} from the gut
- stimulating reabsorption of Ca^{2+} through the proximal convoluted tubule in the kidney
- promoting movement of Ca^{2+} from the skeleton into the plasma

Vitamin D_3 and calcitonin are also involved with calcium homeostasis.

Total calcium is made up of the following parts:

- Ionised calcium is the biologically active portion and accounts for approximately 50% of the total calcium.
- Protein-bound calcium is the portion that is mainly bound to albumin and accounts for approximately 40% of the total calcium.
- Calcium salts, such as calcium phosphate, account for approximately 10% of the total calcium.

The normal reference range of calcium is 2–3 mmol/l in the dog and 1.8–3 mmol/l in the cat.

An increase in plasma calcium (**hypercalcaemia**) can be caused by:

- pseudohyperparathyroidism (caused by some tumours)
- primary hyperparathyroidism
- bone lysis (often cause by bone tumours)
- hypervitaminosis D
- renal failure
- dehydration
- status epilepticus.

A decrease in plasma calcium (**hypocalcaemia**) can be caused by:

- eclampsia
- hypoparathyroidism
- ethylene glycol (antifreeze) toxicity.

Milder hypocalcaemia can also be caused by:

- secondary hyperparathyroidism (renal/nutritional)
- pancreatitis
- malabsorption

• hypoalbuminaemia.

Phosphate

Phosphate in the body is known as plasma inorganic phosphate.

The normal reference range of phosphate is 0.8–1.6 mmol/l in the dog (but can be double this in normal young dogs) and 1.3–2.6 mmol/l in the cat.

Phosphate is derived from the diet, and is present in bones and teeth. Phosphate homeostasis is regulated by parathyroid hormone.

Increases in plasma inorganic phosphate levels (**hyperphosphataemia**) are caused by:

• youth
• renal failure
• bladder rupture
• hypervitaminosis D bone lysis
• hypoparathyroidism
• feline hyperthyroidism.

Decreases in plasma inorganic phosphate levels (**hypophosphataemia**) are caused by:

• malabsorption
• primary hyperparathyroidism or pseudohyperparathyroidism
• diuresis
• steroid treatment
• hyperadrenocorticism
• rickets.

Sodium

The normal reference range of sodium is 140–155 mmol/l in dogs and 145–157 mmol/l in cats.

Sodium is present in the extracellular fluid and sodium levels are carefully controlled by the kidneys.

Increased plasma sodium levels (**hypernatraemia**) are caused by:

• increased sodium intake
• decreased water intake
• excessive water loss.

Decreased plasma sodium levels (**hyponatraemia**) are caused by:

• increased sodium loss (renal failure, vomiting, diarrhoea, diuretics)
• over-hydration.

Low sodium diets alone rarely cause hyponatraemia.

Potassium

The normal reference range of potassium is 3.6–5.8 mmol/l in dogs and 3.6–5.5 mmol/l in cats.

Potassium is mainly present in the intracellular fluid; less than 2% of the potassium is in the extracellular fluid.

Increased plasma potassium (**hyperkalaemia**) can be caused by reduced potassium excretion (hypoadrenocorticism, low sodium intake, bladder rupture) or movement of potassium from ICF to ICF (metabolic acidosis, tissue damage, some drugs).

Hyperkalaemia can cause abnormalities in the heart beat and is potentially very dangerous.

Decreased plasma potassium (**hypokalaemia**) can be caused by:

- decreased potassium intake
- increased potassium loss (chronic vomiting or diarrhoea, liver disease, hyperadrenocorticism)
- movement of potassium from the extracellular to the intracellular fluid (insulin therapy and alkalosis).

Chloride

The normal reference range for chloride is 100–120 mmol/l in the dog and 115–130 mmol/l in the cat.

Increases in plasma chloride levels can be caused by:

- metabolic acidosis
- conditions which cause hypernatraemia.

Decreases in plasma chloride levels can be caused by:

- metabolic alkalosis
- conditions which cause hyponatraemia.

Hormones – tests for thyroid function

Thyroxine (T4)

The normal reference range for thyroxine is 17–46 nmol/l in dogs and 12–52 nmol/l in cats.

Thyroxine production and release are regulated by thyrotropin-releasing hormone (TRH) from the hypothalamus and thyroid-stimulating hormone (TSH) from the pituitary gland.

Increased plasma thyroxine can be caused by:

- youth
- hyperthyroidism

• oestrus and pregnancy.

Decreased plasma thyroxine can be caused by:

• hypothyroidism
• hyperadrenocorticism
• chronic illness such as diabetes mellitus, renal, liver or heart failure (known as *sick euthyroid syndrome*)
• thyroxine treatment
• iodine deficiency.

TSH/T$_4$ ratio

The ratio of TSH to T$_4$ is used to diagnose hypothyroidism in dogs. Hypothyroid dogs normally have a low T$_4$ but a high TSH.

TSH stimulation test

The TSH stimulation test is used to distinguish hypothyroid animals from those with falsely low T$_4$ levels (such as those with sick euthyroid syndrome).

Basal T$_4$ levels are measured with a blood sample. The dog is then injected with TSH, and a second blood sample is taken after six hours.

• The TSH injection has little effect on the T$_4$ levels of hypothyroid dogs because there is little functional thyroid gland for the TSH to stimulate.
• Animals that have a low T$_4$ but are not hypothyroid show a rise in T$_4$ after the TSH injection.

Hormones – tests for adrenal cortex function

Tests for adrenal cortex function are used for diagnosis.

• An excess of glucocorticoid production is known as **hyperadrenocorticism** (Cushing's disease). Cushing's disease can be caused by a pituitary tumour, which secretes adrenocorticotrophic hormone (ACTH), or by a neoplasm in the adrenal gland, which secretes cortisol.
• A lack of glucocorticoids (and sometimes mineralocorticoids) is known as **hypoadrenocorticism** (Addison's disease). Addison's disease is usually caused by damage to the adrenal cortex.

ACTH stimulation test

An ACTH stimulation test is used to test for adrenal cortex function.

• A blood sample is taken to assess baseline cortisol levels.
• A synthetic form of ACTH is given by intravenous injection to

stimulate the release of cortisol from the adrenal cortex.

- Two hours later a second blood sample is taken to assess the response to ACTH.
- Very high post-injection cortisol levels suggest that the animal is suffering from Cushing's disease.
- Animals with Addison's disease show very little increase in cortisol levels post-injection.

There is often difficulty interpreting whether lower results are significant, so further diagnostic tests are often necessary.

Low-dose dexamethasone test

The low-dose dexamethasone test is used to screen for hyperadrenocorticism (Cushing's disease).

- A blood sample is taken to assess baseline cortisol levels.
- A low dose of dexamethasone is injected intravenously (0.01 mg/kg).
- After eight hours a second blood sample is taken to assess the response to dexamethasone.
- In normal animals the dexamethasone injection suppresses the release of ACTH by negative feedback therefore reducing cortisol levels.
- In animals with Cushing's disease the dexamethasone is not able to suppress the release of ACTH and cortisol levels remain higher.

High-dose dexamethasone test

The high-dose dexamethasone test is used to distinguish between animals which have pituitary-dependent Cushing's disease and those which have non-pituitary-dependent Cushing's disease (ie those which have neoplasia in the adrenal cortex).

- A blood sample is taken to assess baseline cortisol levels.
- A higher dose of dexamethasone is injected intravenously (0.1 mg/kg).
- Further blood samples are taken three and eight hours after the injection to assess the response to dexamethasone.
- In normal dogs both post-injection samples are below the baseline cortisol levels.
- In pituitary-dependent Cushing's disease one of the post-injection samples is below the baseline cortisol value.
- In non-pituitary-dependent Cushing's disease there is very little suppression and both cortisol values are above the baseline value.

Hormones – insulin

The normal reference range for fasting insulin levels in both dogs and cats is 36–180 pmol/l (pmol/l = picomoles per litre; where 1 picomole is 10^{-9} moles).

Insulin assays are used to diagnose type II (insulin-resistant) diabetes mellitus, and to detect insulin-producing tumours (**insulinomas**).

- A persistently high plasma insulin level in the presence of low blood glucose is suggestive of an insulin-producing tumour.
- A high plasma insulin level in the presence of very high blood glucose is suggestive of insulin-resistant (type II) diabetes mellitus.
- A low plasma insulin level can be caused by type I (insulin-dependent) diabetes mellitus, or severe trauma.

3.5.14   Urine – collection and preparation of samples

What you need to learn

- You need to be able to describe sterile and non-sterile methods used for the collection of urine in the dog and cat by:
  - free-catch sampling
  - catheter
  - cystocentesis.
- Explain why midstream samples are preferable if a non-sterile technique is used.
- Describe the effects of storage on a urine sample and outline the preservatives which can be used for urine:
  - boric acid
  - refrigeration
  - thymol
  - toluene or HCl
  - formalin.

Urine analysis can be extremely useful in veterinary medicine for the diagnosis and monitoring of a wide range of diseases. Urine collection is usually non-invasive, and many of the tests performed on urine can be carried out immediately in the veterinary practice.

Gloves should always be worn when performing or handling urine samples as zoonotic organisms such as *Leptospira* may be present. Collection containers should be thoroughly disinfected or, if disposable, placed in the clinical waste bins.

Urine can be collected in a number of ways

- free-catch urine sampling
- catheterisation
- cystocentesis.

Free-catch urine sampling

The simplest method of urine sampling is the collection of a free-catch urine sample. This can be performed when the animal is passing urine normally, or when the bladder is expressed manually.

- The urine passes through the lower part of the genito-urinary tract and usually comes into contact with some skin and hair as it leaves the body.
- For this reason free-catch urine samples are non-sterile, and are usually contaminated with bacteria, cells and cellular debris (and often sperm in entire males).
- For most purposes the sample should be taken from the **midstream** flow of urine. This is because the first portion of urine will have flushed most of the bacteria and debris from the tract, reducing the contamination of the mid-stream flow.
- The first part of the urine stream can be useful for the detection of lesions in the distal urinary tract, such as urethral plugs, crystals, or infectious agents.
- The last part of the urine stream can be useful for detection of lesions in the bladder wall (as material such as blood clots may have formed a sediment in the bladder) or prostate gland.
- The free-catch urine sample should be collected into a sterile receptacle such as a bowl or kidney dish. As much urine as possible should be collected so that various tests can be performed.

Catheterisation

A sterile urinary catheter is inserted into the urethra, and advanced slowly and gently into the bladder so that a urine sample can be obtained directly from the bladder.

A urine sample obtained with a catheter is usually cleaner than a free-catch sample but can still be contaminated with bacteria from the lower urinary tract.

The disadvantages of catheterisation are:

- It is more invasive than free-catch and can cause trauma to the urethra.
- It usually requires sedation or anaesthesia in bitches and cats although many male dogs will tolerate catheterisation when fully conscious.

• The procedure can push bacteria from the lower urinary tract up into the bladder as the catheter is advanced.

Cystocentesis

The urine sample is obtained by passing a needle, through aseptically prepared skin of the abdominal wall, directly into the bladder.

• Cystocentesis provides the least contaminated urine sample and is therefore very useful for bacterial culture and sensitivity tests.
• Cystocentesis is invasive but is tolerated by most fully conscious animals.
• There is often contamination of the sample with blood from the damage to the bladder wall by the needle.
• Great care must be taken if cystocentesis is to be performed in a severely distended bladder. The procedure is often necessary to relieve pressure in an obstructed bladder prior to correction of the condition.
• Cystocentesis should not be performed in animals with ascites or clotting disorders.
• Ultrasound guidance can be useful if the bladder is small or difficult to palpate (overweight animals).

Storage and preservation of the urine sample

Once the urine sample has been obtained it is important to perform diagnostic tests as soon as possible as the quality of the sample can deteriorate quickly. If the sample is to be sent to an external laboratory appropriate preservatives should be used.

• Urine samples can be refrigerated at 4°C for up to 24 hours after collection if there is any delay before testing. The sample must be allowed to warm to room temperature before testing as crystals are more likely to form in cold urine.
• Freezing can only be used if physical or chemical tests only are to be performed as sediment containing bacteria and cells will be destroyed.
• If the sample is being sent for bacterial culture a substance which preserves the bacteria should be used. **Boric acid** is an example of such a preservative.
• Preservatives such as **formalin, thymol, toluene,** or **hydrochloric acid** (HCl) can be used but these will destroy bacteria and can affect the outcome of some tests.

3.5.15   Laboratory tests – physical examination

What you need to learn

☙ You need to be able to describe the variations in colour and odour of urine and outline pathological and physiological conditions which may affect urine colour and odour:

☙ dogs

☙ cats

☙ rodents

☙ lagomorphs

☙ reptiles.

Physical examination of the urine should be performed as soon as the sample is available. Physical examination includes:

• volume
• colour
• turbidity
• odour.

Volume

Normal urine production in dogs ranges between 20 and 40 ml/kg/day; and for cats between 18 and 25 ml/kg/day. Urine output varies normally with changes in food and fluid intake.

An **increase** in the volume of urine produced (**polyuria**) can be caused by:

• impaired secretion or action of anti-diuretic hormone (ADH); this occurs with diabetes insipidus, over-hydration with intravenous fluids, Cushing's disease, hypercalcaemia and some drugs
• excess solute in the plasma: increased salt intake, diabetes mellitus, kidney failure
• other diuretic effects: from diuretic drugs such as frusemide and spironalactone.

A decrease in the volume of urine produced (< 7 ml/kg/day) (**oliguria**) can be caused by:

• early stages of acute renal failure
• end-stage chronic renal failure.

Colour

Normal urine appears pale yellow in colour; the more concentrated the urine, the deeper the yellow colour.

Changes in the colour of urine can indicate a number of conditions.

Causes of colour change in urine are listed in Table 5.9.

Table 5.9 Causes of colour change in urine

Colour	Causes
Red/pink	blood (**haematuria**) haemoglobin (**haemoglobinuria**)
Dark red/dark brown	myoglobin (pigment released from damaged muscle) methaemoglobin (forms from haemoglobin in stale samples)
Yellow, yellow/orange	bilirubin urobilinogen some drugs (such as sulphasalazine)
Blue	some drugs (such as ampicillin) cause slight blue tinge
Green	biliverdin (from stale samples containing bilirubin) infection with *Pseudomonas aeruginosa*.

Turbidity

Turbidity describes how transparent the urine sample is. Normal urine is clear (transparent). Cloudiness (turbidity) may be caused by:

- crystals
- cells and cellular debris
- bacteria
- secretions from the urinary tract (such as semen, mucus, prostatic fluid and pus).

Examination of the sediment will help to identify the cause of the turbidity.

Odour

Normal urine has a distinctive smell with which the nurse will be familiar. Normal variations in urine odour are caused by the presence of pheromones (especially in the entire tom cat), or food metabolites such as fish or food containing volatile fatty acids.

Abnormal odours can indicate a number of disorders:

- **Ammonia** – A smell of ammonia indicates the presence of a urinary tract infection if the sample is fresh or suggests the sample is stale.
- **Sweet solvent smell** – Diabetic ketoacidosis will produce a sweet solvent smell (which comes from ketones).
- **Putrefaction** – The breakdown of proteins in the urinary tract, as can occur in severe cystitis, will give an odour of putrefaction.
- **Drugs** – Penicillins cause a distinctive smell in the urine.

Urinary sediments seen in exotic species

Birds and reptiles excrete the majority of nitrogenous waste as **uric acid** and **urates** (compared with most mammals that excrete their nitrogenous waste as urea). These urates form the normal white crystals which are seen in the urine of birds and reptiles.

There is great variation in the colour of normal rabbit urine. The variation in colour is caused by a variety of pigments which come from plant material and can range from white through to dark red. Rabbits excrete excess calcium via the urine as calcium carbonate. This results in creamy urine. Struvite crystals can also be found in small amounts in normal rabbit urine.

Other herbivorous rodents, such as guinea-pigs, can show a similar range of colour for normal urine.

3.5.16   Laboratory tests – specific gravity

What you need to learn

☙ You need to be able to define specific gravity (SG), state the SG of water and the normal parameters of SG of urine.
☙ Outline the equipment and method for estimation of SG in dogs and cats
　☙ dip stick
　☙ refractometer.

Specific gravity is a ratio which compares the density of a liquid with the density of distilled water. Distilled water has a specific gravity of 1.000. Normal reference ranges for the specific gravity of urine are:

• dog: 1.015–1.045
• cat: 1.020–1.040

When plasma is filtered at the glomerulus, the specific gravity of the glomerular filtrate is the same as that of plasma: 1.008–1.012. This is known as **isosthenuria**. The kidneys then modify this filtrate according to the amount of water and solutes present in the body.

Dilute urine has a specific gravity which is lower than isosthenuria. Concentrated urine has a specific gravity which is higher than isosthenuria.

Specific gravity can be measured using a commercially available **dipstick**. Most test strips were designed for use in humans and are not very accurate for measurement of specific gravity.

A more accurate measurement of urine specific gravity can be obtained using a **refractometer**. This instrument measures the refractive index of the liquid. (The refractive index is a measure of how much light bends as it passes through the material. The more material there is dissolved in a liquid, the higher its refractive index.)

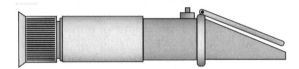

Figure 5.6 Refractometer.

Following calibration, a few drops of urine at room temperature are placed on the glass sample site and the lid is closed. The instrument is then held up to the light, and the scale is viewed through the eyepiece. A reading of specific gravity can be seen as a line on the scale.

3.5.17   Laboratory tests – chemical tests

What you need to learn

* You need to be able to describe the methods available for the testing of urine:
    * dipstick
* Outline common chemical tests on urine:
    * pH
    * blood
    * protein
    * glucose
    * ketones
    * bilirubin.
* State the normal parameters of these tests.
* Outline factors which can lead to abnormal results:
    * condition of animals
    * sample collection
    * storage
    * processing of sample.

A number of chemical tests can easily be performed on urine in the practice laboratory. Most of these are performed using commercially available dipsticks. Dipsticks should only be used with fresh urine samples.

The dipstick is a strip of plastic with a variable number of sample pads. A spot of urine is placed onto each pad and after the designated period of time the colour change present is compared with a scale to give readings.

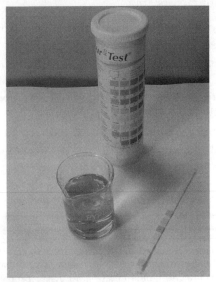

Figure 5.7 Urine dipstick.

Parameters measured include the pH. The normal reference range for the pH of urine for both dogs and cats is 5.5–7. Urine pH depends greatly on the diet. High protein diets (carnivorous diets) produce an acidic urine. Plant foodstuffs cause a slightly more alkaline pH.

A **decrease** in pH (ie increased acidity) can be caused by:

• respiratory acidosis
• hypoxia
• shock
• diabetic ketoacidosis
• severe diarrhoea
• acidifying drugs or diets
• toxicity (metaldehyde or ethylene glycol).

An **increase** in urine pH (ie increased alkalinity) can be caused by:

• respiratory alkalosis
• vomiting
• alkalinising drugs or diets
• some urinary tract infections
• urinary retention
• post-prandial alkaline tide
• stale urine sample.

The presence of substances which are not found in normal urine can also be detected using a dipstick and are listed in Table 5.10.

Improper storage and handling of urine samples leads to inaccurate results from urinalysis.

The most important factors are:

- All necessary steps should be taken to prevent contamination when collecting the specimen.
- There should be correct storage and use of preservatives if necessary.
- The period of time between collecting samples and performing diagnostic tests should be as short as possible.
- A full clinical history should be recorded for each patient as many factors will affect the outcome of urinalysis, such as diet, medication and concurrent medical conditions.

Table 5.10 Indicators of disease and injury in urine measured by dip stick

Substance	Presence indicates:
Blood	Blood loss from part of the urogenitary tract. Can be physiological cause such as oestrus or pathological cause such as infection, inflammation, toxicity, trauma, neoplasia, or a clotting disorder.
Protein	Protein (usually albumin) can come from the kidneys (renal failure or glomerular disease) or from other sources (inflammation, haemoglobinuria, haematuria, myoglobinuria, hyperproteinaemia, natural secretions)
Glucose	Can occur with hyperglycaemia (diabetes mellitus, severe stress, acute pancreatitis, seizures) or without hyperglycaemia (some hereditary renal disorders, renal failure).
Ketones	Mainly occurs in diabetes mellitus, occasionally seen with low carbohydrate/high fat diets, and following severe trauma.
Bilirubin	Impaired liver function, acute haemolysis or biliary obstruction.
Urobilinogen	Unreliable test in dogs and cats Acute haemolysis, impaired liver function, alkaline urine.
Nitrites	Unreliable test in dogs and cats Significant bacterial infection in urine.
Leucocytes	Urinary tract infection/inflammation, pyometra, prostatitis, pylonephritis.

3.5.18 Laboratory tests – microscopic examination

What you need to learn

- You need to be able to describe the method of preparing a urinary sediment:
  - wet and dry preparations
  - stains.
- Describe the preparation of urinary sediment for microscopic examination.
- Describe and define microscopic components that may be seen in urine sediment

- casts – hyaline, cellular, granular, waxy
- epithelial cells
- leucocytes
- erythrocytes
- bacteria
- spermatozoa
- crystals
- mucous strands.

- Explain the reasons for the formation of crystals in urine and state the types of crystals which occur in normal urine.
- Outline the pathological conditions in which increased numbers of crystals occur:
  - infection
  - metabolic
  - dietary.
- Describe and identify the types of urinary crystals:
  - struvite
  - oxalate
  - urate
  - cysteine.
- Describe urinary calculi and outline how urinary calculi may be analysed:
  - qualitative
  - quantitative.

Examination of urine sediment is a vital part of urinalysis and can contribute greatly to the understanding of a patient's condition. The urine sediment should be examined in fresh samples as any cells will become damaged as the urine becomes more stale.

Urine can be prepared as a wet or dry preparation.

To make a **wet preparation**:

- A sample of urine is placed in a sterile tube and spun in the centrifuge so that the sediment sinks to the bottom of the sample.
- The supernatant (liquid on top of the sediment) is carefully decanted using a pipette so that only the sediment is left in the tube.
- A few drops of sediment stain (such as Sedi-stain®) are added to the tube and the mixture is gently agitated so that the stain spreads through the sediment.
- A single drop of stained sediment is placed on a fresh microscope slide and covered with a cover-slip.

To make a **dry preparation**:

- A sample of urine is placed in a sterile tube and spun in the centrifuge so that the sediment sinks to the bottom of the sample.

- The supernatant (liquid on top of the sediment) is carefully decanted using a pipette so that sediment only is left in the tube.
- The sediment is gently agitated to re-suspend the deposit in the few remaining drops of liquid.
- A single drop of the deposit is placed on a fresh microscope slide.
- The slide is allowed to air dry.
- A stain, such as Leishman's stain or Diff-Quik®, can then be applied to the slide in the normal manner.

Once prepared the slide should be viewed under the microscope as described for other samples. The slide should be viewed at low power first, moving up to higher power for closer examination of any areas of interest.

Features of urinary sediment

Cells

- **Red blood cells** – see haematuria.
- **White blood cells** – Small numbers of leukocytes are seen in normal urine but large numbers suggest inflammation in the urinary/genital tract.
- **Epithelial cells**
  - **Renal tubular cells** – These are small round or comma-shaped cells which are difficult to identify. They are not usually significant unless present in casts.
  - **Transitional cells** – Transitional epithelium lines the renal pelvis, ureters, bladder and proximal urethra. These cells are often present in clumps or sheets but their appearance varies depending on their origin. Small numbers are seen in normal urine but large numbers are suggestive of inflammation or neoplasia.
  - **Squamous cells** – Squamous epithelial cells line the distal urethra and the lower genital tract. They are large cells with a small central nucleus, and may be present in sheets. Small numbers are seen in normal urine but large numbers are suggestive of inflammation or neoplasia. During oestrus there are increased numbers of squamous cells shed from the genital tract. These may therefore be seen in higher numbers in a urine sample.

Casts

These are tubular structures which originate from the renal tubules. They are all based on a mucoprotein which is secreted in the nephron. The presence of casts in the urine indicates disease of some kind in the renal tubules.

See Figure 5.8 for hyaline, cellular, granular and waxy casts.

- **Hyaline** – These consist of mucoprotein alone. They dissolve rapidly in alkaline urine and indicate inflammation in the renal tubules.

- **Cellular** – Cells are present within the mucoprotein cast. Cells present can include erythrocytes, leukocytes, and tubular epithelial cells. The presence of cellular casts indicates acute tubular damage such as pyelonephritis, glomerulonephritis and acute renal failure.

- **Granular** – These are a degenerate form of cellular casts. The cells present may be disintegrated and crystals may be incorporated into the cast. Granular cells start off coarsely granular and become more finely granular as they degenerate further. Granular casts in the urine indicate chronic renal damage.

- **Waxy** – Waxy casts are the most degenerate form of cast and suggest that the damage has been present for a while. Waxy casts are pale and amorphous.

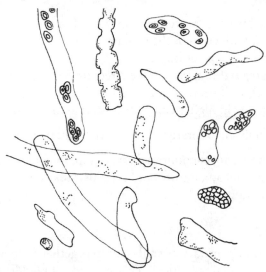

Figure 5.8 Casts.

Bacteria

A small number of bacteria may be seen in normal urine and their presence is usually the result of contamination. Large numbers of bacteria are suggestive of urinary tract infection and culture/sensitivity should be performed on an appropriately preserved sample (boric acid).

Bacteria appear as rods or cocci under high-power magnification.

Sperm

These are a normal finding in the urine of uncastrated males.

Mucus

Strings of mucus may be seen in normal animals. Large amounts of mucus can be seen during oestrus. Large amounts of mucus at other times suggest irritation and inflammation of the urinary/genital tract.

Crystals

Normal urine contains very few crystals, although crystals may precipitate out of normal urine as it cools. The presence of increased numbers of crystals depends on the concentration of the urine, its pH and the solubility of salts in the urine.

Many conditions can favour the production of crystals in the urine, such as:

- diets which cause alteration in the pH of the urine
- bacterial infection in the urinary tract
- genetic predisposition
- breed (eg dalmatians often excrete uric acid in their urine)
- concurrent illnesses (where metabolites or drugs are excreted from the kidney in higher concentration than normal).

Commonly encountered crystals are listed in Table 5.11.

Less commonly encountered crystals include phosphate, carbonate, bilirubin, silica, xanthine and crystals caused by drugs such as sulphonamides.

Calculi

Occasionally urinary crystals clump together to form stones or **calculi** (singular: calculus). The presence of bladder stones (**cystic calculi**) is always abnormal. Stones in the urinary tract can also be referred to as **uroliths**.

Calculi may pass out of the bladder into the urethra. Some may pass out in the urine but it is possible for calculi to become lodged in the urethra and cause an obstruction.

Causes and appearances of calculi are given in Table 5.12.

Urinary calculi are usually sent to an external laboratory for identification. The laboratory will identify the type of stone. This is a **qualitative** analysis.

The laboratory will also report the frequency with which the stones crystals appear in the sample. This is a **quantitative** analysis.

Table 5.11 Urine crystals

Type of crystal	Composition and appearance	Examples of causes
Struvite	Magnesium ammonium phosphate Often known as triple phosphate crystals Coffin lid shaped	Bacterial infection Alkaline urine (but can occur at any pH) Can occur in small numbers in normal animals.
Calcium oxalate	Octahedral or pyramidal in shape	Ethylene glycol poisoning Acidic urine (but can occur at any pH) Genetic defects. Small numbers can occur in normal animals.
Urate	Spindle or diamond-shaped	Acidic urine Portosytemic shunt Bacterial infection Occur mostly in Dalmations.
Cysteine	Flat, hexagonal shape. Colourless	Genetic defects Acidic urine

Table 5.12 Urine calculi

Type of calculus	Causes	Radiographic appearance
Struvite	Alkaline urine Most commonly encountered calculus Sedentary animals predisposed	Radiodense, smooth, round stones
Oxalate	Ethylene glycol poisoning Acidic urine (but can occur at any pH) Genetic defects	Radiodense, rough round stone, often sharp edges.
Urate	Acidic urine Portosytemic shunt Bacterial infection	Radiolucent, smooth, round, brown or green
Cysteine	Acidic urine Genetic defects	Fairly radiolucent, round or oval, smooth.

3.5.19   Elementary parasitology

What you need to learn

❧ You need to be able to identify the term parasite and understand the meaning of ectoparasite and endoparasite.

A **parasite** is an organism which lives on or within another animal (the **host**). The parasite obtains its nutrition from the host. Often the parasite lives at the expense of, and causes some harm to, the host.

Parasites which live on the surface of the host are called **ectoparasites**; examples are fleas, ticks, lice and mites.

Parasites which live inside the host are called **endoparasites**; examples are roundworms, tapeworms and flukes.

Parasites which live with the host throughout their lifecycle are called permanent parasites.

Transmission (the passage from one host to another) occurs when animals come into close contact, eg lice can only survive for a very short period away from the host.

The **final/definitive host** is the host in/on which sexual reproduction takes place.

The **intermediate host** is a host (other than the definitive host) in/on which part of the development of the parasite takes place.

The **paratenic host** is a host entered by the parasite but on/in which no development takes place. Often the parasite is waiting for its paratenic host to be eaten by its final host. An example of this is *Toxocara cati* in the mouse.

A **transport host** carries the parasite from one area to another, or from one animal to another.

A **vector** is usually an invertebrate which spreads disease organisms. An example of a vector is the mosquito which transmits malaria.

A **host-specific parasite** is one which has a narrow range of potential hosts, often just one species. Some parasites have a wide range of potential hosts, such as the cat flea (*Ctenocephalides felis*).

A **parasitic zoonosis** is a parasitic infection which can be transmitted to humans. An example is *Sarcoptes scabei*, which causes sarcoptic mange in dogs and scabies in humans.

3.5.20   Ectoparasites

What you need to learn

❧ You need to be able to describe the appearance and identify common ectoparasites:
  ❧ *Linognathus setosus*
  ❧ *Trichodectes canis*
  ❧ *Felicola subrostratus*
  ❧ *Ctenocephalides*
  ❧ *Ixodes* spp.
  ❧ dipteran larvae
  ❧ *Sarcoptes scabiei*
  ❧ *Otodectes cynotis*
  ❧ *Cheyletiella* spp.
  ❧ *Notoedres cati*
  ❧ *Trombicula autumnalis*
  ❧ *Demodex canis*.
❧ Explain which ectoparasites are temporary and which are permanent.
❧ Outline the significance of host specific and zoonotic ectoparasites.
❧ Describe the life cycle of specified ectoparasites:
  ❧ *Ctenocephalides*
  ❧ *Linognathus*
  ❧ *Trichodectes*
  ❧ *Ixodes*.
❧ Explain how ectoparasites act as disease vectors
❧ Describe and identify flea, flea droppings, flea larvae and the 'wet paper' test.

Lice

Lice are small (a few mm) wingless insects. Each species is host specific and is a permanent parasite. Infestation with lice is called **pediculosis**. Severe pediculosis is often associated with neglect.

Lice are divided into two groups:

• the biting lice (which feed on scales, feathers, scabs and loose epithelium)
• the sucking lice (which have piercing mouth parts and feed on blood and tissue fluids).

The lifecycle of the louse

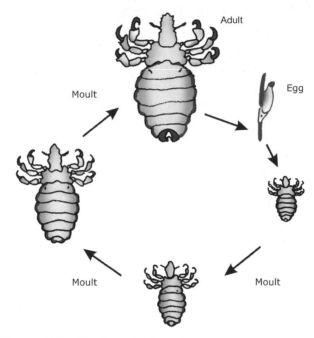

Figure 5.9 The louse's lifecycle.

Adult lays eggs (**nits**) which are cemented to the animal's hair. A **nymph** hatches out of the egg. The nymph moults several times before becoming an adult. The whole lifecycle takes two to three weeks.

Linognathus setosus

This is a sucking louse. It occurs on the dog.

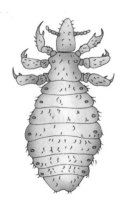

Figure 5.10 *Linognathus setosus.*

The head is long and narrow with piercing mouth parts. The nits are dark in colour and often difficult to see.

Trichodectes canis

This is a biting louse. It occurs on the dog. The head is shorter and rounded. *Trichodectes* is lighter in colour than *Linognathus*. *Trichodectes* can be a vector for the tapeworm *Dipylidium caninum*.

Felicola subrostratus

This is a biting louse. It occurs on the cat.

Fleas

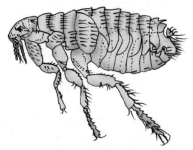

Figure 5.11   Flea (*Ctenocephalides* spp.).

Fleas are wingless insects which feed exclusively on blood as adults. Severe infestation can result in anaemia. Hypersensitivity reactions can occur to both flea saliva and faeces.

Fleas act as the intermediate host for the tapeworm *Dipylidium caninum*. Fleas can act as a vector for other diseases. Examples are cat scratch disease and myxomatosis in rabbits.

Fleas have a laterally compressed body which aids movement between the hairs on an animal's coat.

Species of fleas found include:

• *Ctenocephalides felis* (the cat flea) – This is the commonest flea on both dogs and cats. It will also bite humans.
• *Ctenocephalides canis* (the dog flea) – This flea is fairly uncommon, and is host specific.
• *Pulex irritans* (the human flea) – This flea is fortunately now rare in the UK.

The lifecycle of Ctenocephalides spp.

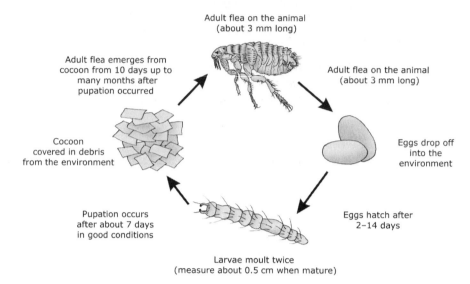

Adult flea on the animal
(about 3 mm long)

Adult flea emerges from
cocoon from 10 days up to
many months after
pupation occurred

Adult flea on the animal
(about 3 mm long)

Cocoon
covered in debris
from the environment

Eggs drop off
into the
environment

Pupation occurs
after about 7 days
in good conditions

Eggs hatch after
2–14 days

Larvae moult twice
(measure about 0.5 cm when mature)

Figure 5.12 *Ctenocephalides* spp. life cycle.

The adult flea finds its host using changes in light intensity, temperature and carbon dioxide. Once it has found a host the adult flea feeds frequently on blood. It produces large quantities of faeces.

After one or two days the adult flea starts to lay eggs. These are white and 0.5 mm in length. The eggs drop off the host onto the ground. The larva is a 2–5 mm long maggot-like creature which prefers dark areas, and feeds on flea dirt and skin flakes on the floor. The larvae pupate to form cocoons (5 mm long). Adult fleas hatch from the pupae and start the cycle again. The whole lifecycle takes three to four weeks, but can be quicker in warm weather.

It is important to understand that 95% of the flea population consists of eggs, larvae, pupae and newly hatched adults in the environment. Only 5% of the flea population is actually on the host.

Detection of flea dirt can be performed using the 'wet paper' test. Coat brushings are collected onto a piece of white tissue paper or cotton wool. This is then moistened. Flea dirt (which is mainly digested blood) will leach red/brown colouring onto the moist tissue. Presence of flea dirt in the coat is a clear indication that flea treatment is necessary.

Ticks

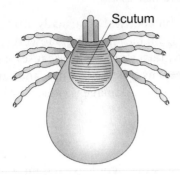

Figure 5.13 *Ixodes* spp.

Ticks are arachnids (possessing eight legs). They are wingless and do not possess antennae.

There are two groups of ticks; the hard ticks which have a chitinous **scutum,** and the soft ticks which lack this scutum.

Most of the lifecycle of the tick is spent away from the host, ie they are temporary parasites.

Ticks can act as vectors for a number of diseases, such as Lyme disease and tick-borne fever.

Ticks sink their mouth parts into the host and secrete agents which prevent the blood in the local area from clotting, and cause inflammation. When removing a tick from its host great care must be taken to completely remove the mouth parts as infection often results from the mouth parts being left behind.

The body of the tick swells as it drinks blood.

Ixodes ricinus

This is the commonest tick present in the UK. *Ixodes* has a wide host range and is commonly seen in dogs. It has a lifecycle involving three hosts, one for each stage of development through larva, nymph and adult.

Other ticks encountered in the UK are *Ixodes canisuga* (an uncommon dog tick), and *Ixodes hexagonus* (the hedgehog tick).

Flies (Diptera)

Many flies are temporary parasites on animals, but the most important flies in veterinary practice are those which are capable of causing fly-strike (**myiasis**). Myiasis is caused by the adult fly laying eggs on the host. The larvae (maggots) hatch out and feed on the host, causing great damage and distress.

Blowflies (greenbottles, bluebottles) are usually attracted by the smell from an injury or from faecal soiling. However, some species can penetrate otherwise intact skin. Myiasis causes severe skin damage; extends and deepens existing injuries, and causes secondary bacterial infections. **NB** All the damage is caused by the fly larvae rather than the adult flies.

Mites

Mites are arachnids (possessing eight legs) and most are very small (< 0.3 mm). They spend most of their lifecycle on the host. Mites can be divided into two groups: the burrowing and non-burrowing mites.

Burrowing mites

Burrowing mites usually have short legs.

Sarcoptes scabei

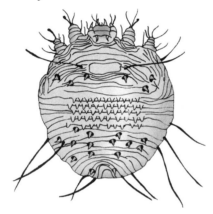

Figure 5.14 *Sarcoptes scabiei.*

This is a small round mite with short legs and dorsal pegs. Infestation with this mite is called **sarcoptic mange**. Symptoms of sarcoptic mange are intense pruritus, erythema and papule formation. The skin becomes scabbed, thickened and wrinkled, and hair loss becomes marked. Sarcoptic mange is common in dogs but rare in cats. It is zoonotic and causes scabies in people.

Notoedres cati

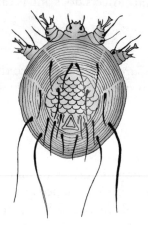

Figure 5.15 *Notoedres cati.*

This mite is similar in appearance to *Sarcoptes*. It has a characteristic thumbprint on its dorsum. *Notoedres* is very rare in the UK and tends to infect cats and rabbits.

Demodex

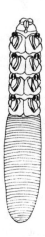

Figure 5.16 *Demodex canis.*

This mite is cigar-shaped and possesses four pairs of very short legs. It is often a commensal organism in the hair follicles and sebaceous glands of most animals. It is transmitted from the bitch to the puppies during suckling. In some animals, such as the immunosuppressed or predisposed animals, *Demodex* can cause disease.

Disease caused by Demodex is called **demodectic mange**. Clinical signs are dry, crusty skin lesions with hair loss. The condition can be localised (small area only affected) or generalised (whole animal affected). The condition mainly affects dogs and is rare in cats.

Trixacarus caviae

Trixacarus is very similar to *Sarcoptes* but is approximately half the size. It causes severe mange in small mammals such as rats, mice and guinea-pigs.

Cnemidocoptes pilae

Cnemidocoptes is the only group of burrowing mite which affects birds. It is a small round mite with a U-shaped bar behind its head. *Cnemidocoptes pilae* causes scaly face/beak in caged birds.

Non-burrowing mites

Otodectes cynotis

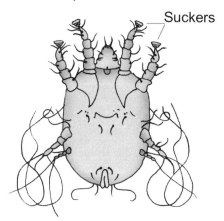

Figure 5.17 *Otodectes cynotis.*

Otodectes inhabits the external ear and is the commonest mite in dogs and cats. It is usually identified by its location although closed bars can be seen on its underside on microscopy and suckers can be seen on the ends of the legs.

The mites are transmitted from a mother to her offspring during suckling. The presence of the mites causes production of a brown waxy discharge which can be followed by secondary bacterial and fungal infections.

Affected animals often shake their heads, scratch their ears and can develop aural haematomas through self-trauma.

Cheyletiella spp.

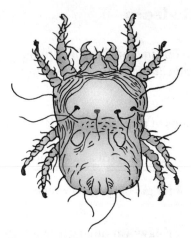

Figure 5.18 *Cheyletiella* mite.

Different types of *Cheyletiella* can be found on dogs, cats, rabbits and occasionally humans. The mite has long legs and a waist and has combs on the end of each leg.

Cheyletiella infestation is often called 'walking dandruff' as movement of the mites can just be seen with the naked eye against a dark background.

Trombicula autumnalis

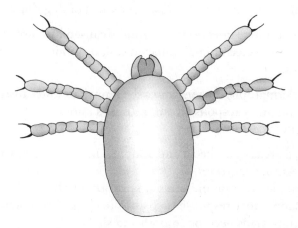

Figure 5.19 *Trombicula autumnalis* larva.

This is the harvest mite. It is bright orange and is hairy. It is only parasitic as a larva. The parasite can affect any animal including humans, and causes irritation and hypersensitivity.

3.5.21   Dermatophytes

What you need to learn

* What you need to learn
* You need to be able to outline the two main fungal organisms common in the dog and cat that cause ringworm:
  * *Microsporum canis*
  * *Trichophyton* spp.
* Describe the clinical signs of ringworm and malassezia in the dog and cat.
* Outline the significance of ringworm as a zoonotic infection.

There are two groups of fungal pathogens which cause skin disease in small animals:

* The dermatophytes or ringworm fungi cause infection of the skin, hair or nails. The species most commonly encountered are *Microsporum* and *Trichophyton*
* The yeasts such as *Malassezia pachydermatis,* and occasionally *Candida albicans* can cause skin disease in dogs and sometimes cats.

Dermatophytosis (ringworm)

The dermatophytes digest keratinous debris in the skin, hair and nails but rarely invade living tissues. The commonest species encountered are *Microsporum canis* (which causes nearly all cat ringworm and two-thirds of dog ringworm cases), and *Trichphyton mentagrophytes* (which causes one-third of dog ringworm cases).

Dermatophyte infections are usually caused by coming into contact with an infected animal, infected soil, or fomites containing fungal spores.

The dermatophytes penetrates the hair shaft and causes an inflammatory response from the host's immune system. The symptoms are:

* focal areas of alopecia and scaling which spread outwards as the infection progresses
* variable pruritus and often no pruritus at all
* inflammatory response such as folliculitis or furunculosis
* healing areas become smooth and shiny
* condition usually resolves spontaneously after a few weeks.

It is extremely important to be aware that dermatophytosis is a potential zoonotic (ie it can be passed on to humans, causing similar lesions to those seen in cats and dogs).

Diagnosis of dermatophytosis can be achieved by

- **Microscopy** – Fungal spores or hyphae can be seen from skin scrapings and hair plucks.
- **Wood's lamp examination** – The lesions of about half of the animals infected with *M. canis* will show bright green fluorescence with a Wood's lamp. **NB** Failure to fluoresce under a Wood's lamp does not exclude a diagnosis of dermatophytosis.
- **Fungal culture** -Skin scrapings and hair plucks are placed on a commercially available dermatophyte culture kit and allowed to grow for 7–14 days. Dermatophytes usually produce white colonies which change the colour of the culture medium from yellow to red.
- **Biopsy** – Conclusive proof of dermatophytosis is provided by demonstration of fungal hyphae invading the skin in a biopsy sample.

Malassezia pachydermatis

Malassezia pachydermatis is a yeast which is found on the skin of healthy animals. It has only fairly recently been recognised as causing skin disease in dogs (and rarely, cats). In affected animals the population of yeast becomes overwhelming and causes clinical signs such as:

- erythema (reddening of the skin) with alopecia and scaling
- greasy exudate which matts the coat
- hyperpigmentation and lichenification of the skin in chronic cases
- otitis externa.

Commonly affected sites include the ventral neck, interdigital skin and the axillae and inguinal areas.

It is thought that *Malassezia* is often a secondary invader when other skin disease is present such as atopy and keratinisation defects. There is usually concurrent infection with bacteria such as *Staphylococcus aureus*.

Diagnosis of *Malassezia* infection can be achieved by:

- **Microscopy** – This is the most useful method. Examination of tape strips, and direct smears from affected areas show increased numbers of *Malassezia* yeasts.
- **Culture**
- **Biopsy** (not a sensitive test).

3.5.22 Skin and hair – collection of specimens

What you need to learn

☙ You need to be able to describe the methods used to obtain samples of hair and skin:
  ☙ hair plucks
  ☙ hair brushings
  ☙ sellotape impressions
  ☙ skin scrapings.
☙ Outline the precautions which must be taken in obtaining such samples (zoonotic cases):
  ☙ ringworm
  ☙ sarcoptes
  ☙ patient contact/restraint.
☙ Outline the effective storage and transport of skin and hair samples.

Laboratory tests are of great importance in the diagnosis of dermatological conditions. Most of the tests necessary can be performed within the practice laboratory.

Hair plucks

Hair plucks are used in the diagnosis of ectoparasites, dermatophytes, and to examine the structure of the hair.

Hairs from the sample site are plucked using forceps. The hairs can then be examined under a microscope or used for the culture of micro-organisms.

Hair brushings

Hair brushings are used to detect the presence of ectoparasites.

A small brush or a toothbrush should be used. The coat is brushed thoroughly while a piece of plain paper is placed underneath the back end of the patient. Loose material in the coat will be brushed out and can be collected on the paper for examination.

Tape impressions

Tape impressions are used to detect ectoparasites and some superficial micro-organisms such as *Malassezia* yeasts.

A strip of clear, colourless adhesive tape is placed on the sample site and then pulled away, taking any loose material from the coat and skin surface. This strip can then be examined and stained as necessary.

Skin scrapings

Skin scrapings are used to diagnose ectoparasites (in particular the burrowing mites), dermatophytes and nematodes (such as *Uncinaria*, the hookworm).

The procedure involves scraping the surface layer of skin away, allowing collection of any pathogens which may be concealed in the superficial skin layer.

Care must be taken when handling animals with skin disease. A number of dermatological conditions can be passed to humans (ie they are zoonotic). Examples of zoonotic skin conditions are:

• sarcoptic mange
• ringworm
• *Cheyletiella* infestation.

If there are any symptoms which could be suggestive of these conditions the animal must be handled carefully to avoid cross-infection.

• Gloves and aprons should be used when handling the animal.
• The owners must be warned about the risk of infection.
• As few people as possible must come into contact with the patient, and care should be taken to avoid contact with other animals.
• Care must also be taken during procedures such as skin scrapes and hair plucks that the animal is suitably restrained, as these procedures can occasionally be uncomfortable.

Once obtained the hair and skin samples must be handled and stored with care to prevent deterioration and also to prevent cross-infection. Samples intended for external laboratories (some bacterial and viral cultures, biopsies) must be packaged carefully as described later (see 3.5.33) in appropriately labelled containers. Samples should be processed as soon as possible to avoid deterioration in quality. Samples which are being used for culture in the practice laboratory must be stored and treated as described by the manufacturer of the test materials; taking care to perform the tests at the correct temperature and for the correct length of time.

3.5.23   Skin and hair – examination procedures

What you need to learn

❧ You need to be able to describe the method of obtaining and preparing samples for direct examination on a microscope slide:
  ❧ skin scrapings

    ❧ pustular contents
    ❧ ear wax
    ❧ hair samples.
❧ Outline the significance of ectoparasites and describe the clinical signs and distribution of any lesions caused by the parasite:
    ❧ common parasites as in 3.5.20.
❧ Describe the principles and methods for using a Wood's lamp, and the colour produced, when recognising ringworm:
❧ Outline other substances which fluoresce under a Wood's lamp and the colour of the fluorescence:
❧ Outline precautions which must be taken when using a Wood's lamp.
❧ Describe how to make a preparation of hairs for examination of ringworm.
❧ Describe a method for culturing hair samples for ringworm.
❧ Identify ringworm spores microscopically and recognise fungal/yeast cultures and possible media colour changes.

Preparing a sample for microscopy

Skin scrapes

- An area of skin is selected which represents the lesions being examined.
- A drop of liquid paraffin can be applied to the skin before performing the skin scrape.
- The skin is squeezed gently between the fingers so that any material within the hair follicles is pushed towards the surface.
- A sterile scalpel blade is held at right angles to the skin and drawn across the sample site, in the direction of the hair growth.
- This action is performed repeatedly until there is slight oozing of blood from the superficial skin capillaries.
- The debris which has been collected on the scalpel blade is transferred to a slide or sample container.
- A drop of liquid paraffin or potassium hydroxide can be used to suspend the clump of debris.
- A coverslip can be placed over the sample.

Pustular contents

- A sample of pus from a pustule is collected using a sterile swab, or a sterile needle, taking care not to touch the surrounding skin.
- If the sample is to be sent for culture it should be placed in an appropriate transport medium and despatched to the laboratory as soon as possible.
- If the sample is to be examined in the practice laboratory the material should be smeared thinly onto a clean microscope slide.

- The sample should be air-dried and then an appropriate stain should be used to highlight the cells and micro-organisms.

Ear wax

- A sample of the ear wax is collected using a sterile cotton bud or swab.
- The sample is then transferred onto a clean microscope slide.

Hair samples

- Individual hairs should be plucked from the sample area using sterile forceps. Where possible the root of the hair should be intact.
- In cases of ringworm and alopecia the samples should be taken from the edge of the lesion as this is where active infection is usually occurring.
- If the sample is to be sent for culture it should be placed in an appropriate transport medium and despatched to the laboratory as soon as possible.
- If the sample is to be examined in the practice laboratory it should be placed on a clean microscope slide.

Ectoparasites in dermatological investigation

Ectoparasites are involved with most of the skin disease seen in general practice.

A summary of the organisms involved and the symptoms of infestation is given in Table 5.13.

Use of the Wood's lamp

Hairs infected with *Microsporum canis* often fluoresce an apple-green colour when illuminated with an ultraviolet lamp called a Wood's lamp.

The Wood's lamp must be switched on and allowed to warm up before the examination takes place. The animal should be examined in a dark room so that fluorescence can be seen clearly. **NB** skin scales and dirt can appear to fluoresce. Beware!

Many detergents and dust particles fluoresce a pale blue colour and should not be confused with *M canis*. It should also be noted that only about half of *M. canis* cases fluoresce with a Wood's lamp, and most dermatophytes do not fluoresce at all. A diagnosis of ringworm cannot therefore be ruled out by a negative result from a Wood's lamp.

Wood's lamps emit ultraviolet light which can be damaging to the

Table 5.13 A summary of the organisms involved and the symptoms of infestation

Ectoparasite	Symptoms	Distribution of lesions
Lice	Biting lice cause pruritus and self-trauma, sucking lice can cause anaemia in large numbers.	Can be found anywhere but often pinnae, axillae, inguinal areas
Fleas	Skin disease usually *only* seen in hypersensitive or heavily infested animals. Pruritus, erythema, anaemia if heavy burden. Can cause symmetrical ventral alopecia in cats	Flea allergy dermatitis (FAD) usually affects rump, thighs, abdomen and flanks.
Ticks	Seldom cause skin problems, bites occasionally become infected.	Can attach anywhere, often seen on head and face.
Dipteran larvae (myiasis)	Moist soft skin, maceration, deep ulcers filled with maggots, strong smell. Animal usually debilitated.	Pressure points, perineum, under matted coat or any wounds.
Mites *Sarcoptes scabiei*	Severe pruritus, small papules/ pustules. Self-trauma causing hair loss. If untreated leads to weight loss, lymphadenopathy, depression and secondary infections.	Edge of pinnae, elbows, hocks and ventral thorax. Prefers lightly haired areas.
Notoedres cati	Pruritus, crusting, skin thickening. Very rare in UK.	Lesions worst on head.
Demodex	Usually non-pruritic, alopecia, thickening of skin, scaling. Pruritus occurs with secondary infections.	**Localised** often forelimb or head (usually benign and resolves without treatment) or **Generalised** affecting various parts of body, usually including the feet (this form of the disease is very serious and difficult to treat).
Trixacarus caviae	Severe pruritus, erythema and alopecia in guinea-pigs.	Mainly affects dorsum and pinnae
Cnemidocoptes pilae	Affects parakeets such as budgies and cockatiels. Scaling on beak and cere, beak can become distorted. Mild pruritus only.	Beak and cere mainly affected. Other lightly feathered areas such as neck, legs and feet can be affected.
Otodectes cynotis	Mild to severe pruritus; head shaking; canal filled with thick brown wax. Often inflammation and secondary changes in ear canal.	Almost always external ear but occasionally found at different sites (especially in cats).
Cheyletiella spp.	Heavy scaling of skin, 'walking dandruff', variable pruritus.	Mainly dorsum in dogs and rabbits, can be localised or generalised in cats.
Trombicula autumnalis	Moderate pruritus, often red larvae can be seen.	Feet, face, ears and ventrum

skin and eyes of the handler if exposure is prolonged. For this reason the Wood's lamp should be used for short periods only, and the handler should not look directly at the light.

Animals which are suspected of being infected with dermatophytes should be handled carefully because of the risk of transmission of this potentially zoonotic disease to the human handler.

Preparation of a hair sample

When making a preparation of hair for examination of ringworm the following procedure should be followed:

- Hairs should be sampled from the edge of the lesion as this is where active infection is usually occurring.
- The hairs should be placed on a clean microscope slide with a drop of potassium hydroxide. A coverslip is then placed over the sample.
- The slide can be gently heated to speed drying if necessary.
- The slide can then be viewed under the microscope to identify fungal hyphae and spores.

Fungal culture

It is easier to identify dermatophytes if they can be grown in a culture prior to microscopic examination. If culturing a hair sample for examination of ringworm this procedure should be followed:

- The plucked hair sample is placed onto a medium designed to encourage growth of dermatophytes. The medium usually used is called Sabouraud's dextrose agar.
- Kits impregnated with this medium are commercially available. These kits are also impregnated with a dye which changes colour if the dermatophyte produces alkali (as dermatophytes often do).
- Once the sample has been placed on the surface of the medium the test is sealed to prevent contamination, and incubated at room temperature (25°C) for 10–14 days.
- At the end of this time the kit should be examined for the presence of fungal colonies. The colour and shape of the colonies should be noted, along with any change in the colour of the medium:
  - *Microsporum canis* – The colony is white to yellow and is flat in appearance. The medium changes colour from yellow to red.
  - *Trichophyton mentagrophytes* – The colony has a fluffy appearance and is white to tan in colour, darker on the underside of the colony. The medium changes colour from yellow to red.

Microscopic appearance of dermatophytes

Species	Pattern of spores on hair shaft	Cultural characteristics	
		Colony Morphology	Colour of colony
Microsporum canis	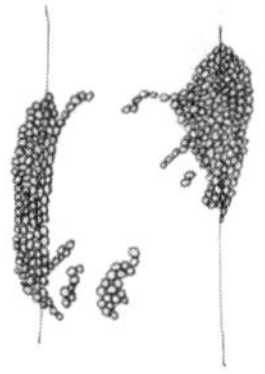	Yellow, orange with a downy surface	Yellow, orange
Trichophyton mentagrophytes	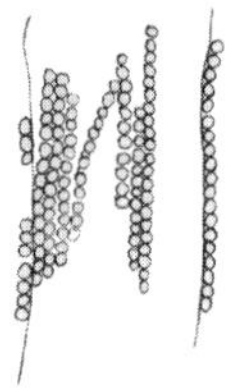	Cream to red powdery to granular surface	Cream to red

Figure 5.20 The most common dermatophytes.

3.5.24 Endoparasites

What you need to learn

☙ You need to be able to describe types of host and explain the terms:
  ☙ final/definitive
  ☙ intermediate
  ☙ paratenic
  ☙ transport host.
☙ Describe the general characteristics of nematodes and cestodes.
☙ Identify the common nematode and cestodes:
  ☙ *Toxocara canis*
  ☙ *Toxocaria cati*
  ☙ *Toxascaris leonina*
  ☙ *Uncinaria stenocephala*
  ☙ *Trichuris vulpis*
  ☙ *Aelurostrongylus abstrusus*
  ☙ *Dipylidium caninum*
  ☙ *Taenia* spp.
  ☙ *Echinococcus granulosus*
  ☙ *Filaroides osleri.*
☙ Describe the life cycles of important nemotodes

- *Toxocara canis*
- *Toxocara cati*
- *Toxascaris leonina.*
- Describe the life cycles of important cestodes:
  - *Echinococcus granulosus*
  - *Dipylidium caninum*
  - *Taenia hydatigena.*
- Describe and identify the terms:
  - scolex
  - strobilla
  - rostellum
  - proglottid
  - onchosphere
  - cysticercus
  - cysticercoid
  - coernurus
  - hydatid cyst.
- Identify round and tapeworm eggs in faeces.
- Describe the important parasitic protozoa of the dog and cat:
  - *Toxoplasma gondii*
  - *Coccidia* spp.
  - *Hammondia* spp.
  - *Sarcocystis*
  - *Giardia.*
- Describe the life cycle of Toxoplasma gondii.
- Describe the treatment and control of Toxoplasma gondi.
- Identify coccidiosis, describe its treatment and control in the rabbit.
- Explain the public health risk of endoparasites and provide appropriate advise for owners:
  - *Toxoplasma*
  - *Toxocara*
  - *Echinococcus*
  - *Giardia.*
- Outline anthelmintic and parasiticide giving appropriate examples.

Parasites which live inside the host are called **endoparasites**; examples are roundworms, tapeworms and flukes.

The two main types of endoparasites encountered in small animal veterinary practice are the **cestodes** (tapeworms) and the **nematodes** (roundworms).

Cestodes

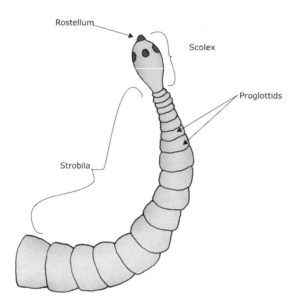

Figure 5.21 Cestode.

A cestode (or tapeworm) is a chain, or **strobila** of reproductive units (segments or **proglottids**) which progressively mature as they reach the tail. When a proglottid has fully matured it contains a uterus packed with eggs, or **onchospheres**, within shells. The head end or **scolex** is anchored to the intestinal wall of the host. The anterior part of the scolex, called the **rostellum**, is often covered with hooks to aid anchorage to the host.

The larval stage of the tapeworm, which takes place in the intermediate host, is called the **metacestode**. There are a number of different types of metacestode:

- The **cysticercus** is a fluid-filled bladder with one inverted scolex.
- The **cysticercoid** is only found in invertebrates (such as fleas and lice). It resembles a cysticercus but the bladder is a virtual space and the scolex is not inverted.
- The **coenurus** is a fluid-filled bladder but has many inverted scolices.
- The hydatid cyst is a fluid-filled bladder which can grow very large. It contains many scolices, some floating freely and some within **brood capsules**. The contents of a hydatid cyst are often called **hydatid sand**.

Some important cestodes are listed.

Dipylidium caninum

This is a very common parasite of dogs and cats. The adult worm lives in the small intestine of its host and can grow up to 50 cm long. The scolex has a protruding rostellum which holds four or five rows of hooks.

It rarely causes disease unless there is a heavy burden.

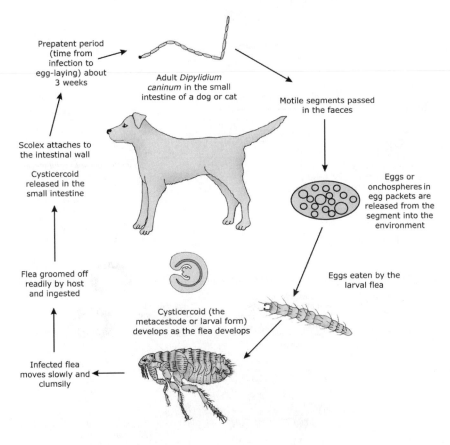

Prepatent period (time from infection to egg-laying) about 3 weeks

Adult *Dipylidium caninum* in the small intestine of a dog or cat

Motile segments passed in the faeces

Scolex attaches to the intestinal wall

Cysticercoid released in the small intestine

Eggs or onchospheres in egg packets are released from the segment into the environment

Flea groomed off readily by host and ingested

Eggs eaten by the larval flea

Cysticercoid (the metacestode or larval form) develops as the flea develops

Infected flea moves slowly and clumsily

Figure 5.22 Lifecycle of *Dipylidium caninum.*

- The proglottids are motile when they emerge from the anus. This can upset owners. The proglottids are oval and have an opening on each side. They resemble a grain of rice.
- As the mobile proglottid moves about it sheds egg packets filled with onchospheres. The onchospheres are often eaten by flea larvae (*Ctenocephalides felis* or *C. canis*) or by lice (*Trichodectes canis*) which act as the intermediate host.
- Once ingested the onchospheres develop into a cysticercoid.
- The final host (dog or cat) ingests the intermediate host which contains the cysticercoids. These then develop into adult worms in the small intestine.

Control of *Dipylidium caninum* relies on control of the intermediate hosts (fleas and lice).

Taenia spp.

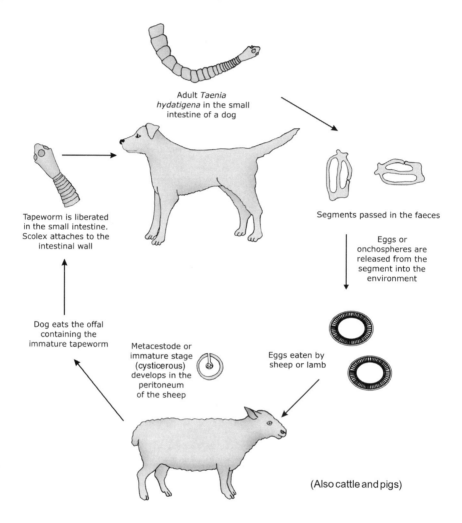

Adult *Taenia hydatigena* in the small intestine of a dog

Segments passed in the faeces

Eggs or onchospheres are released from the segment into the environment

Tapeworm is liberated in the small intestine. Scolex attaches to the intestinal wall

Dog eats the offal containing the immature tapeworm

Metacestode or immature stage (cysticerous) develops in the peritoneum of the sheep

Eggs eaten by sheep or lamb

(Also cattle and pigs)

Figure 5.23 Lifecycle of *Taenia hydatigena*.

There are a number of species of *Taenia* which affect dogs, namely *T. hydatigena*, *T. pisiformis*, *T. multiceps*, *T. serialis* and *T. ovis*, and *T. taeniformis* which affects the cat.

The adult worms rarely cause clinical disease unless there is a heavy burden. Various animals act as the intermediate hosts. In some intermediate hosts the metacestode can cause disease.

The adult tapeworm lives in the small intestine of the dog (and occasionally the fox). The proglottids are rectangular and have just one opening. The onchospheres are not contained in egg packets.

Taenia hydatigena is the commonest *Taenia* species in the UK.

- The onchosphere is consumed by the intermediate host, which for *T. hydatigena* is the sheep. The ingested onchosphere hatches in the sheep's small intestine, and travels to the liver via the hepatic portal system.
- The onchospheres develop into cysticerci and grow rapidly as they migrate through the liver. They emerge into the peritoneal cavity and when fully matured the cysticercus is 8 cm in length and is attached to the peritoneum of the intermediate host.
- The final host (the dog) must eat a cysticercus to become infected. This usually involves the dog eating raw or improperly cooked meat. The cysticercus travels to the dog's small intestine where it develops into the adult worm.
- The adult worm produces eggs which are shed in the faeces, often infecting large areas of land. Infection is much more common therefore in farming areas.

Control is based on preventing dogs from eating carcasses or uncooked meat.

Echinococcus granulosus

This tapeworm is an important zoonotic agent because its metacestode is the hydatid cyst, which can develop in a number of intermediate hosts including man. The hydatid cyst can grow to the size of a football in man. The final host is the dog or fox.

The adult tapeworm is about 6 mm long. It consists of a scolex and three or four proglottids. The last proglottid is larger than the others. Proglottids are shed approximately once a week in the faeces of the final host; these look exactly like other *Taenia* eggs.

Echinococcus granulosus is an uncommon parasite in the UK but occurs mainly in Wales and the Hebrides.

Hydatid disease in humans can involve the development of hydatid cysts in the liver, lungs, brain, or bones.

Control of this parasite relies on preventing dogs from eating carcasses or uncooked meat, regular worming of farm dogs in affected areas and reduction of the number of stray dogs.

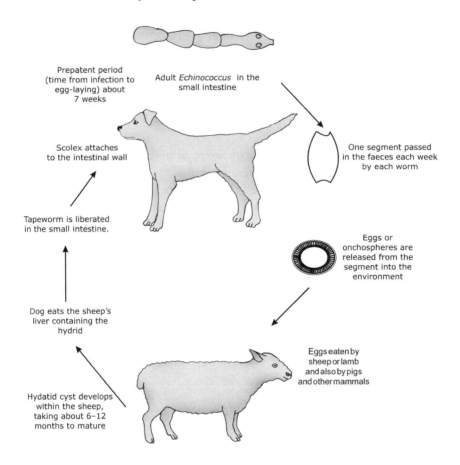

Figure 5.24 Lifecycle of *Echinicoccus granulosus*.

- The onchosphere is ingested by the intermediate host (usually sheep, pig or man).
- It escapes through the intestinal wall and migrates in the blood to the liver or in the lymph to the lungs.
- The onchosphere then matures into a hydatid cyst over 6–12 months.
- The final host (the dog) must eat a hydatid cyst to become infected. This usually involves the dog eating raw or improperly cooked meat.
- The hydatid cyst travels to the small intestine and develops into adult worms.
- The adult worm rarely causes disease unless there is a very heavy burden.
- The adult worms then shed proglottids which pass out of the body in the faeces.

Nematodes

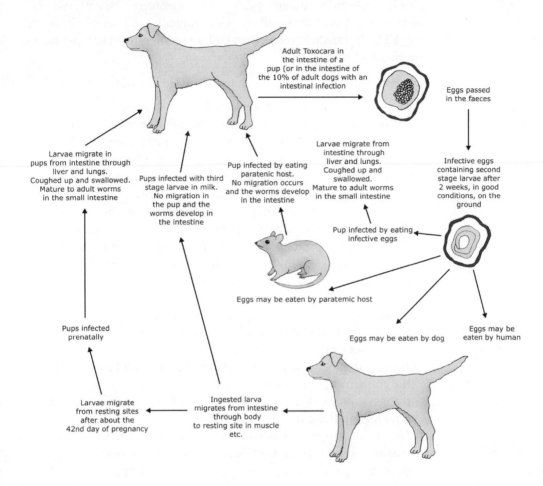

Figure 5.25 Lifecycle of *Toxocara canis*.

The nematodes are the most important roundworms in veterinary medicine in the UK. They have a tough outer cuticle and a muscular digestive system. The sexes are separate. The lifecycle of nematodes follows the basic lifecycle pattern of:

Egg → L1 → L2 → L3 → L4 → Adult

Where L1–L4 are the stages of larval development.

There are variations in lifecycle between species.

Some important nematodes are listed.

Toxocara canis (ascarid worm)

This is a common parasite in dogs. The large (up to 10 cm), white, adult worms live in the small intestine. Stages L1–L2 occur within the egg. L2 is the infective stage. If an L2 larva is ingested it hatches out in the small intestine.

The behaviour of the parasite depends on the age of the host:

- **In pups younger than ~12 weeks** – The L2 larvae migrate via the hepato-tracheal route: (gut → liver → lungs (coughed up and swallowed) → small intestine). The larvae mature into adults in the small intestine. Burdens of *T. canis* cause a pot-bellied appearance, diarrhoea, vomiting and weight loss in young puppies.
- **In older dogs** there is **somatic migration** of larvae. More and more larvae fail to reach the lungs and are distributed throughout the body, ending up in the muscle, brain, kidneys, heart and liver.
  - These L2 larvae remain dormant (do not develop further) until there is a suitable stimulus (usually pregnancy). The dormant larvae are protected by a thick shell, or cyst. If a bitch becomes pregnant these encysted larvae become activated (on approximately the 42nd day of pregnancy).
  - Nearly all of these activated larvae pass across the placenta into the fetuses (this is called **transplacental infection**).
  - A small number also travel to the mammary gland and pass into the colostrum, to be ingested by the puppies (this is called **transmammary infection**). There is no migration of larvae in the final host in this case.
  - Nearly all puppies are born infected with *T. canis*. This is the reason behind careful worming of the bitch throughout pregnancy, and of the puppies when they are born.

Toxocara canis is a potentially zoonotic parasite. L2 eggs which are ingested by a human migrate as in dogs. Larvae which invade the tissues are called **visceral larval migrans** (VLM) while those which migrate to the eye are called **ocular larval migrans** (OLM) and can cause unilateral impairment of vision.

Birds and rodents can act as paratenic hosts of *T. canis* if they ingest the L2 larvae. The larvae migrate to the host's tissues and wait to be eaten by the final host. There is no migration of larvae in the final host in this case.

Toxocara cati (ascarid worm)

This is a common parasite in cats. The large, white adult worms live in the small intestine.

The lifecycle is similar to that of *T. canis* except that there is no prenatal transmission. Infection is usually through milk, or through ingestion of the paratenic hosts.

The zoonotic importance of this worm is not known.

Toxascaris leonina (ascarid worm)

This is a common parasite in *both* cats and dogs.

The lifecycle is similar to that of *T. canis* except that there is no prenatal or transmammary transmission, and there is no hepato-tracheal migration. Infection occurs through ingestion of the L2 larvae within its egg, or by eating the paratenic host (containing the encysted larvae). Further development takes place in the small intestine of the final host. Once mature the adult worm produces eggs which pass out in the faeces.

Uncinaria stenocephala (hookworm)

These worms are less common parasites of dogs than the ascarids. They are 1 cm long and are most frequently encountered in racing greyhounds and hunt kennels. They have teeth within a large buccal cavity, which are used to attach firmly to the host's small intestine.

Infection is caused by ingestion or by penetration of the skin by the L3 larva. Hypersensitivity and moist dermatitis can occur at the site of skin penetration (usually the feet).

Heavy infestations can cause protein-losing enteropathy, with diarrhoea and weight loss.

Trichuris vulpis (whipworm)

The adult worms are 5–6 cm long and inhabit the caecum of dogs.

Infection is caused by ingestion of the L1 larva within its egg. The larva hatches in the caecum and resides in the glands within the caecal mucosa. Once mature the adult worm releases eggs which pass out in the faeces.

Infestations cause intermittent diarrhoea.

Aelurostrongylus abstrusus (lungworm)

This is the lungworm which affects the cat.

Infestation is often asymptomatic, but may cause respiratory compromise in immunosuppressed animals.

The L1 larva enters molluscs (through the fleshy foot) and matures into L3. The mollusc is eaten by the paratenic host (bird or rodent).

Infestation of the final host is through ingestion of the paratenic host.

Filaroides osleri (Oslerus osleri-lungworm)

This is the lungworm which affects the dog.

Infestation is often asymptomatic but can result in respiratory compromise or poor performance in racing greyhounds.

Eggs hatch in the trachea and are coughed up and swallowed, passing out in the faeces. Infection is caused by ingestion of the L1 larva (often from the bitch licking her pups). This passes into the small intestine and develops into an L2 larva which then migrates to the lungs via the blood. The adults live in nodules on the tracheal wall.

Identification of worm eggs in faeces

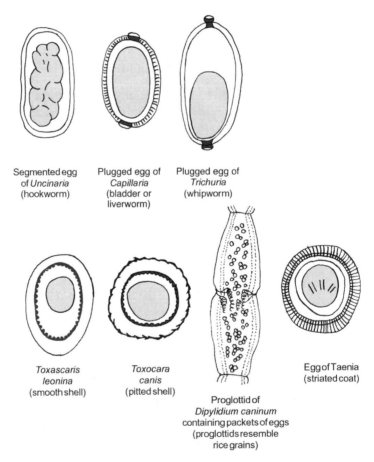

Segmented egg of *Uncinaria* (hookworm)

Plugged egg of *Capillaria* (bladder or liverworm)

Plugged egg of *Trichuria* (whipworm)

Toxascaris leonina (smooth shell)

Toxocara canis (pitted shell)

Proglottid of *Dipylidium caninum* containing packets of eggs (proglottids resemble rice grains)

Egg of Taenia (striated coat)

Figure 5.26 Worm eggs in faeces.

Protozoal parasites

Protozoa are motile, single-celled eukaryotic organisms. Many are free-living but a number are parasitic and can cause disease. Protozoa of importance in small animal veterinary practice include:

- **The Coccidia** (*Eimeria in particular in small animals*)
- **The tissue cyst-forming coccidia**
  - *Toxoplasma gondii* – which is found in cats.
  - *Neospora caninum* – which causes neuromuscular disorders in young puppies.
  - *Sarcocystis* – which is often non-pathogenic in the final host (dogs and cats) although can cause mild diarrhoea.
  - *Hammondia hammondi* - which can infect dogs and cats but are rarely pathogenic. The oocysts are detected in faeces and are very similar to those of toxoplasma.
- **The Microspora**
  - *Encephalitozoon cuniculi* -is an important and fairly common parasite of lagomorphs. Symptoms include neurological disorders, cataracts, renal failure. Infective spores are passed in the urine and many rabbits are infected *in utero*.
- **The flagellate protozoa**
  - *Giardia* – is a flagellate protozoan (it possesses a flagellum which is used for locomotion). It causes chronic diarrhoea and can affect man. Diagnosis is by demonstration of the organisms in faeces.

Toxoplasma gondii in cats

Toxoplasma is a cyst-forming coccidian. It causes serious disease in a number of species including man. The final host is the cat and other felids. The intermediate host can be any warm-blooded animal.

Most cats become infected by ingesting animals (usually birds or rodents) infected with *Toxoplasma* tissue cysts. Direct transmission through ingestion of oocysts can also occur.

- Once ingested the cyst wall is digested and asexual reproduction (**schizogony**), then sexual reproduction (**gametogony**) occur until oocysts are produced. These are shed in the faeces for one to two weeks.
- Further asexual reproduction occurs in the oocyst (known as **sporulation**). Sporulated oocysts (**sporocysts**) contain four **sporozoites**.
- Sporulated oocysts are ingested by the intermediate host and pass through the intestinal wall into the blood stream.

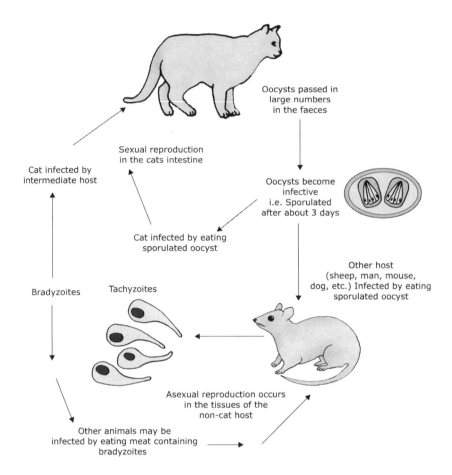

Oocysts passed in
large numbers
in the faeces

Sexual reproduction
in the cats intestine

Cat infected by
intermediate host

Oocysts become
infective
i.e. Sporulated
after about 3 days

Cat infected by eating
sporulated oocyst

Other host
(sheep, man, mouse,
dog, etc.) Infected by eating
sporulated oocyst

Bradyzoites   Tachyzoites

Asexual reproduction occurs
in the tissues of the
non-cat host

Other animals may be
infected by eating meat containing
bradyzoites

Figure 5.27 Lifecycle of *Toxoplasma gondii*.

- The liberated sporozoites are either **tachyzoites** or **bradyzoites**.
- In the **acute phase** of *Toxoplasma* infection the tachyzoites spread in the blood and infect other cells. This acute phase lasts for about two weeks, by which time the host has mounted an immune response and the infection enters the chronic phase.
- In the **chronic phase** of infection the bradyzoites become walled off in cysts in the host's tissues. These cysts remain viable for a long time and can cause acute infection if the host's immunity wanes at any time.

Prevention of *Toxoplasma* infection is impossible if cats are allowed outside as infection is caused by hunting and eating the intermediate hosts. Diagnosis of toxoplasmosis is made by serological testing. Oocysts can also be identified in faecal samples but shedding is intermittent. Treatment is with antibiotics such as clindamycin.

Control involves avoiding contact with cat faeces by using good hygiene (daily emptying of cat litter trays, wearing gloves when gardening) and avoiding feeding raw meat to cats.

Toxoplasma poses a risk to human health.

- Humans can be infected by ingesting oocysts from the environment, eating cysts in tissues of intermediate hosts, or across the placenta.
- Most infections are sub-clinical and self-limiting, however:
  - *Toxoplasma* infection in pregnant women can cause abortion, stillbirth and fetal abnormalities.
  - *Toxoplasma* infection is dangerous in immunosuppressed individuals, including the very young or elderly, and people suffering from AIDS.

Coccidiosis in rabbits

There are three pathogenic species of coccidia in rabbits, two of which occur in the caecum (*Eimeria intestinalis* and *E. flavescens*), and one in the bile duct (*Eimeria steidae*).

Coccidia causes serious disease in both pet and farmed rabbits. Symptoms include diarrhoea and weight loss. The bile duct form can also cause ascites and polyuria.

Diagnosis can be made by demonstration of the oocysts in faeces, or by post-mortem examination.

Treatment involves the use of suitable anti-coccidial drugs in the drinking water and control involves good hygiene and regular cleaning.

Endoparasites and public health

As described, a number of endoparasites pose a threat to human health. It is important that guidelines are followed to reduce the risk of infection with these organisms, and to be able to recognise and treat infestations in pets.

Toxoplasma gondii

Toxoplasma gondii causes disease in pregnant women, and in immunocompromised people. Ingestion of oocysts can be avoided by:

- washing potentially contaminated raw food (such as salad)
- wearing gloves when gardening and washing hands thoroughly afterwards
- washing hands after handling cats, especially before eating

• cleaning litter trays daily (before the oocysts sporulate).

Ingestion of the tissue cysts can be avoided by:

• ensuring that meat is thoroughly cooked
• washing hands after handling raw meat
• taking care when dealing with sheep at lambing time (sheep are an important intermediate host).

Toxocara canis

Humans are infected by swallowing embryonated eggs from the environment or from the coats of infected dogs. Prevention of infection involves reducing the environmental burden of eggs. This is done by:

• worming bitches from day 40–42 of pregnancy and during lactation
• worming puppies at regular intervals from the age of two weeks
• clearing up dog faeces so that environmental contamination is minimised
• washing hands (particularly those of children) after playing in areas where there is a risk of contact with dog faeces (eg public parks).

Echinococcus granulosus

The metacestode of *E. granulosus* causes hydatid disease in humans. Control is based on:

• education of owners and farmers in areas where *E. granulosus* is prevalent
• registration and regular worming of all dogs
• reduction of the number of stray dogs
• ensuring that dogs do not have access to raw food, including carcasses.

In countries where hydatid disease is a problem there is often legislation to enforce these guidelines.

Giardia

This is the commonest cause of protozoal diarrhoea in man (approximately 5000 cases each year). Infection can be avoided by:

• maintaining careful hygiene,
• avoiding uncooked foodstuffs
• boiling or sterilising water in parts of the world where water supplies are affected by *Giardia*.

Anthelmintic and parasiticide treatments

Treatments used to treat ectoparasites are listed in Table 5.14.

Table 5.14 Examples of treatments used to treat ectoparasites

Product	Treats	Comments
Fipronil	Fleas, ticks, lice, some mites (cheyletiella,	Spot-on and spray formulations
Selamectin	Fleas, ticks, lice, some mites (otodectes, cheyletiella, sarcoptes)	Spot-on formulation, sarcoptes requires repeat treatment after 30 days
Ivermectin	Many ectoparasites	**Not licensed**, MUST NOT be used in collie or part collie dogs. Toxic in chelonians.
Lufenuron	Fleas	Insect growth inhibitor, does not kill adult fleas but renders them infertile.
Imidacloprid	Fleas	Spot-on formulation
Amitraz	Sarcoptes, Demodex	Weekly baths. Organophosphate so must be handled with great care.

A parasiticide is a drug that is used to kill parasites. An anthelmintic is a drug that is used to kill helminth parasites (ie kills worms). See Table 5.15.

Table 5.15 Examples of drugs used to treat endoparasites

Product	Treats	Comments
Levamisole	Roundworms	Used more in large animals and exotic species. Usually given by injection or pour on formulation.
Ivermectin	Many ectoparasites; all stages of development for most roundworms. Inactive against tapeworms.	Must not be used in collies or part collies, toxic in chelonians. Usually given by injection.
Selamectin	Many ectoparasites; roundworms. Inactive against tapeworms.	Available as spot-on formulation.
Fenbendazole	Treats roundworms and has some activity against tapeworms. Also can be used to treat Giardia.	Available as oral paste, liquid or granules. Can be used in young animals.
Praziquantel	Kills round worms and tapeworms effectively.	Available as oral tablet.

3.5.25 Faeces – collection of specimens

What you need to learn

* You need to be able to explain the collection and storage and preservation of freshly passed faeces in dog and cats:
  * newly passed faeces
  * digitally extracted specimens.

☙ Describe the precautions which should be taken when obtaining a rectal sample:
  ☙ health and safety
  ☙ patient safety.

Examination of fresh faeces can provide a great deal of information about the health status of the patient.

Faeces should always be placed in a sterile container (such as a plastic faecal pot or a glass wide-mouth jar) to prevent contamination. Samples can be obtained in the following ways:

• The sample should be as fresh as possible. A lubricated, gloved finger can be used to remove faeces directly from the rectum.
• Alternatively freshly deposited faeces can be lifted as soon as it has been produced, again using a gloved hand or sterile scoop.
• The sample pot should be as full as possible to reduce the amount of air in the container.
• Examination should be performed as soon as possible as the sample will deteriorate and ferment quickly.
• Samples should be kept at room temperature and away from direct sunlight.

A number of zoonotic diseases can be passed on in the faeces, including *Giardia, Toxocara canis, Salmonella, Escherichia coli*, and *Campylobacter*. For this reason great care must be taken when collecting faeces to minimise the risk to the handler.

• Gloves should always be worn, and the hands should be washed thoroughly at the end of the procedure.
• Care must also be taken to minimise the risk of injury from the patient. Many animals resent rectal examination and will bite or scratch. An assistant should be used to restrain the animal and muzzles should be used where necessary.
• There is a risk of damaging the rectal mucosa when digitally extracting a faecal sample. Lubrication should be used and the fingernails should be short and smooth within the gloves.

3.5.26 Faecal examination

What you need to learn

☙ What you need to learn
☙ You need to be able to describe the macroscopic examination of a faecal sample. Observations include:
  ☙ consistency
  ☙ colour

☘ odour
☘ presence of visible blood
☘ mucus
☘ fat
☘ ascarid worms
☘ tapeworm segments and oocysts
☘ hair
☘ bone
☘ foreign bodies.
☘ Describe the preparation of a direct faecal smear.
☘ Describe the preparation of a faecal sediment.
☘ Describe the method for examination of a faecal sample for parasitic ova using flotation solution. The fluids include:
☘ saturated salt/sugar solution
☘ zinc sulphate
☘ sodium nitrate.
☘ Describe and identify parasitic ova from the dog and cat:
☘ common endoparasites.

Macroscopic appearance

The macroscopic appearance of the faeces can provide information about the patient (Table 5.16).

Preparation of a direct faecal smear

A direct smear can be used to examine faeces under a microscope and check for worm eggs, protozoan oocysts, or undigested food.

• A drop of saline is placed on the microscope slide.
• A similar volume of faeces is added and thoroughly mixed with the saline.
• A coverslip is placed over the suspension.
• The sample is viewed at low power first, checking for worm eggs.
• The sample is then viewed at higher power to check for oocysts.

Preparation of a faecal sediment

A faecal sediment can be used to concentrate, and therefore improve chances of detection of worm eggs in the faeces.

• A small faecal sample (2–3 g) is mixed thoroughly with distilled water.
• The resulting fluid is sieved to remove large particles.
• The sieved fluid is placed in a centrifuge and spun for approximately 90 seconds.
• The supernatant is decanted.

Table 5.16 Information provided by the macroscopic appearance of faeces

	Normal	Physiological	Pathological
Consistency	Firm, segmented	Firmer on low residue diet or if eating small bones (eg hunting cats) Looser following change in diet	Constipation – hard faeces Diarrhoea – loose or watery faeces
Colour	Mid-brown	Lighter colour on high fat diet or when eating bones Darker colour if on diet with +++ red meat	White – malabsorption Black(melaena) – digested blood Red – undigested blood Yellow – increased bile pigments
Odour		Depends on diet	Rancid – increased fat in stool Strong sweet smell accompanies haemorrhagic diarrhoea (as in parvovirus)
Blood	None		If digested – proximal gut (stomach/small intestine) disorder If fresh and on surface of stool – colon or rectal disorder
Mucus	None		Suggests inflammation of distal gut (colon and rectum)
Fat	None		Malabsorption
Parasites	None		Tapeworm segments, ascarids
Hair	Very occasional		Overgrooming for example with flea allergies
Bone	None		Improper diet
Foreign bodies	None	Parts of prey in cats	Grass, string, paper, plastic, bones, elastic bands commonly found

- A drop of the sediment is transferred to a microscope slide and a coverslip is placed on top.
- This is viewed under low power to check for worm eggs.

Preparation of faecal flotation

This method relies on suspending faecal samples in special solutions which allow worm eggs to float while other faecal matter sinks.

Flotation fluids have a specific gravity which is higher than that of the worm eggs so that the eggs will float. Examples of flotation fluids are concentrated sugar or salt solution, zinc sulphate and sodium nitrate.

- A 2–3 g faecal sample is mixed thoroughly with the flotation fluid.
- The resulting fluid is sieved to remove large particles.
- The sieved solution is then used to fill a test tube completely so that a meniscus forms at the very top of the tube.
- A coverslip is placed on the meniscus at the top of the tube.
- The sample is left for 25–30 minutes during which time any worm eggs float upwards and become adherent to the coverslip.
- After this time the coverslip is carefully lifted off the tube and placed onto a clean microscope slide, trapping any worm eggs between the slide and coverslip.
- The slide is examined under low power.

For identification of worm eggs in faeces – See 3.5.24.

3.5.27   Elementary microbiology

What you need to learn

- You need to be able to outline and list micro-organisms:
  - viruses
  - bacteria
  - algae
  - protozoa
  - yeast/fungi.
- Describe terms associated with micro-organisms:
  - saprophyte
  - parasite
  - pathogen
  - symbiont.
- Explain the units of measurement of size of micro organisms:
  - μm (micrometre/micron)
  - nm (nanometre).
- Tabulate the major similarities and differences between types of micro organisms.
- Describe the basic bacterial cell structure:
  - cell wall
  - cell membrane
  - cytoplasm
  - flagella
  - capsule and slime layer
  - chromosome
  - plasmids

* pili/fimbriae.
* Describe the classification of bacteria according to shape and to Gram stain:
  * see Introduction to bacteriology.
* Understand the meaning of aerobic and anaerobic bacteria.
* Outline the modes of reproduction of bacteria:
  * binary fission
  * conjugation.
* Describe spore reproduction.
* Describe and select appropriate media suitable for bacterial growth:
  * simple
  * enriched
  * selective
  * biochemical.
* Define virulence and explain the significance of toxin production.
* Describe endotoxin and exotoxin and their actions.
* Describe the basic structure and components of viruses:
  * genome capsid
  * capsomeres
  * envelope
  * spikes.
* Describe the mode of reproduction of the virus and its relationship with the host cell.
* Describe the basic classification of fungi.
* Define the term infection and describe how micro organisms cause disorders within the animal body
* Explain terms:
  * bacteraemia
  * septicaemia
  * toxaemia
  * viraemia
  * pyaemia
  * endemic disease
  * epidemic disease
  * zoonotic disease.

Micro-organisms are organisms which can only be seen using microscopy techniques. A number of micro-organisms are of veterinary importance. These include:

• bacteria
• viruses
• fungi and yeasts
• protozoa
• algae.

Table 5.17 Major similarities and differences between types of micro-organisms

Type	Size	Structure	Nutrition	Motility
Bacteria	0.5-5 μm	Prokaryotic (no membrane-bound nucleus), unicellular, cell wall	Mainly heterotrophic, saprophytic or parasitic	Some are motile
Virus	20-300 nm	Central core of DNA or RNA, protein coat (**capsid**), often has a lipoprotein membrane	Heterotrophic. Obligate parasites, require machinery of host cell to survive and reproduce	
Fungi	Variable	Uni- or multi-cellular, chitinous cell wall, (membrane-bound nucleus)	Heterotrophic; saprophytic or parasitic	Non-motile except for some spores
Protozoa	10–200 μm	Unicellular, eukaryotic, no cell wall	Heterotrophic; saprophytic or parasitic	All are motile
Algae	0.5–20 μm	Uni- or multi-cellular, cellulose cell wall, eukaryotic	Autotrophic	Some are motile

Some micro-organisms, such as algae, are **autotrophs** (they are able to synthesise their own food). However most micro-organisms of veterinary importance are **heterotrophs** (they gain their nutrition from their environment).

Heterotrophs can obtain their food from decaying organic material. These organisms are called **saprophytes** and include many fungi. Heterotrophs can also obtain food from other organisms, usually by living on or within them as a **parasite**.

Those parasitic micro-organisms which cause disease (infection) in the host are called **pathogenic micro-organisms**, or **pathogens**.

Many parasitic micro-organisms cause no damage to the host. These are called commensals.

Some commensals can cause disease if they are present in high numbers, or if the host's immune system is weakened. These are called **potential pathogens** or **opportunists**. **Symbiosis** is a close association between two organisms of a different species.

A symbiotic relationship can therefore be:

• parasitic
• commensal
• mutualistic (where both parties benefit – an example is bacteria in the rumen of the cow which are vital for digestion of cellulose).

Often the partners in a mutualistic relationship cannot live without one another.

Micro-organisms are extremely small. They are measured using very small units. Small organisms such as bacteria are usually measured in **micrometres** (μm). Micrometres are sometimes called **microns**.

- Most bacteria measure between 0.5 and 5 μm.
- One micrometre is 1/1000th of a millimetre.
- A micrometre can also be expressed as 1×10^{-6} metres (0.000001 m).
- Even smaller organisms such as viruses are measured in **nanometres** (nm).
- Most viruses measure between 20 and 300 nm.
- One nanometre is 1/1,000,000th (one-millionth) of a millimetre.
- A nanometre can also be expressed as 1×10^{-9} metres (0.000000001 m).

Bacteria

Bacteria are **prokaryotic**, which means that their nucleus is not surrounded by a nuclear membrane. There is no nucleolus, mitotic spindle or separate chromosomes. Prokaryotic cells are usually much smaller than eukaryotic cells.

- The cytoplasm is bounded by a thin, semi-permeable **cell membrane**. This membrane is supported by a more rigid **cell wall**. The cytoplasm contains the DNA which is organised into a single circular **chromosome**.
- Smaller extra packages of DNA called **plasmids** are also suspended in the cytoplasm. Plasmids are important for the development of resistance to antibiotics which is seen in bacteria.
- Ribosomes and their associated RNA are also suspended within the cytoplasm.
- Many bacteria are also surrounded by a thick gelatinous **capsule**. In some species the capsule is less gelatinous and is called a **slime layer**. The function of this extra layer is to help the bacterium to evade the host's immune system.
- A number of appendages can be found on the surface of bacteria.
- A **flagellum** is a whip-like projection which rotates and propels the bacterium along.
- **Fimbrae** or **pilae** are much thinner and shorter than flagellae. Their function is to allow the bacterium to adhere to a surface.
- Specialised pilae known as **sex pilae** are involved with the transfer of genetic material from one bacterium to another during a process known as **conjugation**.

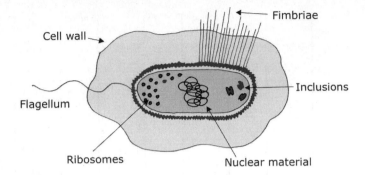

Figure 5.28 Typical bacterial cell.

Classification of bacteria according to shape and Gram stain

Bacteria have characteristic shapes. They are usually:

- Spherical (*cocci*)
- Rod-shaped (*bacilli*)
- Spiral (for example, the spirochaetes)
- Bacteria also have characteristic arrangements which may aid in their identification.
- Cocci are usually bunched (eg Staphylococci) or in chains (eg Streptococci).
- Bacilli can be individual or paired (eg *E. coli*); in chains (eg *Bacillus*); or curved (eg *Campylobacter*).

Unstained bacteria are very difficult to see under a light microscope. Stains are used to make the bacteria more visible. Bacteria often take up the stains in different ways and this can be used to identify the bacteria.

- **Gram's stain** is a differential stain (ie it contains a number of dye substances).
- Some bacteria take up both of the dyes in Gram's stain and show up purple under the microscope – these are called **Gram-positive** organisms.
- Other bacteria just take up the second dye and show up a red/pink colour under the microscope – these are called **Gram negative** organisms.

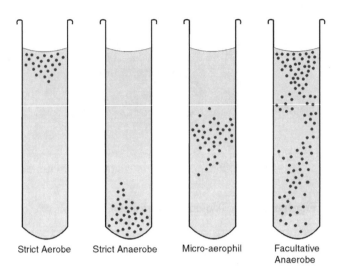

Strict Aerobe Strict Anaerobe Micro-aerophil Facultative
Anaerobe

Figure 5.29 Gaseous requirements of bacteria.

The gaseous requirements of bacteria

Many bacteria grow well in air. Some cannot survive without oxygen. These are known as *strict*, or **obligate aerobes**. Others cannot tolerate the presence of oxygen and must grow in an air-free environment. These are called the **obligate anaerobes**.

Some bacteria grow well in air but can manage to metabolise anaerobically if necessary. These are called the **facultative anaerobes.**

Another group of bacteria require a lower amount of oxygen than in normal air but cannot survive without any oxygen. These are called the **microaerophiles**.

Reproduction in bacteria

Most bacteria multiply by dividing in two. This is called **binary fission**. As the cell grows in size the bacterial chromosome replicates. A septum or cross-wall forms across the cell.

The protoplasm is cleaved by growth of the cross-wall and the two daughter cells are formed.

With some species the daughter cells remain attached in a characteristic arrangement (eg staphylococci remain clustered in bunches; streptococci are attached in chains).

Growth of a colony of bacteria occurs in a number of phases.

• As the bacteria adjust to their new environment there is a **lag phase**. See Figure 5.31.

- The bacteria then enter a **log** or **exponential growth phase** where there is regular doubling in bacterial numbers. During this phase there is a good supply of nutrients and conditions are optimal.
- When nutrients become exhausted or a toxic metabolite begins to inhibit growth, the colony enters a **stationary phase**. The birth rate equals the death rate at this point.
- The final phase is the **decline phase** where bacteria begin to die. This is usually because the conditions have become incompatible with bacterial survival (eg nutrients exhausted, temperature unsuitable, toxin present, or oxygen tension unsuitable).

Most bacteria grow best in the pH range 7.2–7.6 but many are able to tolerate variation in pH. Most pathogenic bacteria grow best at 37°C but are able to survive and reproduce at temperatures between 15°C and 45°C.

In some species a process called **conjugation** occurs.

Conjugation involves the transfer of DNA from one cell (the **donor**) to another (the **recipient**).

The two cells are drawn together by the sex pilus on the donor cell. Once in contact, the cell membranes of the two cells fuse allowing transfer of a package of DNA (a **plasmid**) from the donor to the recipient.

Under certain conditions two genera of bacteria (*Clostridia* and *Bacillus*) are able to form **spores**.

Spores (or **endospores**) are a resting or dormant form of the bacterium.

They usually form when conditions are unsuitable for bacterial growth, for example when nutrients are scarce, or temperature is unsuitable.

- Spores are not reproductive as only one spore is produced per bacterium and only one bacterium is formed when the spore germinates.
- Spores form within the bacterial cell.

Spores are very resistant to heat, desiccation, cold, radiation and chemical treatment which would kill the growing (**vegetative**) form of the bacterium. They can therefore survive in the environment for many years. This ability makes spores very difficult to kill with normal cleaning techniques.

Spore formation is important in the spread of diseases caused by *Clostridia* (such as tetanus and botulism) and *Bacillus* (such as anthrax).

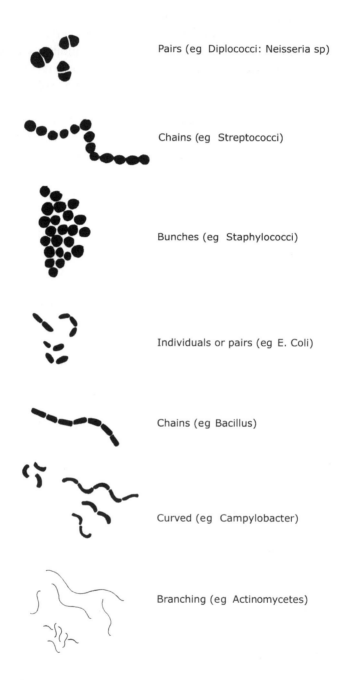

Pairs (eg Diplococci: Neisseria sp)

Chains (eg Streptococci)

Bunches (eg Staphylococci)

Individuals or pairs (eg E. Coli)

Chains (eg Bacillus)

Curved (eg Campylobacter)

Branching (eg Actinomycetes)

Figure 5.30 Common shapes and configurations of bacteria.

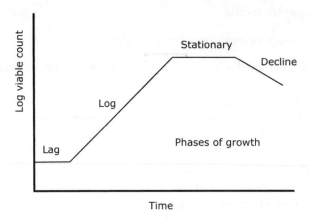

Growth curve for batch culture

Figure 5.31   Bacterial growth curve.

When favourable conditions return the spores germinate and become vegetative bacteria again.

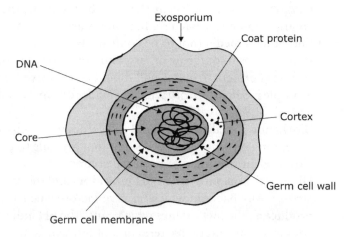

Figure 5.32   Spore structure.

Media used for bacterial growth

A **medium** is a substance within or upon which a colony of bacteria can grow. Different bacteria have different nutritional requirements and so not all bacteria will grow on a particular medium. Media can be liquid (**broth**) or solid (based on **agar**). Before use a medium must be sterile. Media can be classified as:

• **Simple** media contain a mixture of substances (such as ammonia, glucose and phosphate buffer) which provides the basic

requirements for undemanding species of bacteria such as *Escherichia coli*.
• **Complex** media

The complex media can be further divided into:

• **Enriched media** have substances added to them to encourage the growth of more demanding species. Most mammalian pathogens are able to grow in these enriched media. Examples are:
  • *Blood agar*, containing 7% horse, sheep or calf blood
  • *Heated blood agar* (*chocolate agar*), containing blood which has been heated to 85°C to coagulate and denature blood proteins.
• **Selective media** are complex media that contain substances which inhibit the growth of certain organisms while encouraging the growth of others. Examples are:
  • *MacConkey's agar/broth* to which bile salts are added that suppress non-intestinal bacteria but allow intestinal bacteria to grow freely.
  • *Sabouraud's agar* which has a low pH and a high glucose content that encourages the growth of fungi.
  • *Deoxycholate citrate agar (DCA)* which inhibits the growth of many non-enteric bacteria but allows growth of *Salmonella*.
• **Enrichment media** (not to be confused with enriched media) allow some species to outgrow others, and are used when the required species is present in very small numbers in a mixed sample. An example is *Selenite broth* which provides optimal conditions for the growth of *Salmonella*.
• **Biochemical media** contain pH indicators which change colour depending on which types of sugar that are able to ferment. This aids in identification of a bacterial colony.
• **Differential media** contain pH indicators and the carbohydrate lactose. Any bacteria which ferment lactose (such as *E. coli*) produce acidic metabolites which cause the pH indicator to change colour. Many enteric bacteria do not ferment lactose and therefore do not cause any colour change.

Micro-organisms and disease

Micro-organisms do not all cause disease. Those which cause disease are called **pathogens**. Some bacteria are opportunistic pathogens and will only cause disease when the immune system is weakened. The presence of pathogens does not necessarily result in disease.

The ability of pathogens to cause disease varies greatly. The **virulence** of a pathogen is a measure of the pathogen's ability to cause disease. The ability of the host's immune system to resist infection also affects whether a pathogen causes disease. The virulence of a pathogen depends on its **invasiveness** (ability to invade tissues and cells) and its **toxigenicity** (ability to produce toxins which cause further damage).

Toxins produced by micro-organisms

Micro-organisms damage the host either with the production of toxins, or simply by being in the body and causing a severe reaction from the host immune system. The presence of toxins in the blood is called **toxaemia**.

Exotoxins are protein toxins that are produced by mainly Gram-positive organisms such as *Staphylococcus* and *Clostridia*.

- They are released into the bacteria's immediate environment.
- Exotoxins can have a **local** action, or a **systemic** action (such as the neurological toxin produced by *Clostridium tetani*).
- Exotoxins also cause food poisoning when ingested.
- Recently, many exotoxins have been discovered which are produced by Gram-negative bacteria such as *E. coli* enterotoxins, *Pseudomonas* and *Bordetella* toxins.
- The host immune system often produces antibodies to these toxins which render them harmless.
- Exotoxins are heat labile (ie degraded at high temperatures) and are therefore destroyed when food is properly heated.

Endotoxin is the lipopolysacharidecomponent of the bacterial cell wall and is found in Gram-negative bacteria only.

- Endotoxin is thought to be released when the bacterial cell wall is degraded after cell death.
- Endotoxin has numerous systemic effects ranging from pyrexia, hypotension and leukopenia to impaired organ perfusion, disseminated intravascular coagulation, shock and death.
- The effects of endotoxin are often as a result of the immune response rather than of the toxin itself.

Fungi are also able to produce toxins. For example aflatoxin is produced by *Aspergillus flavus* and can be fatal if ingested from spoiled grain and nuts.

Viruses

Viruses are obligate parasites which require the host cell for reproduction and development. They are very small, ranging from 20 to 300 nm. *Parvovirus* is an example of a very small virus (*parvo* coming from the Latin word for small).

Viruses cannot be grown on conventional culture media because they are only able to multiply within other cells. Instead they are grown on sheets of specially grown animal cells. These are called **tissue cultures**.

Viruses consist of:

- A **genome** contained in a central core of nucleic acid. The nucleic acid can be DNA or RNA
- A protein coat, or **capsid**, which is made up of polypeptides called **capsomeres**. The capsid provides protection for the nucleic acid core, and gives the virus its shape (usually **icosahedral** (20-sided), **helical**, or **complex**).
- Many viruses also possess an outer **envelope** made of lipoprotein. The envelope is sometimes penetrated by **spikes**, which are involved with attachment of the virus to the host cells.

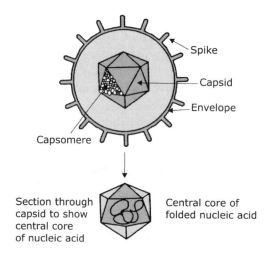

Figure 5.33 Virus structure.

Viruses reproduce themselves by **replication** within the host cell.

- The virus particle attaches itself to receptor sites on the surface of the host cell.
- The whole virus, or sometimes just the nucleic acid core, passes through the cell membrane into the cytoplasm.
- The virus then 'hijacks' the cell, and redirects its metabolic activity so that many copies of the viral components are produced.
- These components are then assembled into virus particles and released (either through the cell membrane, or by lysis of the infected cell).
- The host cell may be destroyed by this activity but in many cases the cell continues to grow and divide, and may show no obvious ill-effects.

Viruses are very hard to treat because it is very difficult for a drug to gain entry to a cell and kill the virus without also killing the host cells.

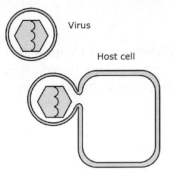

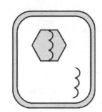

1. The virus attaches to receptor sites on the host cell membrane and fuses with it.

2. The virus enters the host cell and the protein coat (capsid) breaks down to release the viral nucleic acid.

3. The viral nucleic acid replicates (either in the host cell cytoplasm or nucleus) and directs the host cell metabolism to make new virus material.

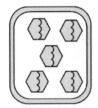

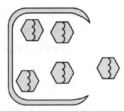

4. The new viruses are assembled.

5. They leave the host cell either by budding through or rupture of the cell membrane.

Figure 5.34 Viral replication.

The presence of receptor sites on the host cell surface varies between individuals, and could account for the variation in susceptibility to viral infection. Currently the most effective method of virus control is through education, avoidance and vaccination rather than treatment of the infected animal.

Some anti-viral drug treatments are becoming available (such as **aciclovir**) and a great deal of research into the treatment of viruses is underway.

Viral diseases of importance in small animal veterinary medicine include:

- canine parvovirus
- canine distemper virus
- infectious canine hepatitis (caused by canine adenoviruses 1 and 2)
- feline leukaemia virus
- feline immunodeficiency virus
- feline infectious peritonitis (caused by feline coronavirus)
- cat flu (caused by feline herpes virus 1 and feline calicivirus)
- rabies.

Fungi

Fungi are basically very primitive plants. They are eukaryotic but lack chlorophyll. To obtain nutrients they are saprophytes, parasites, or in symbiotic relationships with other organisms. Very few fungi cause disease.

The cell wall is a very rigid structure which determines the shape and volume of the cell. The cell membrane lies just within the cell wall and is selectively permeable. The cell may have more than one nucleus. The cytoplasm also contains fats, glycogen and protein stores, and vacuoles, as in other eukaryotic cells.

The fungi can be divided into three morphological groups (ie based on shape):

• yeasts
• moulds (or filamentous fungi)
• dimorphic fungi.

The yeasts

Yeasts are unicellular and are usually ovoid in shape. They reproduce by budding. Daughter yeast cells form as buds from the parent cell. These can remain attached so that chains of yeast cells form.

Examples of yeasts are *Candida albicans* (which causes **candidiasis** or **thrush**) and *Malassezia pachydermatis* (which is commonly implicated in skin disease and otitis).

The moulds (or filamentous fungi)

Mould colonies consist of a mass of interlacing cylindrical tubes called **hyphae**. The hyphae grow at the apex, where new cell wall material is constantly being laid down. Some hyphae have cross walls called **septa** along their length. Others do not have septa and are called **aseptate**.

The moulds reproduce sexually or asexually by spore formation.

Examples of moulds are the dermatophytes such as *Microsporum canis* and *Trichophyton mentagrophytes*; *Aspergillus fumigatus* (which usually causes respiratory disease); and *Saprolegnia* (which causes disease in fish and amphibians).

The dimorphic fungi

These show both a yeast-like unicellular phase and a filamentous phase. An example is *Histoplasma* (a notifiable disease in the UK).

Infection with micro-organisms

When an organism enters a host's body and is able to multiply, the host is described as being **infected** with that organism. To be pathogenic an organism must:

• gain entry to the host
• survive and multiply
• avoid/resist the host defences
• damage host tissues.

Disease caused by infection with a micro-organism occurs if the organism is pathogenic. The severity of the disease depends on the virulence of the pathogen. Damage to the host can be caused by:

• toxin production
• over-reaction of the host's immune system to the presence of the organism
• tissue damage
  • viruses often damage tissues through interference with normal cell metabolism)
  • many bacteria produce toxic enzymes such as **hyaluronidase** (which facilitates penetration of the host tissues by breaking down bonds between cells).

Effects of infection can be:

• **Systemic** – when the organism is able to spread, either in the blood or lymphatic system
• **Localised** – when the infection is restricted to one tissue, organ, or location (such as an abscess).

Terms used when describing microbiological infections

• **Bacteraemia** is the presence of bacteria in the blood which are not multiplying.
• **Septicaemia** is the presence of bacteria in the blood which are actively multiplying.
• **Toxaemia** describes the presence of toxins in the blood.
• **Viraemia** describes the presence of virus in the blood.
• **Pyaemia** is the presence of pus in the blood
• An **endemic disease** (sometimes called enzootic disease) is a disease which is present in the population and causes intermittent disease, eg feline leukaemia virus and feline immunodeficiency virus are endemic in the British domestic cat population.
• An **epidemic disease** (sometimes called epizootic disease) occurs

when there is a sudden steep rise in the incidence of infection with a particular disease. The recent outbreak of foot and mouth disease in the UK can be described as an epidemic, as could an outbreak of parvovirus in a kennel block.

- **Pandemic disease** describes a disease which is present worldwide. An example is the virus which causes human influenza.
- A **zoonotic disease** is a disease which can be passed from animals to humans. Examples are *Salmonella*, sarcoptic mange, toxoplasmosis and *Toxocara canis* infection.

3.5.28   Introduction to bacteriological examination

What you need to learn

- You need to be able to outline correct method for collecting and storing bacteriology samples:
  - swabs
  - blood culture
  - urine culture.
- Describe how to make a bacterial smear from a swab, a culture plate or body fluids observing health and safety principles.
- Identify the reasons for fixing bacterial smears using methylene blue and grams stains techniques. Use the following terms:
  - primary stain
  - mordant
  - decolouriser
  - counter stain.
- Explain why staining with methylene blue should be carried out prior to the use of other methods of staining.
- Describe and identify types of bacteria which can be identified on a bacterial smear:
  - cocci
  - bacilli
  - diplococci
  - staphylococci
  - Gram+ve/Gram-ve, acid fast bacilli.
- Explain why bacteria take up stains in different ways.
- Describe the difference between Lugol's iodine and Gram's iodine.

During investigation of an illness it may be necessary to determine whether bacteria are involved. If bacterial infection is suspected it is also important to identify which species are present. Aseptic sampling techniques are important to minimise contamination of the samples taken.

Direct swabs can be taken from a surface such as a wound or an orifice (mouth, nose, ear, prepuce, vagina, etc). A sterile swab should be used and care must be taken to only touch the surface being tested to avoid contamination. Once collected the swab should be placed in transport medium (usually provided by the laboratory) and despatched as soon as possible. Alternatively the swab can be used to inoculate a culture medium for in-house bacterial cultivation.

Blood samples intended for bacterial culture should be collected aseptically as described earlier, and transferred to an appropriate container.

Urine samples can be collected by free-catch, catheterisation, or cystocentesis. An aseptically collected cystocentesis sample is preferable for bacteriology as this method is the least likely to result in contamination of the sample. Urine intended for bacteriology should be transferred into a sample pot containing boric acid as this will preserve the bacteria during transport to the laboratory.

When making smears for bacteriology it is extremely important to obey health and safety principles. All bacteria should be treated as potential agents of disease.

Smears can be made in a variety of ways:

• Direct smears can be made from a swab by rolling the swab across the surface of a clean microscope slide.
• Smears can also be made directly from the surface being tested. For example, a clean microscope slide can be pressed lightly onto an area of infected skin, or a burst abscess.
• Smears from body fluid samples can be made by placing a single drop of fluid onto a clean microscope slide and allowing it to air dry. A sterile pipette or a cooled, flamed wire loop should be used to transfer the fluid sample aseptically.
• Smears can be made from colonies which have been cultivated on an agar plate. A cooled, flamed wire loop is used to lift a small portion of the colony from the surface of the plate. Care is taken to avoid lifting any agar. The sample can be smeared directly onto a clean microscope slide, or mixed with a drop of sterile water before air drying.

Once the sample has been air-dried on the slide it is **fixed** by passing it two or three times briefly through the flame of a Bunsen burner. This kills the cells but retains their morphology so that further examination can take place. It also helps the cells to adhere to the slide so that they are not washed off during the staining process.

The fixed sample can be stained in a number of ways.

- **Methylene blue:**
  - Methylene blue is a simple stain, using a single dye solution.
  - Staining with methylene blueallows the general morphology of the bacteria to be examined.
  - The prepared slide is flooded with methylene blue solution and left for 2-3 minutes.
  - The stain is then washed off using distilled water and the slide is allowed to dry.
  - This staining should be carried out before using other stains because other stains can be used on top of the methylene blue.
- **Gram's stain:**
  - Gram's stain is a differential stain (involving a number of different dyes).
  - The slide is flooded with the **primary stain**, which is a purple stain called crystal violet.
  - This is then washed away and a **mordant** (iodine solution) is added. The mordant causes the crystal violet stain to become chemically bound to the bacterial cell. (**NB** The iodine used in Gram's stain is less concentrated than Lugol's iodine. Sometimes Lugol's iodine is used as a mordant to provide a darker stain which is more difficult to decolourise.)
  - The mordant is removed and a **decolourising agent** is added (usually acetone). This removes the purple stain from Gram-negative bacteria only. Gram-positive bacteria retain the purple stain.
  - A **counterstain** (usually carbol fuschin) is then used to stain the Gram-negative organisms so that they too can be seen under the microscope. This counterstain does not affect the colour of the Gram-positive bacteria.
  - Gram-positive organisms therefore stain purple while Gram-negative organisms stain pink/red.
  - The Gram stain is an important stain for differentiating species of bacteria. The Gram-negative and Gram-positive organisms differ in a number of ways, including the structure of their cell wall, nutritional requirements, toxin type and resistance to certain drugs.
- **Ziehl-Neelsen stain:**
  - This is used to distinguish bacteria which are **acid-fast**. This means that they have a waxy component in their cell wall and resist most stains.
  - Hot, strong carbol fuschin is used to penetrate the waxy cell wall. The bacteria then hold the stain firmly and resist decolourising solutions.
  - Acid is used to decolourise the rest of the smear, and a counterstain is used to highlight the background so that the slide can be viewed.

- Acid-fast bacteria include the *Mycobacteria* which cause tuberculosis.

Useful information can be obtained by viewing the bacteria after treatment with these stains:

- Morphological information can be obtained.
- Cocci can be distinguished from bacilli by their shape.
- The arrangement of cocci can provide information about the species. *Staphylococci* appear in bunches, *Diplococci* are present in pairs and *Streptococci* occur as chains.
- Gram-negative bacteria can be distinguished from Gram-positive bacteria based on the uptake of the Gram's stain.
- Acid-fast bacteria can be identified using the Ziehl-Neelsen stain.

3.5.29   Collection of body fluids

What you need to learn

- You need to be able to describe how to collect body fluids for laboratory examination:
  - cerebrospinal fluid
  - synovial fluid
  - thoracic fluid
  - abdominal fluid.
- Explain patient and equipment preparation.

Blood and urine collection techniques are described in 3.5.07 and 3.5.14.

Cerebrospinal fluid (CSF)

The examination of CSF can be invaluable in the investigation of neurological disease, particularly when inflammatory changes are suspected. CSF sampling is therefore indicated in cases involving neck pain, seizures which fail to respond to treatment, neurological deficits or following identification of a spinal lesion by myelography or magnetic resonance imaging.

CSF sampling should not be performed if a fracture of the spine is suspected, if there is raised intracranial pressure, or if the animal cannot be anaesthetised. The patient should be under general anaesthesia so that there is no movement and to avoid causing pain during the procedure. The main site for sampling CSF is the cisterna magna, but the lumbar subarachnoid space can also be used.

- The animal is normally placed in lateral recumbency and the area being sampled should be clipped and prepared aseptically.

- The patient's neck is flexed and parallel to the table surface. Care is taken to avoid kinking the endotracheal tube.
- A spinal needle is inserted into the cisterna magna and when the stylet is removed CSF can be seen in the hub.
- The CSF sample is allowed to drip into the sample containers (plain and EDTA).
- A maximum of 1 ml per 5 kg body weight can be safely withdrawn.
- The cells in the sample will deteriorate quickly so some of the sample should be used to produce a smear immediately.
- CSF should be examined for physical appearance, red and white blood cell numbers, protein concentration and cytology.

Synovial fluid

The examination of synovial fluid can be invaluable in the investigation of joint disease. It is particularly useful when more than one joint is affected (polyarthropathies).

The patient should normally be under general anaesthesia so that there is no movement, and to avoid causing pain during the procedure.

- The area being sampled should be clipped and prepared aseptically.
- A sterile hypodermic needle is inserted into the synovial space and the fluid is allowed to drip into the sample containers (plain and EDTA).
- Occasionally synovial fluid can clot as a result of the presence of elevated levels of fibrinogen.
- Smears should be prepared immediately.
- Synovial fluid should be examined for physical appearance, cytology, protein content, microbiological examination and immunological analysis.

Thoracic fluid

Thoracic fluid should be sampled where possible in animals with a pleural effusion. As the patient is usually dyspnoeic the procedure is performed in a conscious patient.

- The area should be clipped and prepared aseptically. The commonest site used is the seventh or eighth intercostal space just ventral to the costochondral junction.
- Local anaesthetic is instilled into the skin and intercostal muscles.
- A catheter attached to a three-way tap and syringe is passed into the pleural cavity and the sample is drawn into a syringe. The procedure is often used to relieve dyspnoea so a large sample of fluid is usually available.

Table 5.18 Fluid characteristics

Type of effusion	Appearance	Protein (g/l)	Cell count (×10⁹/l)	Types of Cell
Transudate	Clear, colourless	5–10	0.5–1.0	Mesothelial, occasional WBCs
Modified transudate	Clear or slightly turbid; red/orange	15–30	1.0–5.0	Mesothelial, neutrophils, macrophages, occasional RBCs.
Exudate	Turbid, variable colour	>25	>25	Degenerate neutrophils, micro-organisms, mesothelial cells, macrophages. **NB** can be sterile.
Chylous	Milky, white or pink	30–80	varies	Small lymphocytes
Haemorrhagic	Dark red, bloody	40–80	N/A	RBCs, WBCs.
Neoplastic	Variable.	30–80	varies	Mesothelial cells, occasional neoplastic cells and WBCs.

RBCs = red blood cells, WBCs = white blood cells.

- A smear of the fluid should be made immediately.
- The fluid should be examined for physical appearance, protein content, specific gravity, cytology, biochemistry (triglyceride, cholesterol and glucose in particular).

This information allows the effusion to be characterised as indicated in Table 5.18.

Additional information can be gained from haematology, serology (feline leukaemia virus, feline immunodeficiency virus and feline coronavirus, in particular), and clotting function (when effusion is haemorrhagic).

Abdominal fluid

Abdominal fluid can be sampled in animals with ascites or when an abdominal haemorrhage is suspected. The procedure is not particularly painful and can usually be performed in the restrained conscious patient.
- The animal is normally standing or in lateral recumbency.
- The area to be sampled on the ventral abdomen is clipped and prepared aseptically. The usual site for sampling is 1-2 cm caudal to the umbilicus.
- A sterile needle attached to a three-way tap and syringe is inserted and fluid is withdrawn.

- A smear should be made immediately.
- The sample should be examined for physical appearance, protein content, specific gravity, cytology, and if necessary, biochemistry.

This information allows the effusion to be characterised as a transudate, a modified transudate, an exudate or a haemorrhage as described in Table 5.18.

3.5.30   Tissue samples and body organs

What you need to learn

❧ You need to be able to describe the methods used for the preservation and storage of specimens for histopathology:
  - ❧ tissue samples
  - ❧ tumours
  - ❧ body organs
  - ❧ body fluids.
❧ Explain why only small pieces of organs or tumours should preferably be stored rather than whole tumour or entire organ.
❧ Explain the importance of selecting correct container for specimens:
  - ❧ size
  - ❧ strength
  - ❧ sealable.
❧ Define formalin, formal saline and neutral buffered formalin and differentiate between them.

Often a tissue sample is necessary to identify a lesion. The microscopic examination of tissue samples is called histopathology. There are two ways in which tissue samples can be obtained for examination.

- **Antemortem** – in a **biopsy** a sample of tissue is taken from the live animal.
- **Postmortem** or **necropsy** samples are removed from a deceased patient.

Once removed from the patient the tissue sample must be correctly preserved and transported to prevent deterioration.

Biopsies can be **incisional** (where a sample area of a lesion or organ is removed for examination), or **excisional** (where the whole lesion or, where possible, organ is removed for examination).

The tissue sample is normally placed in a preservative solution before transport to the laboratory. The preservative solution prevents necrosis and degradation of the sample. The sample must be no more than 2-3 cm thick so that the preservative is able to penetrate the whole sample.

When deciding which part of a tissue sample to send it is important to include the border between diseased and normal tissue. The centre of a large lesion is often necrotic and of little diagnostic value.

When an excisional biopsy has been taken it is important to send the normal margins for histopathology. This is necessary for determining whether the whole lesion has been removed. If the lesion is a malignant tumour this information is vital for providing prognosis.

If a whole organ has been removed (usually the spleen, kidney or a gland or lymph node) small (< 2 cm) representative samples only must be preserved and sent for histopathology.

Body fluids can be preserved by making a fixed smear as described earlier; or by adding a drop of formal saline to 1 ml of fluid. This preserves the morphology of any cells.

When collecting samples for histopathology care must be taken when selecting a container for transport. A suitable container must be large enough to contain the sample and the preservative fluid. Wide-necked containers allow easy removal of the sample. The container must be sealable, so that liquid will not escape when the container is inverted, and strong enough to withstand reasonable handling. Fragile or easily breakable containers must be avoided (such as glass or brittle plastic).

Preservatives which are commonly used in veterinary practice include:

- **Formalin** – this is a 40% solution of dissolved formaldehyde gas. It fixes, or hardens, tissue samples. Formalin is irritant and COSHH rules must be followed when handling it.
- **Formal saline** – this is more commonly used than formalin. It consists of a 10% solution of formalin in a saline solution
- **Neutral buffered formalin** – this is also a 10% solution of formalin in saline but is buffered to protect against changes in pH. This protects the sample from damage caused by changing acidity.

3.5.31   Specimens for toxicological examination

What you need to learn

🐾 You need to be able to outline the special precautions which must be taken when collecting and preparing pathological samples for toxicological examination.

When investigating the cause of a suspected poisoning, various samples can be collected and sent for laboratory analysis. Samples should be labelled with details of the owner and animal, date, type of sample and the practice details. Details of the case must be carefully recorded in case any legal action is taken. Samples should always be collected aseptically to prevent contamination and erroneous results. Suspected poisons can also be toxic to the handler so precautions, such as the wearing of plastic gloves, should be taken when obtaining samples.

Samples can be taken pre or postmortem:

- Whole blood should be sent in an EDTA or heparin tube (eg heavy metal toxicity).
- Serum should be sent following decanting from a clotting tube (eg chocolate toxicity).
- Brain, kidney and liver samples from a postmortem should be frozen before transport to the laboratory.
- Stomach contents (or gastric lavage fluid) can be collected in a waterproof bag or vial. This can then be frozen if necessary.
- Foodstuffs and water can be sent in a watertight container. These should be refrigerated or frozen.
- Environmental samples (bedding or soil samples) should also be collected if they are indicated in a poisoning case.

3.5.32   Records required for pathological samples

What you need to learn

❧ You need to be able to outline the information which should be included on a report form if a pathological sample is to be examined either in the practice laboratory or is being sent away for examination.

When a pathological sample is sent to an external laboratory it is very important that the correct details are sent with the sample.

- Detailed information about the patient's condition should be provided. This helps the pathologists to interpret their findings.
- Pathology request forms are usually provided by the laboratory. These should be filled in fully. Information required includes:
  - details of the owner
  - details of the patient, including species, breed, age, and whether the animal is neutered or not
  - date (and if possible time) of sampling
  - clinical history, including any recent treatment, and previous pathology results
  - site of sampling for tissue samples, and whether the whole lesion has been submitted
  - test(s) required.

When a sample is being examined in the practice laboratory it is important to label the sample carefully with the above details. This prevents samples from getting mixed up and anomalous results being obtained.

3.5.33   Despatch of pathological material to laboratories

What you need to learn

- ☙ You need to be able to describe how to pack samples if they are being sent away for examination:
  - ☙ blood
  - ☙ serum
  - ☙ urine
  - ☙ other body fluids
  - ☙ faeces
  - ☙ hair
  - ☙ coat brushings
  - ☙ skin scrapings
  - ☙ tissues
  - ☙ tumours
  - ☙ organs
  - ☙ samples for virology.
- ☙ Outline the postal regulations in the UK for pathological specimens:
  - ☙ packaging
  - ☙ labelling.
- ☙ State the other considerations that you should bear in mind before despatching a sample:
  - ☙ transit time
  - ☙ weekends/holidays
  - ☙ sample durability.
- ☙ Describe the types of spoilages which can occur with pathological samples and give reasons for their occurrence:
  - ☙ haemolysis
  - ☙ dehydration
  - ☙ autolysis.
- ☙ Describe how post mortem samples and cadavers should be sent to a laboratory for examination and use the term autolysis.

Pathological samples are potentially hazardous materials which are being handled by members of the public (in the postal service). For this reason all pathological samples must be correctly packaged and labelled. Careful packaging also avoids damage to the samples through spillage and contamination. Postal services will not accept improperly labelled or packaged pathology samples.

Postal regulations are outlined.

- Faeces or any sample containing fluid, such as blood, serum, urine, tissue samples and body fluids, should be placed in an appropriate sample tube.
  - The tube should be sealed (usually with a fully tightened screw-on lid).
  - The sample tube should then be wrapped in enough absorbent material (often paper towel) to soak up all of the sample if the container breaks.
  - This should then be placed in a sealed leak-proof plastic bag.
  - This bag should then be placed in an appropriate container for posting. This could be a cardboard, plastic or metal box; or a padded envelope.
- Dry samples such as dried smears, coat brushings, hair plucks and skin scrapings should be placed in an appropriate sealed container. Plastic slide holders are usually used for smears; sealed plastic bags can be used for coat brushings and hair samples. These are then packaged as described.
- Pathology samples should be labelled with the term 'pathological specimen' and 'biohazard'. The biohazard symbol should be clearly visible. The package should also be marked 'Fragile – Handle with Care'.
- Improperly packaged or labelled pathology samples will not be handled by the postal services.

Before sending a sample remember to consider how long the sample will be in the post before being received by the pathologist. It is preferable to send samples well before a weekend or public holiday as these cause a delay in processing samples.

Some samples will deteriorate very quickly (for example, bacteriology specimens and urine crystals). These should always be sent First Class. Fixing or freezing samples helps to reduce deterioration of the sample. (**NB** Samples intended for histopathology should not be frozen as the ice crystals damage the cells.)

When deciding on which external laboratory to use choose the nearest suitable laboratory to reduce sample transit time.

Pathological samples can spoil in a number of ways:

- **Haemolysis** Under some circumstances red blood cells rupture and release their haemoglobin. This is called haemolysis. It occurs when blood is exposed to low or high temperatures, or when blood is shaken. Care should be taken when packaging blood samples that the sample is protected from changes in temperature (by using an insulating layer (usually bubble wrap in padded envelopes) in the packaging. The sample should also be padded well enough to prevent physical damage.

- **Dehydration** This occurs when water is allowed to evaporate from the sample. This can affect blood samples (usually resulting in falsely elevated results). It can also cause desiccation of tissue samples. To avoid dehydration all sample containers should have an airtight seal. Swift transfer to the laboratory helps reduce the possibility of dehydration of the sample.
- **Autolysis** This occurs when samples are improperly preserved. Autolysis begins as soon as the tissue leaves the body. Cell lysis occurs and the tissue degrades. Bacteria in the sample hasten the process. Autolysis affects any tests performed on the sample. These changes occur more quickly in warm, humid conditions.

If a whole cadaver is to be sent to the laboratory (for postmortem examination) it should be refrigerated prior to transport. This slows down the process of autolysis. (**NB** specimens for histopathology should not be frozen as this damages the cells.) The laboratory should be informed that the specimen is on its way. Postal services are usually too slow for sending cadavers so courier services should be used. In this way the journey takes hours rather than days.

Tissue samples from an in-house postmortem should be preserved and packaged as described earlier.

3.5.34   Specimens for virology

What you need to learn

- You need to be able to outline the importance of liasing with the laboratory to identify types of sample required.
- Describe commonly required samples:
    - blood
    - tissues
    - swabs
    - body fluids.
- Describe reasons for sample collection:
    - diagnosis
    - disease eradication
    - vaccine efficacy.
- Describe applications for the common ELISA tests and the principles of the test procedure:
    - FELV
    - FIV.

When sending samples for virology it is useful to discuss with the laboratory which specimens should be sent. This is because different laboratories identify viruses in various ways.

- Blood is used to test for viruses such as feline leukaemia virus, feline immunodeficiency virus and feline coronavirus.
- Faecal samples can be used to test for parvovirus.
- Swabs can be used to test for viruses which affect oro-nasal and ocular areas, such as feline herpes virus, feline calicivirus and canine distemper virus.
- Body fluids can be used to test for other viruses, for example ascitic fluid can be examined for feline coronavirus, the agent which causes the effusive (wet) form of feline infectious peritonitis.

Samples may be tested for viruses for a number of reasons:

- diagnosis of disease
- to check antibody titres in vaccinated animals. (This is performed routinely to check the rabies antibody titre of animals vaccinated against rabies for the pet travel scheme (PETS).)
- to eradicate disease. (For example, the owners of breeding cats should have all incoming cats tested for feline leukaemia virus, feline immunodeficiency virus and feline coronavirus to avoid bringing those diseases into their colony.)

It is possible to test for some viruses in the practice laboratory. The interaction between an antibody and a specific antigen is used in in-house laboratory tests to check whether an animal is infected with a particular organism. Descriptions of some of these tests have been given in 3.5.06.

3.5.35   Communicating test results

What you need to learn

☙ You need to be able to identify correct procedures to record and communicate laboratory test results:
- ☙ within veterinary practice
- ☙ external laboratories.

Details of laboratory tests performed in-house should be recorded. They should include the owner and the patient's details and the date.

Results should be made available to the veterinary surgeon as soon as they are received. Results should also be recorded in the patient's records. It is useful to keep a file of printed laboratory results in case the patent's records are lost or damages (eg through a computer crash).

Any problem with the results (eg poor sample quality, analyser failures) should be reported to the veterinary surgeon involved as soon as possible.

Records should be kept of any samples which have been sent to an external laboratory. This should include the date on which the sample was sent and the veterinary surgeon responsible for the patient. If results are not received when expected there should be communication with the laboratory to ensure that there is not a problem with the sample. Results from an external laboratory should be made available to the veterinary surgeon as soon as they are received. Results should also be recorded in the patient's records.

3.5.36 Communicating advice to owners

What you need to learn

🐾 You need to be able to communicate effectively to owners the principles of parasitic control:
  🐾 ectoparasites
  🐾 endoparasites.

Owners will regularly request information about parasite control. It is important to be familiar with the parasiticide treatments used by the practice, along with the indications and contraindications for use.

When giving advice about endoparasiticides it is important to know:

• How old must the animal be before the treatment can be used.
• What dose should be used.
• How the product should be administered (usually orally, with food; occasionally spot-on preparations are used).
• How often the treatment should be used.
• Which parasites are killed using the product.
• What the possible side-effects are.

When giving advice about ectoparasiticides it is important to know:

• How old must the animal be before the treatment can be used.
• What dose should be used.
• How the product should be administered (usually sprays or spot-ons, occasionally orally or in baths)
• How often the treatment should be used.
• Which parasites are killed using the product.
• What the possible side-effects are.
• Any handling precautions (eg Amitraz is an organophosphate and must be handed with care; some spot-ons and sprays contain flammable liquids, etc)

• Whether any environmental treatment is necessary (it is usually necessary to treat the environment if a flea infestation is suspected).
• How long the product will take to work.

Multiple choice questions

1. The main legislation covering the control of risk to staff from exposure to harmful substances at work including those found in a practice laboratory is:
   - ☐ A Reporting of Injuries, Diseases and Dangerous Occurrences Regulations (RIDDOR) (1995)
   - ☐ B The Health and Safety at Work Act (1974)
   - ☐ C The Control of Substances Hazardous to Health Regulations (COSHH) (1998)
   - ☐ D Collection and Disposal of Waste Regulations(1998)

2. The equation used to calculate the total magnification of a specimen viewed under a microscope is the magnification of the objective lens in use:
   - ☐ A ÷ magnification of the eye-piece
   - ☐ B × magnification of the eye-piece
   - ☐ C + magnification of the eye-piece
   - ☐ D – magnification of the eye-piece

3. Faulty collection of an anticoagulated blood sample can result in haemolysis. The colour of the plasma above such a sample would present as:
   - ☐ A milky
   - ☐ B yellow
   - ☐ C clear
   - ☐ D pink

4. The normal range of PCV in a cat is:
   - ☐ A 30–45%
   - ☐ B 37–55%
   - ☐ C 42–65%
   - ☐ D 60–70%

5. The anticoagulant of choice for performing routine haematology is:
   - ☐ A Heparin
   - ☐ B EDTA
   - ☐ C Sodium citrate
   - ☐ D Fluoride oxalate

6. The most suitable anticoagulant for performing a glucose estimation is:
   - ☐ A Heparin
   - ☐ B EDTA
   - ☐ C Sodium citrate
   - ☐ D Fluoride oxalate

7. The most numerous type of leucocytes in canine blood are:
   - ☐ A Monocytes
   - ☐ B Neutrophils
   - ☐ C Lymphocytes
   - ☐ D Eosinophils

8. Hyperkalaemia is increased plasma:
   - ☐ A calcium
   - ☐ B sodium
   - ☐ C potassium
   - ☐ D phosphate

9. The plasma enzyme which is almost completely liver-specific in the dog is:
   - ☐ A AST
   - ☐ B ALT
   - ☐ C ALKP
   - ☐ D Amylase

10. The test used to distinguish between animals which have pituitary-dependent Cushing's disease and those which have non-dependent Cushing's disease is a:
    - ☐ A ACTH Stimulation Test
    - ☐ B TSH Stimulation Test
    - ☐ C Low Dose Dexamethasone Test
    - ☐ D High Dose Dexamethasone Test

11. The specific gravity of a urine sample is a comparison between the density of the urine and distilled water. The normal range of specific gravity in the dog is:
    - ☐ A 1.000–1.020
    - ☐ B 1.015–1.045
    - ☐ C 1.020–1.040
    - ☐ D 1.050–1.075

12. The urinary crystals illustrated in the diagram are:
    - ☐ A cysteine
    - ☐ B uric acid
    - ☐ C calcium oxalate
    - ☐ D struvite (triple phosphate)

13. The sucking louse of the dog is:
    - ☐ A Felicola subrostratus
    - ☐ B Trichodectes canis
    - ☐ C Linognathus setosus
    - ☐ D Trixacarus caviae

14. The endoparasite involved in the lifecycle of Ctenocephalides felis is:
    - ☐ A Toxocara canis
    - ☐ B Toxascaris leonina
    - ☐ C Dipylidium caninum
    - ☐ D Taenia hydatigena

15. The strobila of a cestode consists of:
    - ☐ A scolices
    - ☐ B proglottids
    - ☐ C onchospheres
    - ☐ D rostellum

16. The tapeworm whose metacestode stage causes hydatidosis in man is:
    - ☐ A Taenia taeniaformis
    - ☐ B Dipylidium caninum
    - ☐ C Echinococcus granulosus
    - ☐ D Trichuris vulpis

17. The bacterial shape illustrated in the diagram is:
    - ☐ A Staphylococci
    - ☐ B Streptococci
    - ☐ C Bacilli
    - ☐ D Campylobacter

18. Bacteria which grow well in air but can survive in anaerobic conditions are known as:
    - ☐ A obligate anaerobes
    - ☐ B microaerophiles
    - ☐ C facultative anaerobes
    - ☐ D obligate aerobes

19. A selective bacterial media contains substances which inhibit the growth of certain organisms but facilitate the growth of others. An example of such a media is:
    - ☐ A Desoxycholate citrate agar
    - ☐ B Chocolate agar
    - ☐ C Blood agar
    - ☐ D Nutrient agar

20. The most suitable preservative for a histological sample is:
    - ☐ A   Methylated spirit
    - ☐ B   Formol saline
    - ☐ C   Potassium hydroxide solution
    - ☐ D   Boric acid

Level 3: Unit 6
Medical nursing

What you need to learn

- You need to be able to outline the pathogenesis and clinical signs of the common infectious diseases:
    - common infectious diseases – see general range statement
    - dogs
    - cats
- Describe the causal agents of infectious diseases:
    - viruses
    - bacteria
    - ectoparasites
    - endoparasites
    - fungal
    - protozoa.
- Describe the principles of nursing animals with infectious diseases:
    - nursing methods
    - barrier
    - isolation
    - quarantine.
- Define 'incubation period' and give examples of the incubation periods of the common infectious diseases:
    - common infectious diseases – see range.

Common infectious diseases

Distemper

The causal agent is a morbillivirus.

Its pathogenesis involves spread by inhalation, direct contact by all body fluids and by fomites. It multiplies in the lymph nodes of the respiratory tract and targets epithelial cells in the gastrointestinal tact and respiratory tract.

Clinical signs are:

• sub-acute – viraemia, depression, anorexia, pyrexia

• acute – initial viraemia, dysphagic temperature, vomiting and dehydration (plus subsequent dehydration), respiratory, ocular and nasal discharges, hyperkeratosis of the skin, fits.

Infectious canine hepatitis (ICH)

The causal agent is adenovirus 1.

Its pathogenesis involves spread by direct and indirect contact, usually by ingestion (environmental contamination). It can be excreted for up to six months. It multiplies in the lymph nodes of the throat and targets the liver, lymphoid tissue and vascular endothelium.

Clinical signs are:

• sub-acute – corneal oedema (blue eye), nephritis
• acute – anorexia, pyrexia, jaundice, enlarged lymph nodes, petechial haemorrhage, enlarged liver, painful cranial abdomen, thrombocytopenia.

Sudden death is seen in young puppies. You may observe anorexia, pyrexia, abdominal pain and crying followed by collapse, shock and death.

Kennel cough complex

The causal agents are adenovirus 2, parainfluenza virus and *Bordetella bronchiseptica*. Pathogenesis involves spread by inhalation. The infecting organisms multiply in the lymph nodes of the upper respiratory tract and target the upper respiratory tract.

Clinical signs are:

• cough (dry/hacking, may retch and produce white froth), swollen cells at the back of the throat, sometimes there are nasal and ocular discharges.

Leptospira canicola

The causal agent is a *Leptospira* aerobic spirochaete bacterium. Pathogenesis involves spread by direct contact with the urine of infected dogs and rats. Transient bacteria in the blood target the kidney.

Clinical signs are:

• polydipsia, vomiting, oliguria, uraemia, oral ulceration, renal and hepatic damage.

Leptospira icterohaemorrhagiae

The causal agent is a *Leptospira* aerobic spirochaete bacterium.

Pathogenesis involves spread by direct contact with the urine of infected dogs and rats. Transient bacteria in the blood target the liver, and the vascular endothelium of the gastrointestinal and respiratory tracts.

Clinical signs are:

• vomiting, haemorrhagic diarrhoea, petechial haemorrhage, jaundice, dehydration, hepatocellular destruction, perivascular haemorrhage.

Lyme disease

The causal agent is *Borrelia burgdorferi*, a spirochaete bacterium.

Following a tick bite there is a local skin infection which progresses to infection of the connective tissues, joints, muscles and lymph nodes.

Clinical signs are:

• acute arthritis, pyrexia, anorexia, depression.

Parvovirus

The causal agents are parvoviruses 1 and 2.

Pathogenesis involves direct contact via fomites or ingestion of faeces. It multiplies in the lymph nodes of the throat and tonsils and targets rapidly dividing cells in the lymphoid tissue, bone marrow, gastrointestinal tract and myocardium in the very young.

Clinical signs

• in young puppies – myocarditis which leads to sudden death
• in older puppies and adults – anorexia, pyrexia, depression, vomiting, haemorrhagic diarrhoea.

Rabies

The causal agent is a rhabdovirus.

Pathogenesis involves spread by direct contact (biting). Initially the virus multiplies at the site of the bite then moves along peripheral nerves into the central nervous system (CNS).

Clinical signs are:

- once the virus is in the CNS ataxia develops
- once the virus is in the brain hydrophobia, laryngeal spasm causing dyspnoea and fits (as a result of high ammonia levels) develop.

Death occurs within five to seven days of the virus reaching the CNS.

Salmonellosis

The causal agents are many different serotypes of *Salmonella* Gram-negative bacteria. The bacteria adhere to and invade the small intestine and multiply in the lymph nodes.

Clinical signs are:

- vomiting, diarrhoea, pyrexia, anorexia, and severe cases will develop septicaemia, abortion.

Chlamydiosis

The causal agent is the *Chlamydia psittaci* bacterium.

Pathogenesis involves spread by ocular discharges from an infected cat. It commonly affects cats between five and twelve weeks of age. Initially it may only affect one eye but the infection rapidly spreads to both eyes.

Clinical signs are:

- uni- and then bilateral ocular discharge, becoming mucopurulent as a result of secondary infection
- mild rhinitis occasionally.

Feline leukaemia virus (FeLV)

The causal agent is a retrovirus. Pathogenesis involves spread by direct or indirect contact. The virus multiplies in the lymph nodes of the throat and tonsils and then moves onto other lymphoid tissue. It replicates in the bone marrow and crypt cells of the intestines and releases infected neutrophils into the circulation.

Clinical signs are:

- anorexia, depression, lethargy, non-regenerative anaemia.

Feline infectious anaemia (FIA)

The causal agents are the *Haemobartonella felis* and *Rickettsia elmeria* intracellular bacteria.

Pathogenesis involves spread through blood (bites, fleas, transfusions and instruments), *in utero* and by mating. The bacteria multiply in the red blood cells, causing them to rupture.

Clinical signs are:

• anaemia, anorexia, weakness, tachycardia, tachypnoea, splenomegaly.

Feline infectious peritonitis (FIP)

The causal agent is a coronavirus. The infection is spread by direct and indirect contact (urine and faeces). Spread can also be transplacental. The virus multiplies in the intestines.

Clinical signs are:

• dry FIP – pyrexia, anorexia, weight loss, diarrhoea
• wet FIP – enlarged abdomen due to ascitic fluid.

Feline immunodeficiency virus (FIV)

The causal agent is a lentivirus. Pathogenesis entails direct contact with saliva (bite wounds). Initially there is a neutropaenia and lymphadenopathy which can remain dormant for many years until signs of immunodeficiency develop. Acts on lymph nodes and bone marrow.

Clinical signs are:

• pyrexia, weight loss, lethargy, anaemia, chronic gingivitis, nail bed infections, diarrhoea, respiratory infections.

Feline upper respiratory tract disease (FURTD)

The causal agents are the feline calicivirus and feline herpes virus type 1. Pathogenesis involves spread by inhalation. The virus multiplies in local lymph nodes before affecting the epithelial cells of the respiratory tract and conjunctiva.

Clinical signs are:

- sneezing, conjunctivitis, ocular and nasal discharges, ulceration, anorexia, pyrexia, depression, coughing, hypersalivation.

Toxoplasmosis

The causal agents are *Toxoplasma gondii* and *Eimeria* spp., both single-cell coccidian protozoa.

The infection is spread by ingestion of the intermediate host, which contains toxocysts in its tissues. These toxocysts enter the intestines and release merozooites which develop into macrogametes. After fertilisation an oocyst is formed and shed in the faeces.

Clinical signs are:

- no clinical signs or
- diarrhoea, weight loss, anorexia, lethargy.

Causal agents of infectious diseases

Infectious diseases are caused by various types of organism.

- **Viruses** can only be seen with an electron microscope. They have no cell structure and both live and grow within living cells. They contain either RNA or DNA (but not both).
- **Bacteria** are unicellular organisms. They have no distinct nucleus and most have a rigid wall or capsule.
- **Ectoparasites** are parasites that live on the outside of the body.
- **Endoparasites** are parasites that live within the body.
- **Fungi** include both yeasts and moulds. Some are parasites but most are saprophytic and feed on dead and decaying matter.
- **Protozoa** are small single cells. Some are parasitic.

Nursing animals with an infectious disease

Infected animals require specialised nursing methods: barrier, isolation, or quarantine.

Barrier nursing

- use foot baths
- wear separate aprons for each patient
- wear separate gloves for each patient
- wash and dry hands before and after handling patients
- disinfect any equipment used, eg thermometers.

Isolation

- Infectious patients should be housed away from healthy patients, preferably in an isolation unit.

- An isolation unit should have its own feeding and cleaning equipment, storage space and sink.
- Use the same kennel for one patient throughout the patient's illness.
- Use the same feeding bowls, litter trays and other equipment for each patient.
- Sterilise suitable equipment after use.
- Disinfect all surfaces.
- Disinfect the kennel daily.
- Disinfect the floors daily.

Quarantine

Animals entering the country not covered by the pet passport scheme are required to be quarantined for six months to help prevent the transmission of certain infectious agents, eg rabies.

Incubation periods

The incubation period is defined as the time between invasion of the body by an infectious agent and the development of clinical signs. Incubation periods are given below for veterinary diseases.

- distemper – 7–21 days
- ICH – 5–9 days
- kennel cough – 5–7 days
- Leptospirosis (*Leptospira canicola*) – 5–7 days
- Leptospirosis (*Leptospira icterohaemorrhagiae*) – 5–9 days
- Lyme disease 2–5 months
- parvovirus – 3–5 days
- rabies – 2 weeks to 4 months
- salmonellosis – a few days
- chlamydiosis – 4–10 days
- FELV – months to years
- FIA – a few days
- FIP – months
- FIV – months to years
- FURTD – 2–10 days
- Feline panleucopaenia 2–7 days
- toxoplasmosis – variable, from 2–4 weeks to months

3.6.02   Zoonoses

What you need to learn

- You need to be able to define the term.
- Describe the principles of good nursing to reduce the risk of spread of zoonotic disease:

* awareness
* exposure
* hygiene and prophylaxis
* barrier nursing.
* Identify the common zoonotic diseases and which animals commonly carry them:
    * salmonella in reptiles and birds
    * psittacosis in parrots
    * leptospirosis in rodents.
* Identify and explain the principles of zoonotic diseases.

A zoonosis is defined as a disease that can be passed from animal to human.

Reducing the risk of spreading zoonotic infections

* *Awareness* – be aware of which diseases are zoonotic.
* *Exposure* – keep exposure to these patients at a minimum, as far as possible.
* *Hygiene prophylaxis* – pay strict attention to hygiene and take preventative measures, ie wash and dry hands, change clothes.
* *Barrier nursing* – this must be instigated in all patients with zoonotic diseases.

Common zoonotic diseases and their carriers

Common zoonotic diseases in dogs and cats include:

* rabies
* Leptospirosis (*Leptospira canicola*)
* Leptospirosis (*Leptospira icterohaemorrhagiae*)
* dermatophytes, eg *Microsporum canis*
* toxoplasmosis.

Zoonotic diseases found in species other than dogs and cats are listed.

* **Reptiles** – *Salmonella* spp., some parasites
* **Birds** – *Salmonella* spp., pittacosis (chlamydiosis), tuberculosis, some ectoparasites such as the mite *Dermanyssus gallinae*
* **Rodents (such as rats and mice)** – leptospirosis *L. icterohaemorrhagiae* (Weil's disease), some parasites, ringworm, *Salmonella* spp.

Carriers are animals which have ceased showing clinical signs of disease but which still have a latent infection. Carrier animals are a potential source of infection with zoonotic disease.

Birds which are treated for psittacosis can recover their health but remain carriers of the causal agent (*Chlamydia*). Apparently healthy animals can shed the organism intermittently for years.

Reptiles such as tortoises can carry latent *Salmonella* infections and shed the organism intermittently in faeces. The infection can revert to its pathogenic form when the animal becomes stressed (eg by dehydration or concurrent disease).

Principles of zoonotic diseases

Zoonotic diseases are infections or infestations which can be transmitted from animals to humans.

3.6.03   Prevention of the spread of infection

What you need to learn

* You need to be able to describe infectious, non-infectious and contagious diseases, and understand their routes of transmission:
  * viruses
  * bacteria
  * ectoparasites
  * endoparasites
  * fungal
  * protozoa.
* Explain the various routes by which infectious agents gain entry to and are excreted from the body:
  * ingestion
  * inhalation
  * trans dermis
  * via mucous membranes
  * congenital.
* Define the terms associated with transmission of diseases:
  * direct contact
  * indirect contact
  * fomite
  * vector
  * non-biological vector
  * biological vector
  * transport host
  * paratenic host.
* Describe methods of transmission from one animal to another and identify how this transmission can be minimised:
  * dogs
  * cats
  * exotics
  * as above.
* Outline the meaning of 'carrier animal' and define types of carriers:
  * dogs

- ❧ cats
- ❧ exotics
- ❧ latent infection
- ❧ 'healthy carriers'.
- ❧ Briefly describe the various methods used in the prevention of transmission of disease:
  - ❧ disinfectants
  - ❧ nursing methods
  - ❧ isolation
  - ❧ barrier
  - ❧ quarantine
  - ❧ treatments.
- ❧ Outline the importance of personal health and safety with respect to zoonotic diseases.

The term **infection** indicates a disease that has been caused by micro-organisms invading and growing within the host's tissues.

The term **non-infectious** describes a disease that cannot be transmitted to other animals.

The term **contagious** describes a disease that is able to be transmitted from one animal to another, either directly or indirectly.

Infectious agents include:

- viruses, eg parvovirus
- bacteria, eg *Salmonella*
- ectoparasites, eg *Ctenocephalides felis*
- endoparasites, eg *Toxocara canis*
- fungi, eg *Aspergillus*
- protozoa, eg *Toxoplasma gondii*

Routes by which infectious agents gain entry to the body include:

- ingestion, eg by the eating of faeces
- inhalation, ie breathing in
- transdermal, ie through the skin
- via the mucous membranes, ie oral or genital
- congenital, ie born already infected.

Routes by which infectious agents are excreted from the body include:

- urine and faeces
- vomit
- blood
- discharges, eg ocular, nasal, oral
- body fluids, eg milk, semen

• parturition
• dead animals

Transmission of infectious agents

An infectious agent can be transmitted to other patients by several methods which include:

• In the direct method the infection is spread by direct physical contact with the animals.
• In the indirect method the animals are not in physical contact, instead the infection is spread via the environment.
• Spread by fomites involves inanimate objects, eg feeding bowls.
• Spread by vectors requires an invertebrate animal carrier, eg mites.
• Spread by intermediate hosts involves a biological vector, eg fleas
• Transport host – a medium by which infection can travel temporarily
• Spread by aerosols occurs when the infection is carried in water droplets in the air (otherwise known as airborne).
• Spread can be by contact with oral and body fluids.
• Spread can be through contact with contaminated food and water.

Transmission of infectious agents can be minimised.

• Patients should be kept away from one another.
• No fighting should be allowed between patients.
• All urine, faeces, vomit and blood (both inside and outside) should be cleaned up.
• Patients should be isolated if necessary.

Transmission of zoonotic disease in exotics

Many zoonotic diseases can be transmitted in the faeces of exotic animals. Contact with faeces or soiled bedding can result in ingestion of the bacteria and infection. Examples of diseases transmitted by the faecal-oral route are:

• *Salmonella*
• nematode and helminth parasites.

Leptospirosis can be transmitted by contact with urine from an infected animal.

Direct contact or contact with shed skin can result in infection with some skin diseases. Examples are:

• ringworm
• ectoparasites

Inhalation of infectious agents is also a common route of disease transmission. Examples of diseases which are transmitted in this way include:

- psittacosis (chlamydiosis)
- tuberculosis.

Carriers – dogs and cats

A carrier is a patient who has come into contact with an infectious agent and may harbour that agent without showing any clinical signs. A carrier may be a **closed carrier**, ie does not shed the agent into the environment, or an **open carrier**, ie they do shed the agent into the environment.

There are two types of carrier, both of which can be open or closed.

- **Healthy carrier** – This is a patient who has been exposed to the infectious agent but has never shown any clinical signs. They are usually immune to that particular agent.
- **Convalescent carrier** (or latent carrier) – This is a patient who has recovered from the infectious agent.

Prevention of infection

The following methods can be seen to help prevent the transmission of infectious agents.

- **Disinfectants** – All kennels, equipment, floors and surfaces should be cleaned regularly with a suitable disinfectant throughout the day.
- **Isolation** – Patients with known or suspected infections should be housed away from healthy patients; a separate kennel area away from the main ward is ideal for this.
- **Quarantine** – Animals entering the country not covered by the pet passport scheme are required to be quarantined for six months to help prevent transmission of certain infectious agents, eg rabies.
- **Treatments** – Any medications or treatment initiated by the veterinary surgeon should be administered to the animal.
- **Sterilisation** – Any equipment used for both infected patients and those suspected of having infections should be sterilised if possible, eg stainless-steel bowls should be used as these can be easily sterilised after use.

Personal health and safety must always be the first matter considered when dealing with patients carrying zoonotic infections because these diseases can be transmitted to humans, causing the same illness, the same symptoms and even death.

Use all the described methods to maintain high standards of personal health and safety in addition to basic handwashing and personal habits.

What you need to learn

* You need to be able to describe the major concepts of immunity:
  * innate immunity
  * acquired immunity.
* Outline the methods by which infection is prevented from entering the body:
  * innate barriers and systems.
* Outline the ways in which agents overcome these barriers:
  * infectious
  * non-infectious.
* Outline the terms relating to passive and acquired immunity.
* Explain the terms related to humoral and cell-mediated immunity:
  * pathogen
  * antibody
  * T cells
  * B cells.
* Describe the different forms of antibody/antigen reactions ELISA tests for FeLV FIV and other antigens:
  * see lab 3.5.06.
* Describe the methods of how immunity develops and understand the importance of colostrum in the neonate:
  * passive and active immunity (particularly in relation to colostral transfer).

Concepts in immunity

Immunity is the ability to resist infection by pathogens (including bacteria, viruses, unicellular organisms and parasites). Immunity can be divided into **innate** and **acquired** immunity.

Acquired immunity is provided by the action of antibodies in response to exposure to a specific micro-organism.

Innate immunity is the non-specific resistance to disease which is incorporated into many body systems. Examples are:

* physical barriers, such as skin and mucous membranes
* mechanical actions, such as the flushing action of fluid in the gastrointestinal, respiratory and urinary tracts
* chemical barriers, such as the acidity of the stomach conter

enzymes in sweat and tears
• phagocytes which engulf and destroy pathogens in the blood and tissues.

Innate immunity is the first line of defence and prevents a wide range of micro-organisms from gaining access to the body. The innate immune system alerts the acquired immune system that a micro-organism is present.

Micro-organisms have developed a number of ways of overcoming the barriers provided by the innate immune system.

• Some micro-organisms are able to bind tightly with the host's cells and therefore avoid being flushed out.
• Some micro-organisms possess thick capsules which prevent damage by acid and enzymes.
• Some micro-organisms are able to hide from the host defences by moving inside the host's own cells (becoming **intracellular** pathogens). Some viruses are able to hide within nerve ganglia.

Micro-organisms include bacteria, viruses and unicellular organisms such as *Toxoplasma*. They also include **prions** (which are the infectious agents that cause diseases such as bovine spongiform encephalopathy (BSE) and scrapie in farm animals.

Not all micro-organisms are harmful. Those which have the ability to cause disease are known as **pathogens**.

The acquired immune system

The acquired immune system recognises a pathogen and provides a response directed specifically at that pathogen. The acquired immune system has the ability to remember pathogens it has met before and can therefore provide a swift response when the pathogen is encountered again.

Antibodies which are produced in the animal's own body provide **active immunity**.

Antibodies which are passed from the mother to the offspring (through the placenta or milk) provide **passive immunity**.

An **antigen** is any substance which triggers an active immune response. Antigens are usually proteins on the surface of an invading micro-organism. The animal's own cells are coated with **self-antigens**. The animal's immune system normally recognises these self-antigens and does not mount an immune response.

Cell-mediated immunity

Cell mediated immunity occurs in the following manner.

- A foreign antigen is presented at the lymph node.
- **T-lymphocytes** become sensitised to the antigen.
- The sensitised T-cell then divides many times.
- Different types of T-cells have different functions.
  - **Killer T-cells** destroy invading cells.
  - **Helper T-cells** help with the production of antibodies.
  - **Memory T-cells** retain the ability to recognise the invading antigen in the future.

Humoral immunity

Humoral immunity occurs as follows.

- A foreign antigen is presented at the lymph node.
- **B-lymphocytes** become activated and divide many times, becoming **plasma cells**.
- Plasma cells produce large numbers of antibodies.
- Antibodies are **immunoglobulins** which are specific to the foreign antigen which caused the immune response.
- Antibodies then react with the antigen in a number of ways.
  - **Neutralisation** – Viruses, and toxins produced by pathogens are neutralised by the antibodies.
  - **Complement activation** – Antibodies stimulate the activation of the complement cascade. Complement is a collection of proteins in the blood which aid in the destruction of pathogens.
  - Interaction with killer T-cells to destroy the pathogen.

The interaction between an antibody and a specific antigen is used in laboratory tests to check whether an animal is infected with a particular organism. These tests are discussed further in 3.5.06.

- The ELISA (enzyme-linked immunosorbent assay) test is used to test for diseases such as feline leukaemia virus (FeLV) and feline immunodeficiency virus (FIV) in cats or parvovirus in dogs. There are also ELISA tests available which detect whether an animal is suffering from allergy (eg they detect antibodies to fleas, pollen and house-dust mites).
- The FeLV ELISA test detects viral antigens in the blood. The test well is impregnated with antibodies to FeLV. Any viral antigens in the blood sample bind with these antibodies and activate a dye. This produces the coloured line or spot seen in a positive result.
- The FIV ELISA test detects antibodies to FIV in the blood. The test well is impregnated with FIV antigens. Any antibodies in the blood sample bind with these antigen and activate the dye.

The development of immunity

Maternal antibodies are able to cross the placenta into the developing fetus. At birth the fetus has **passive immunity** to disease.

Colostrum also contains antibodies which are absorbed across the neonatal gut during the first 24 hours of life. These antibodies which protect the neonatal animal are therefore known as **maternally derived antibodies** (MDA).

Clearly those neonates which drink plenty of colostrum in their first 24 hours of life will have greater protection against disease. This explains why weaker neonates which take less colostrum tend to be the ones which fail to thrive and are prone to infection.

Maternal immunity also depends on the mother's immune status. A healthy mother which has been fully vaccinated is able to pass on better immunity to her offspring.

This maternal immunity wanes during the first 2–3 months of life as the offspring develops its own immune system (ie **active immunity**).

3.6.05 Vaccination

What you need to learn

- You need to be able to explain the principles behind vaccination:
  - passive immunity
  - active immunity
  - primary response
  - secondary response.
- Describe the terms relating to vaccines:
  - vaccine
  - toxoid
  - antitoxin
  - antisera
  - hyperimmune sera
  - courses of vaccination
  - booster vaccination.
- Describe the difference between live and dead vaccines.
- Outline the effectiveness of live versus dead vaccines.
- State the types of vaccines available for common infectious diseases:
  - dog
  - cat
  - rabbit.
- Describe the method of stock control, storing, reconstituting and administering vaccines, and correct procedure for vaccination certification.

❧ Explain why primary vaccination may be ineffective:
  ❧ effect of maternal immunity
  ❧ incubation period.
❧ Outline why vaccinated animals can suffer vaccine breakdowns:
  ❧ timing of vaccination and boosters.

Antibodies which are produced in the animal's own body provide **active immunity**. Antibodies which are passed from the mother to the offspring (through the placenta or milk) provide **passive immunity**. Vaccination is a way to help the immune system to recognise a pathogen, and to be able to mount an active immune response against that pathogen.

A harmless form of the pathogen is given to the animal (usually by injection or inhalation).

The animal's lymphocytes detect antigens on the surface of the vaccine molecules and a **primary response** occurs. The primary response produces a relatively small number of lymphocytes, some of which attack the antigen and some of which become memory cells.

The memory cells enable the immune system to mount a quick response if the same antigen is encountered again (ie if the animal is exposed to the disease itself). The next time the immune system encounters the antigen it produces a **secondary response**. This is a more marked response than the primary response. The secondary response is quicker and lasts for longer than the primary response. Again lymphocytes are produced which provide humoral and cell-mediated immunity.

Vaccines must present the animal's immune system with recognisable antigens from the pathogen without causing any disease. The pathogen against which the animal is being vaccinated could be a bacterium or a virus. There are a number of ways in which the pathogen can be made safe.

• Harmless strains of pathogen can be used as live vaccines.
• An antigenic portion of the pathogen can be used in dead or inactivated vaccines.
• A **toxoid** is an inactivated form of the toxin produced by a pathogen. An example of a toxoid is Tetanus toxoid.
• An **antitoxin** is an antibody which binds with and neutralises toxins.
• **Hyperimmune serum** contains large amounts of antibody to a particular disease. It can be given to an animal in the face of an outbreak to provide short-lived passive immunity to that disease.

Vaccination courses cannot be given to newborn animals immediately because of the maternally derived antibodies. These antibodies would destroy any vaccine antigens without providing any memory for the immune system. Vaccination courses therefore start in young animals as the maternal immunity wanes (most vaccinations start at 9 weeks in kittens and 6–8 weeks in puppies).

The primary vaccination is usually given as two separate injections. The first vaccination produces some immunity to disease but this is often incomplete because there is still some maternal immunity in the young animal's body. Two to four weeks after the first vaccination a second vaccination is given. This produces a stronger response and should provide the animal with substantial immunity to the diseases.

If the immune system is not exposed to the diseases it has been vaccinated against the number of memory cells starts to wane until eventually the animal's immunity wears off. For this reason **booster vaccinations** are given (usually annually). The booster vaccination contains all the same antigenic components and reminds the immune system of which pathogens to be prepared for.

Live vaccines contain living organisms which are a harmless strain of the pathogen. They are able to multiply in the host, creating a long-lasting active immune response.

Dead or inactivated vaccines contain antigens from the pathogen but are not whole living organisms. The antigens cause an active immune response but this tends to be shorter-lived than the effect seen after vaccination with a live vaccine. Inactivated vaccines usually contain a substance called an **adjuvant** (usually aluminium hydroxide) which enhances the immune response.

Vaccines for common infectious diseases

Diseases which are commonly vaccinated against in dogs are:

- canine parvovirus (CPV)
- canine distemper virus (CDV)
- leptospirosis
- infectious canine hepatitis (canine adenovirus (CAV 1 and 2))
- canine parainfluenza virus
- kennel cough (*Bordetella bronchiseptica*)
- rabies.

Diseases which are commonly vaccinated against in cats are:

- feline herpes virus (FHV-1)
- feline calicivirus (FCV)
- feline panleukopaenia (feline parvovirus)

• feline leukaemia virus (FeLV)
• *Chlamydia*.

Diseases which are commonly vaccinated against in rabbits are:

• haemorrhagic viral disease (HVD)
• myxomatosis.

Vaccine storage, administration and certification

The vaccines should be stored carefully as overheating or cooling can destroy the active components. They should be kept at 2–4°C in a refrigerator. They should not be stored in the door of the fridge as they will be exposed to variations in temperature each time the fridge door is opened. The vaccine stock should be checked regularly to ensure that all vaccines are in date. Old vaccines are less effective. Vaccines should be discarded if they have been reconstituted for more than one hour.

Some vaccines are produced as a small, freeze-dried powder disc with a separate bottle of liquid for reconstitution. The liquid (often sterile water) is drawn out of the bottle using a syringe and needle. This is injected into the bottle containing the freeze-dried disc. The solution is agitated gently until all of the powder has dissolved. The resulting solution is then drawn into the syringe ready for injection into the animal. The vaccine should be reconstituted just before injecting to prevent degradation.

Most vaccines are given by subcutaneous injection. An area with plenty of loose skin should be selected. The scruff of the neck is the commonest injection site.

Some vaccines are given intra-nasally. An example is the kennel cough vaccine in dogs. The vaccine is reconstituted as directed. A nozzle is provided for attachment to the syringe. The dog is restrained by an assistant (a muzzle should be used where necessary). The dog's head should be elevated slightly so that the vaccine liquid does not run straight out of the nose. Half of the liquid is the gently squirted into each nostril. Most dogs experience mild irritation and will sneeze or snort.

The myxomatosis vaccine for rabbits is given by both subcutaneous and intra-dermal injection. The subcutaneous injection is given as described earlier. The intra-dermal portion of the injection can be given by withdrawing the needle slowly through the skin while injecting the last portion of liquid. It is difficult to know how much of the vaccine has been deposited intra-dermally using this method so an alternative method can be used. The intra-dermal portion can be administered using a fine needle (such as an insulin needle) into an area of thick skin such as the base of the ear. The needle is inserted into the skin rather than under the skin. A bleb of fluid should be seen within the skin if the vaccine has been injected correctly.

Vaccine certificates should be filled out for every vaccination performed. This provides the owner with a record of vaccination and also provides proof of vaccination for kennels, shows and transportation. The vaccine certificate should always contain:

- owner's details – including name and address
- animal's details – including breed, age, description and sex of animal, and whether or not it is neutered
- vaccine details – including type of vaccine and batch numbers, date of administration and the suggested time for the next vaccination
- signature of the veterinary surgeon who administered the vaccine.

Reasons for ineffective vaccination

Sometimes vaccination is ineffective in producing immunity. There are a number of reasons for this.

- Vaccinating a young animal which has high levels of maternally derived antibody (MDA) often fails to produce immunity. This is because the passive immunity provided by MDA destroys the vaccine before an active immune response can occur. For this reason primary vaccination courses start as MDA starts to wane, and two doses are given at a 2–4 week interval.
- Vaccination can appear to fail if the young animal suffers from the disease it is being vaccinated against. This is because the animal has been infected with the disease before the immune system has had time to respond to the vaccine. This is therefore not an actual vaccine failure. The incubation period of some diseases can be quite prolonged – for example canine distemper virus can have an incubation period of up to three weeks.
- Vaccination can also fail if the animal is not capable of mounting an immune response. This could occur if the animal is already fighting off disease. For this reason only healthy animals should be vaccinated. Animals on immunosuppressive drugs such as corticosteroids should not be vaccinated as they will not mount an effective immune response.

Vaccine breakdown can occur even if the animal was originally vaccinated correctly. This can happen if immunity has waned because the animal has not had booster vaccinations annually. Immunity to leptospirosis and kennel cough is fairly short-lived and will fail to be protective if the booster vaccinations are missed. Immunity to some of the other diseases is longer lasting but will still wane if the animal misses booster vaccination over a period of years.

Vaccine breakdown can also occur if the animal is exposed to an overwhelming infection. An example would be an animal which is in kennels being repeatedly exposed to high doses of parvovirus from infected animals in the same building.

3.6.06   Nutrition

What you need to learn

* You need to be able to describe the basic nutritional requirements and their functions in healthy animals throughout the animal's life stages:
  * neonate
  * young
  * adult
  * pregnancy
  * geriatric
  * working
  * illness/medical conditions.
* Basic nutritional requirements:
  * protein
  * carbohydrates
  * fats
  * minerals
  * vitamins
  * dietary fibre.
* Describe the functions of the different components of the digestive system for small companion animals normally kept as pets:
  * dogs
  * cats
  * small mammals
  * birds
  * reptiles.

Components of a healthy diet

A complete diet should contain the following:

* **Protein** – are formed by chains of amino acids linked by peptide bonds. Amino acids are divided into non-essential amino acids, of which there are 12, and essential amino acids, of which there are 11. Each protein has its own combination of amino acids. The biological value (BV) of the protein refers to the quality of that protein: the higher the BV the less is needed in the diet as it is utilised well. Protein is needed for tissue growth and repair, for energy production and for the transportation of oxygen. In commercially prepared food protein levels are approximately 15–25%.

- **Carbohydrate** – the main sources of carbohydrates are plants, such as fruit, vegetables and cereals. There are four groups.
  - Monosaccharides – are single-molecule sugars. They are the main carbohydrates used by animals, eg glucose and fructose.
  - Disaccharides – are two sugar molecules linked by an alpha bond, eg lactose and sucrose.
  - Oligosaccharides – are a chain of three to ten monosaccharides (which can be all the same or a mixture).
  - Polysaccharides – are formed from thousands of monosaccharides.
- Carbohydrates provide 40–50% of energy in dogs and 30% of energy in cats. In commercially prepared food, carbohydrates are present at approximately 85% in dog food and 75% in cat food.
- **Fats** (also known as lipids) – are formed from fatty acids and glycerol. Fatty acids are either saturated (no double bonds), unsaturated (one or more double bonds), or polyunsaturated (those unsaturated fats containing more than one double bond). There are three essential fatty acids (EFA):
  - linoleic
  - alpha-linolenic
  - arachidonic acid.
- Fat provides energy, is a carrier for fat-soluble vitamins, increases palatability and provides the essential fatty acids listed.
- **Micro-minerals** (also known as trace elements) – are required to maintain metabolic processes and include iron, zinc and selenium.
- **Vitamins** – can be divided into water-soluble vitamins (vitamins B and C), of which any excess is excreted in the urine, and fat-soluble vitamins (vitamins A, D, E and K), of which any excess is stored within the body.
- **Dietary fibre** (or roughage) – is formed from indigestible polysaccharides, eg cellulose, which are usually plant material. These polysaccharides aid bowel function, provide the faeces with bulk and prevent constipation.
- **Water** – is required on a daily basis to replace the obligate water loss from the body. Intake can be derived from drinking water and from food (70% water content in moist food, 10% water content in dry food). Water is needed to maintain normal electrolyte balance and is essential in the thermoregulation and lubrication of body tissues.

Dietary requirements

A complete diet containing all the above components is required by both dog and cat. Cats have two extra requirements that are added into feline diets. These are:

- taurine – an essential amino acid

• arachidonic acid – an essential fatty acid derived from animal origin.

Cats also require lower levels of carbohydrates as they are unable to metabolise large amounts of carbohydrate. They derive most of their energy from proteins and fats.

Life stages

Neonates

Neonates will normally feed from their mother. If they are orphaned they need to be fed a complete milk substitute diet such as Whelpi® or Cimicat® (not cows' milk as this is too low in protein, fat and calories).

Puppies and kittens

Puppies and kittens require more protein, energy and minerals than adults. They have high requirements but only a small stomach capacity so a puppy or kitten diet should be chosen that is highly digestible and palatable. If the animal is under 8 weeks old the food can be softened with water, gravy or milk.

Large breed puppies should be fed reduced energy and fat, and reduced calcium and phosphorus. This is to prevent excessively fast growth which may result in bone and joint abnormalities. Adults should be fed a complete adult maintenance diet. Supplements should not be necessary.

Pregnancy and lactation

During pregnancy and lactation the mother can be fed a puppy or kitten diet that contains increased protein, energy and minerals.

Geriatric animals

For older animals energy and protein are reduced in their diet. Calcium and phosphorus are also reduced to avoid excessive intake.

Working animals

The diet must be easily digested. Protein must be of high biological value as energy is increased along with nutrient concentration. Faecal output should be reduced as a result of reduced dietary fibre.

Illness and medical conditions

Specific diets are now available for medical conditions. These should be fed wherever possible.

3.6.07   Nutritionally-induced disease

What you need to learn

🐾 You need to be able to describe the diseases resulting from deficiency or excess of dietary components:

🐾 protein
🐾 carbohydrates
🐾 fats
🐾 vitamins
🐾 minerals
🐾 calcium.

Tables 6.1 and 6.2 indicate the results of excesses or deficiencies of the basic nutritional requirements.

Table 6.1

Nutrient	Excess	Deficiency
Protein	Osteochondrosis, cervical spondylomyelopathy	Poor immune response Poor coat Reduction in the transport of oxygen
Carbohydrate	Obesity Diarrhoea (if lactase is in excess)	Lack of energy
Fat	Obesity	Poor absorption of the fat soluble vitamins Lack of energy

Table 6.2 Vitamins and minerals

	Excess	Deficiency
Taurine	Non-toxic	Central retinal degeneration, dilated cardiomyopathy, reduced growth rate
Vitamin B	None reported	Anorexia, skin disorders, neurological disorders
Vitamin C	Non-toxic	Scurvy
Vitamin A	Liver damage, ankylosis of joints especially the cervical vertebrae	Seborrhoeic coat conditions, night blindness, crusting lesions of the external nares and nasal discharge
Calcium and phosphorus	Hip dysplasia, oestochondrosis syndrome Eclampsia (deficient in calcium)	Nutritional secondary hyperparathyroidism

3.6.08   Dietetics in relation to disease

What you need to learn

* You need to be able to describe the dietary requirements of animals in disease:
  * disease conditions
  * general post-operative care
  * diseases of the major body systems as detailed later.
* Describe the different preparations available for feeding animals in disease and advise owners on the feeding of animals with disease conditions:
  * dry, semi-moist and moist diets
  * proprietary therapeutic diets
  * homemade diets.
* Understand the principles of enteral nutritional support with reference to animals in disease:
  * see Level 2, 2.4.16.

Post-operative patients should be fed half the amount of their normal volume of diet for their first meal. It should be palatable and easily digestible with high biological value proteins, eg chicken and rice.

Hospitalised patients should be fed an adult maintenance diet if they are not suffering from disease or injury. These contain maintenance levels of carbohydrates, protein, fat, vitamins and minerals. Maintenance diets with reduced levels of energy and fat are available to control weight or maintain weight loss.

Convalescing patients may need a specific diet relative to their disease or injury, eg a high-quality protein diet for renal failure patients.

Feeding animals with disease

Proprietary therapeutic diets are available for specific conditions. They are normally available in dry and moist forms and should be fed as the patients' only diet.

Home-made diets can used in some conditions such as colitis, eg chicken and rice or pasta is made. However, this is a time-consuming and inaccurate method of feeding a patient.

To introduce a dog or cat to a new diet a small amount of the new diet should be mixed with the patient's old diet. This should be continued, increasing the new and decreasing the old preparation with each meal. The following points can also be used to encourage a patient to eat a new diet.

• add a little melted butter
• add a small amount of salt
• warm or fry the food in meat juice
• add smelly fish such a pilchards in tomato sauce.

It should be explained to owners that the new diet should be the only one fed and that water must be available at all times.

Table 6.3 Food preparations available and their characteristics

Food type	Advantages	Disadvantages
Dry	Convenient Cheap Complete diet Aids dental care Diets available for both dog and cat	Some dogs and cats may not find them palatable Storage May drink more
Semi-moist	Available as a complete diet and as treats or snacks Diets available for both dog and cat More palatable than dry	More expensive than dry Not as convenient as dry Does not aid dental care
Moist	Diets available for both dog and cat Very palatable Available in cans, trays and pouches to promote easy storage Complete diet	Expensive Does not aid dental care Not as convenient as dry

Assisted feeding

There are various levels of assistance with feeding.

• Hand feeding – food should be offered to the patient on clean hands or fingers.
• Syringe feeding – liquefied diets should be used and should be applied into the side of the mouth. Ensure that the animal can swallow and that the head is in a natural position to avoid **aspiration pneumonia.**
• Spoon feeding – this involves feeding the diet into the mouth from a spoon.
• Tube feeding – the techniques for tube feeding are given in Level 2, Unit 2.4.16.

Conditions that lead to a requirement for assisted feeding include:

- Psychological – eg an animal may become depressed from being recumbent for long periods.
- Trauma – eg a road traffic accident can cause a fractured mandibular symphysis, making eating impossible.
- Alimentary surgery – eg during recovery after intestinal surgery.
- Systemic illness – eg an animal with renal failure.
- Medication – eg in some animals assisted feeding may be necessary to administer medication.
- Oral surgery – eg if oral surgery has been performed they may be physically unable to eat.

Enteral nutritional support

(See Level 2, Unit 2.4.16)

Feeding via a tube

The tube should be flushed with 5–10 ml water before and after feeding each time to avoid blockages. If a blockage does occur then Coca-Cola can be used to dislodge it. The cap should be replaced on the tube each time it is removed.

When starting feeding:

- On the first day one-third of the total amount is given.
- On the second day two-thirds of the total amount is given.
- On the third day the total amount is given.
- If using a PEG tube food should be withheld for the first 24 hours.
- Amounts given should be divided between four to six meals a day.

This same process should be repeated in reverse when the tube is to be removed to avoid hypoglycaemia. The food should be warmed to body temperature and given slowly to avoid overload, vomiting and diarrhoea.

Stoma care

The skin and area around the exiting tube should be bathed daily, kept clean and dry. Any soiled/wet bandages should be changed.

Calculations for the basic energy requirement (BER) are as follows:

- over 5 kg – BER = 30 × bodyweight + 70
- under 5 kg – BER = 60 × bodyweight

If disease, injury, or surgery is present then a disease factor needs to be added to the calculation as follows:

- BER × disease factor = daily calorie requirement

The following are the disease factors for various conditions:

- cage rest 1.2
- surgery/trauma 1.3
- multiple surgery 1.5
- sepsis/cancer 1.7
- burns 2.0

Fluids should be maintained at 40–50 ml/kg/day to replace the inevitable losses, eg urinary and other. If the patient is vomiting or has diarrhoea an extra 4 ml/kg/episode should be added.

Complications of tube feeding include:

- occlusion of the tube
- vomiting/diarrhoea
- oedema/haemorrhage
- aspiration of food
- hypoglycaemia
- peritonitis.

3.6.09 Common medical diseases

What you need to learn

- You need to be able to identify common classification of medical diseases:
  - physical
  - metabolic
  - infectious
  - allergic
  - degenerative
  - nutritional
  - congenital
  - poison or drug induced.
- Describe the principles of clinical examination for general health and specific body systems, to include accurate recording of findings:
  - TPR
  - examination of the mucous membranes
  - state of eyes
  - ears
  - skin
  - teeth
  - weight
  - general body condition and specific examination of the body system.
- Describe the relevant diagnostic procedures used in the diagnosis and monitoring of medical conditions.

🐾 See laboratory and radiographic units.

🐾 Outline the basic principles of treatment and nursing of medical conditions with reference to advising owners:

  🐾 medical

  🐾 dietary and other management as specified.

Medical diseases are classified according to their causes.

Physical disorders are diseases caused by a change in the structure of a tissue or organ.

Metabolic diseases are those disorders which result from a change in the way an organ or a system works. Metabolic disorders rarely result in a visible change in the affected organ or tissue but can be detected as a change in blood levels of metabolites such as glucose; plasma ions such as calcium or bicarbonate; hormones, or enzymes.

Infectious diseases are those disorders which are caused by an infectious pathogen such as a bacteria, virus, fungus, protozoa, or parasite.

Allergic diseases are diseases caused by hypersensitivity reactions. Examples are atopy, anaphylactic shock and food allergies.

Degenerative diseases are diseases caused by a failure of the body to renew or repair damaged or worn out tissues. Examples are degenerative joint disease (DJD), degenerative neurological conditions such as chronic degenerative radiculomyelopathy (CDRM), and myxomatous degeneration of the mitral valve which causes congestive heart failure.

Nutritional diseases are those disorders which are caused by improper diet. They include deficiency or excess of substances in the diet. Examples are starvation, obesity, hypovitaminosis or hypervitaminosis, and mineral deficiencies or excesses.

Congenital diseases are those diseases which are present at birth. They are not necessarily inherited diseases. Examples are persistent ductus arteriosus (PDA), cleft palate, hydrocephalus, umbilical and inguinal hernias and atresia ani (imperforate anus).

Toxin- or drug-induced disease are those diseases caused by a toxic dose of a substance or drug which enters the body and causes harm.

There are many ways in which the body changes when an animal is affected by disease. By monitoring various easily measurable parameters it is possible to detect disease and monitor the progress of that disease. Thorough clinical examination is therefore vital to assess the health status of the patient. All the information gained from the examination should be carefully recorded, even if it appears normal. This ensures that any changes in the patient's condition can be recognised.

- The demeanour of the patient should be noted before approaching the animal. Most animals will show some signs of nervousness or excitement in an unusual environment such as at the practice.
- Before approaching the animal it is possible to get an impression of the general body condition and the appearance of the coat.
- The stance and gait can also be assessed before handling the patient.
- The animal should be weighed.
- In hospitalised animals the appetite and thirst should be monitored. Abnormalities in urine and faeces should also be recorded.
- The animal can then be examined more closely. Choose a systematic way of examining an animal so that nothing is missed. Most people find it easiest to start at the nose and work caudally.
- The appearance of the eyes, nose and mouth should be assessed and any abnormalities recorded. When examining the mouth the colour of the mucous membranes and the capillary refill time can be checked. Take care in aggressive animals when examining the face.
- The ears and the coat and skin should be checked. Any signs of parasites should be recorded.
- When examining the body it is useful to assess the animal's condition by palpating the fat covering the ribs. The surface of the whole body including the mammary area should be gently palpated for lumps, hernias and other lesions or injuries.
- This part of the examination should include the limbs. Palpation for swelling or heat over the joints is useful.
- The heart and lungs should be auscultated using a stethoscope. At this point the heart rate and respiratory rate should be recorded. The pulse should be palpated while auscultating the heart in order to check for pulse deficits. The femoral pulse is usually used for this.
- The perineum and prepuce or vulva should be examined and any abnormalities, including discharges, should be recorded. The testicles should be palpated in every entire male.
- The animal's rectal temperature should be taken and recorded.
- Temperature, pulse and respiration should be regularly monitored in any hospitalised patient. This is often referred to as **TPR**.

This initial systematic examination may lead to closer investigation, for example an animal which is bleeding from the rectum or showing prostate pain will need a rectal examination.

Further diagnostic tests may be necessary depending on what information has been acquired during the initial examination. Tests which are commonly used include:

- radiography, including contrast studies

- ultrasound
- urinalysis
- faecal analysis
- blood tests (haematology and biochemistry as well as hormone assays, organ function tests and serology)
- cytology of any fluids or fine-needle aspirates.
- microscopic examinations of samples from skin and hair, including ringworm culture tests.

Treatment of medical diseases often involves careful nursing which may be at the practice or in the owner's home.

Most medical conditions take some time to treat. During this time all aspects of the patient's husbandry must be considered.

The correct diet should be selected and fed at an appropriate rate via an appropriate route. Often this may simply be an ordinary diet fed regularly. Some animals require special diets, or are unable to eat normally (requiring assisted feeding). Appetite is often reduced in poorly animals so these patients must be encouraged to eat.

Medical treatments which have been prescribed by a vet must be administered as instructed. These may take the form of fluid therapy, tablets, injections, enemas, topical applications, or inhalational treatments. These should be stored properly and administered at the correct intervals.

The patient should be kept warm using suitable bedding. Appropriate measures should be taken if the patient's temperature falls or rises.

The patient should also be kept comfortable on suitable bedding material. Recumbent animals need particular attention to prevent ulceration of bony prominences.

The animal should be allowed the opportunity to urinate and defecate regularly. Animals which do this in the kennel must be cleaned out immediately for hygiene purposes. Those animals which have difficulty passing urine or faeces require extra attention. Enemas, manual bladder expression and urinary catheters may be necessary.

The patient must be kept stimulated mentally to avoid depression. This may involve physical contact, such as daily grooming; visits from the owner; regular walks and bedding or toys from home.

If an animal is to be cared for at home during treatment the owner must be made aware of their patient's specific needs. If necessary the owner can be given written instructions following discussion with the vet or nurse. These instructions may include details of the medication and diet required as well as details of how to monitor the animal's condition. The owner should be instructed to contact the nurse or vet if they are unsure of how to proceed at any time.

3.6.10 Upper respiratory system

What you need to learn

- You need to be able to describe the function of the upper respiratory system including terms associated with functional abnormalities:
  - sinusitis
  - rhinitis and epistaxis
  - laryngitis.
- Outline the causes of nasal discharge, epistaxis and sneezing and identify the appropriate diagnostic tests:
  - dogs
  - cats
  - small mammals
  - birds
  - reptiles.

To learn about the diseases which affect the upper respiratory system it is important to have an understanding of this system's anatomy and physiology.

The nasal cavity

See Level 2, 2.3.29.

The **paranasal sinuses** consist of the **frontal sinus** and the **maxillary sinus**. The function of the sinuses is not fully understood but it has been suggested that they may:

- provide insulation for the brain, eyes and nose
- allow development of a larger head without adding extra weight
- act as a resonating chamber for the voice
- protect the brain from blows to the head
- help to keep the nasal mucosa moist by the mucous secretions in the sinuses.

Functional abnormalities of the nasal cavity

Infection and inflammation of the mucous membrane of the nasal cavity is **rhinitis**. Rhinitis often presents as persistent sneezing. It can be caused by bacterial and viral infections, allergy and foreign bodies.

Increased inspiratory noise can be caused by narrow or **stenotic nares**. This is common in brachycephalic breeds.

Infection and inflammation of the paranasal sinuses is called **sinusitis**. Sinusitis can be caused by bacterial, viral and fungal infections.

Infection and inflammation of the naso-lacrimal duct is called **dacryocystitis**. It can cause the duct to become occluded. This condition is common in brachycephalic animals, and is often seen with *Pasteurella* infection and dental disease in rabbits.

Inflammation of these parts of the upper respiratory tract usually results in nasal discharge. The discharge may start off being serous or mucoid but often becomes mucopurulent in the presence of bacterial infection.

Trauma or severe infection to the nasal cavity often results in haemorrhage from the nose. This is called **epistaxis**. Aggressive nasal tumours can erode through blood vessels or become ulcerated, resulting in epistaxis.

It is important to ascertain whether nasal discharge or epistaxis is affecting one or both nostrils. Most viral and bacterial infections affect both nostrils. Fungal infections, such as aspergillosis, and nasal tumours usually just affect one nostril.

Other investigations include:

- Air flow down each nostril should be assessed.
- Culture and sensitivity tests should be performed on swabs taken of nasal discharges in cases which are unresponsive to treatment.
- Radiography is useful if sinusitis or nasal cavity tumours are suspected.
- Biopsies should be taken if a tumour is detected.

The pharynx

See Level 2, 2.3.30.

Functional abnormalities of the pharynx

Inflammation of the pharynx is called **pharyngitis**. Pharyngitis may be caused by bacterial and viral infections, trauma, foreign bodies and excessive coughing. Inflammation of the tonsils is called **tonsillitis**. The tonsils can be affected by neoplasia.

The larynx

See Level 2, 2.3.31.

Functional abnormalities of the larynx

Inflammation of the larynx is called **laryngitis**. Laryngitis may be caused by bacterial and viral infections, trauma, foreign bodies and excessive coughing.

Paralysis of the muscles which control the laryngeal cartilages causes increased inspiratory noise and effort. Laryngeal paralysis often occurs in dogs with hypothyroidism. Animals with laryngeal paralysis are at risk of aspiration pneumonia.

Neoplasia can affect the larynx.

The trachea

See Level 2, 2.3.32.

Functional abnormalities of the trachea

Inflammation of the trachea is called **tracheitis**. Tracheitis may be caused by bacterial and viral infections, trauma, foreign bodies and excessive coughing.

Tracheal collapse is common in some toy breeds of dog, eg the Yorkshire terrier. The C-shaped tracheal cartilages are weak and can collapse, particularly when the dog's respiratory rate is increased. A collapsing trachea usually manifests as a 'honking' cough.

Masses which press on the trachea, such as thyroid masses or abscesses, can also affect respiration.

Birds can suffer from an infestation of the nematode *Syngamus tracheae* (also known as 'gape worm'). The worms can obstruct the trachea and cause respiratory distress.

3.6.11 Lower respiratory tract

What you need to learn

* You need to be able to identify the common causes of acute respiratory failure and describe associated clinical signs in dogs, cats, small mammals, birds and reptiles. The clinical signs include:
  * dyspnoea
  * apnoea
  * tachypnoea
  * orthopnoea.
* Describe the types of treatment/First Aid which may be given following acute obstruction of the airway and the appropriate nursing procedures.

* Describe the causes of chronic pulmonary failure and identify common treatments which include:
  * bronchodilators
  * antitussives.
* Describe the causes and clinical signs of pulmonary failure due to extra-pulmonary causes:
  * pneumothorax
  * haemothorax
  * hydrothorax
  * chylothorax
  * pyothorax.
* Outline the principles and procedure in performing thoracocentesis.

Acute respiratory failure

Acute respiratory failure is the inability of the respiratory system to perform oxygen and carbon dioxide exchange well enough for the blood and tissues to remain adequately oxygenated.

Acute respiratory failure is an emergency situation. Use first-aid measures and medical treatment are necessary to prevent worsening of the condition and death. Symptoms of acute respiratory failure are:

* change in the character of breathing, such as:
  * **dyspnoea** – difficulty breathing
  * **tachypnoea** – increased respiratory rate
  * **orthopnoea** – mouth breathing, often in sternal recumbency with elbows abducted
  * **apnoea** – when breathing has stopped altogether
* cyanosis (as a result of darker coloured, poorly-oxygenated haemoglobin in the circulation)
* tachycardia with a weak, thready pulse
* collapse, unconsciousness and death.

Acute respiratory failure can be caused by:

* airway obstruction – foreign body, neoplasia, laryngeal paralysis
* pleural effusion – blood, air, pus, chyle, other effusions
* trauma
* lung disease (pulmonary parenchymal disease) – pneumonia, pulmonary oedema, pulmonary haemorrhage, neoplasia, fibrosis, asthma, thromboembolism, paraquat poisoning (in birds aspergillosis is a frequent cause of lung disease)
* respiratory muscle paralysis – tetanus, botulism, spinal injury.
* failure of respiratory control centre – brain injury, anaesthetic overdose.

First aid must be provided immediately for any animal in acute respiratory failure.

The animal should be handled with great care as severely dyspnoeic animals have minimal reserve lung capacity and can die if stressed.

The most important action is first aid is to ensure that the patient has a patent airway. This may involve removal of a foreign body, suction of mucus, or intubation. If a patent airway cannot be established an **emergency tracheotomy** may be necessary. A skin incision is made just caudal to the larynx in the ventral midline (there is not usually time for clipping and preparing the site). The trachea should be exposed by bluntly dissecting between the muscles of the ventral neck. An incision is made between two tracheal rings and a tracheotomy tube is placed to hold the airway open. The tube is then secured.

Supplementary oxygen should be provided using an oxygen tent, face mask, nasal catheter or endotracheal tube.

Appropriate medication should be provided depending on the cause of the respiratory failure. This may include diuretics to clear pulmonary oedema; respiratory stimulants; bronchodilators; treatment for heart failure.

Thoracocentesis may be necessary when a pleural effusion is causing the respiratory failure.

The patient's condition should be monitored constantly until it is out of danger. Records of the animal's condition and any medication given should be kept. The owner should be notified of any changes in the animal's condition.

Chronic pulmonary failure

Chronic pulmonary failure is caused by more slowly progressive impairment of the lung function. Symptoms of chronic pulmonary failure are:

• reduced exercise tolerance
• chronic cough
• breathlessness
• increased respiratory noise.

If left untreated chronic pulmonary failure can lead to acute respiratory failure and the symptoms of respiratory distress described earlier. Chronic pulmonary failure can be caused by:

• chronic bronchitis/bronchiectasis
• lungworm

- foreign bodies (which do not cause complete airway occlusion)
- pulmonary oedema
- pulmonary neoplasia
- asthma (in cats)
- pleural effusions
- pneumonia

Treatment of chronic pulmonary failure involves treatment of the underlying problem. It may include the following:

- **Bronchodilators** (eg theophylline, etamphylline, terbutaline, clenbuterol) are useful for dilating the lower airways and allowing removal of any accumulated material such as mucus.
- **Expectorants/mucolytics** (eg bromhexine, ipecacuanha) encourage removal of mucus secretions by stimulating the cough reflex, and also by reducing the viscosity of the mucus.
- **Anti-tussives** (cough suppressants, such as butorphanol or codeine phosphate) can be provided if the cough is non-productive.
  NB Cough suppressants are contraindicated in productive coughs as they prevent the removal of secretions from the lower respiratory tract.
- **Antibacterial, anti-parasitic, or anti fungal agents** are used based on culture and sensitivity of the causative organisms. Long courses are often necessary to clear infections.
- **Corticosteroids** are used to reduce the inflammation in the lungs. They should be avoided where an infection is causing the disease as they suppress the patient's immunity.
- **Changes in the patient's management** can help.
  - Limited exercise may help loosen mucus in the airways. A harness or head collar should be used if there is upper respiratory disease. Excessive exercise and exposure to extremes of temperature should be avoided.
  - A clean atmosphere should be maintained by avoiding dust and cigarette smoke.
  - Humidification of inspired air helps prevent drying of the mucous membranes and aids removal of mucus.
  - Coupage can help loosen mucus.
  - Overweight animals should be encouraged to lose weight as this can significantly improve ventilation.

Extra-pulmonary causes of respiratory failure

Respiratory failure can also be caused by problems in the pleural cavity which prevent the lungs from expanding properly. The commonest extra-pulmonary cause of respiratory failure is pleural effusions. Excess fluid or gas is present in the pleural space. This reduces the lung capacity and can cause the lungs to collapse.

Hydrothorax is the accumulation of liquid in the pleural cavity. There are a number of liquids which can be present.

- **Haemothorax** is the presence of blood in the pleural space. It is usually the result of trauma, a bleeding tumour, or a clotting disorder.
- **Chylothorax** is the presence of chyle in the pleural space. It is caused by rupture of the thoracic duct.
- **Pyothorax** is the presence of pus in the pleural space. It is usually the result of a bacterial infection but can occasionally be sterile.
- **Transudates** (serum-like fluid) can be found in the pleural space, usually as a result of hypoproteinaemia or right-sided heart failure.
- **Exudates** (other than pus) can be found in the pleural space as a result of other pleural diseases such as neoplasia, or effusive feline infectious peritonitis.

Pneumothorax is the presence of air in the pleural space. Damage to the lung tissue can result in air leaking into the pleural cavity. Pneumothorax is a common result of blunt trauma to the chest. As air builds up in the pleural cavity the pressure causes the lungs to collapse, resulting in respiratory distress.

- If a small volume of air has escaped and the animal is not in respiratory distress it is not necessary to drain the air.
- If a large volume of air is leaking the air must be drained from the chest using a needle (**thoracocentesis**). The damaged lung will often seal itself so that repeated thoracocentesis is not necessary. However, if the pneumothorax is recurring a chest drain may need to be placed to allow continuous removal of air.

Pneumothorax can also occur as a result of injuries which penetrate the thoracic wall. In this case the air in the chest comes from outside the body, through the wound and into the pleural cavity. In these cases the wound must be repaired and the air drained as described.

Thoracocentesis can be used to drain any pleural effusion if the animal is in respiratory distress. It is also very useful for obtaining samples of the effusion to diagnose the underlying problem. The thorax can be drained intermittently, or an indwelling chest drain can be used to remove fluid as it is produced or released. The animal must be handled very carefully throughout the procedure as stress can further compromise respiratory function.

The following procedure is used when performing thoracocentesis.

- The patient is usually conscious. Local anaesthesia is used to prevent discomfort.
- A suitable site is selected and the chest wall is clipped and prepared aseptically.

- A commonly used site is the seventh intercostal space at the level of the costochondral junction.
- A needle or catheter is passed through the skin and intercostal muscles into the pleural cavity.
- A three-way tap should be attached to the needle and gentle negative pressure should be used to withdraw the fluid.

3.6.12 Circulatory system

What you need to learn

- You need to be able to describe terminology, including clinical signs, associated with disease of the circulatory system:
  - myocarditis
  - endocarditis
  - endocardiosis
  - tachycardia
  - bradycardia
  - pericarditis.
- Describe normal blood pressure and heart rate and the mechanisms for monitoring and recording:
  - manual pulse
  - electrocardiography
  - pulse oximeters.
- Indirect and direct blood pressure monitoring systems:
  - normal heart rate
  - rhythm
  - pulse quality
  - mucous membrane colour
  - CRT.
- Describe the common congenital heart defects and recognise their long term effects.
- Describe the clinical signs of acute and chronic heart failure.
- State and describe the procedures used to diagnose cardiac disease:
  - use of an ECG machine (electrocardiograph)
  - sonography and ultrasound
  - radiography.
- Outline nursing and long term management of animals with chronic heart failure:
  - weight control/diet
  - exercise regime
  - drugs.

The pericardium

The heart sits within the **pericardium,** a closed sac of serous membrane. A small amount of **pericardial fluid** allows the heart to move easily within the pericardium. The heart and pericardium sit within the mediastinum.

Inflammation of the pericardium is called **pericarditis.** Pericarditis can be caused by bacterial infection, viruses (such as feline infectious peritonitis in cats) or neoplasia.

An increase in the amount of fluid in the pericardium is called a **pericardial effusion.** Pericardial effusions can be haemorrhagic or can be exudates or transudates. They are often associated with neoplasia. Clinical signs of pericardial effusion occur when the pressure in the pericardium exceeds the filling pressure in the right side of the heart. Cardiac output is compromised and the heart sound is muffled on auscultation. The effects of a pericardial effusion on the heart are often called **cardiac tamponade.** The pericardial effusion must be drained and the cause identified.

The heart

The **myocardium** is the muscular wall of the heart. Inflammation of the myocardium is called **myocarditis.** It is associated with infectious diseases such as parvovirus. Disease of the heart muscle is called **cardiomyopathy.** The two commonest types of cardiomyopathy are:

- **Dilated cardiomyopathy** (DCM) is more common in large breeds of dog such as Dobermanns and Great Danes. The myocardium becomes thinner and loses its ability to contract efficiently. The result of DCM is congestive heart failure.
- **Hypertrophic cardiomyopathy**(HCM) is more common in small breeds of dogs, and cats. The myocardium becomes thickened so that the diameter of the heart chambers is reduced. The result of HCM is congestive heart failure.

The **endocardium** is the endothelial layer lining the inner walls of the heart. There are two main diseases of the endocardium:

- **Endocarditis** is inflammation of the endocardium. It is caused by bacterial infections which travel to the heart in the blood. Affected animals are pyrexic and have a murmur. There may be signs of other infections as septic foci can spread from the heart valves to other sites.
- **Endocardiosis** is degeneration of the heart valves which leaves them thickened and nodular. The cause is not known but some breeds, such as Cavalier King Charles Spaniels, are predisposed. The mitral

valve is most commonly affected. Endocardiosis results in insufficiency in the function of the valve and eventually congestive heart failure occurs.

Blood pressure

The pressure of the blood in the arteries after ejection from the ventricles is called **systolic pressure**. It is relatively high. Normal systolic pressure is:

- cats 170–180 mmHg
- dogs 180 mmHg.

The pressure of the blood in the veins which fill the relaxed heart is called **diastolic pressure.** It is relatively low. Normal diastolic pressure is:

- cats 120 mmHg
- dogs 100 mmHg.

Blood pressure is measured by stretch receptors (baroreceptors) in the aortic arch and carotid sinus. When blood pressure changes an appropriate response occurs. An example follows.

An increase in blood pressure is detected by the receptors. The medulla oblongata co-ordinates a response to reduce blood pressure (reduction in cardiac output, dilatation of blood vessels, reduction in circulating blood volume).

Blood pressure can be assessed by palpating peripheral pulses but this only provides a rough guide to the blood pressure. It can be measured using sphygmomanometry. A distal pulse is palpated in a limb and a Doppler receiver is used to detect the pulse. A cuff is used on the proximal part of the limb. This cuff is inflated and occludes the arterial flow to the limb so the distal pulse can no longer be palpated. The cuff is very slowly deflated. The pressure at which the Doppler receiver detects the distal pulse returning is the systolic pressure.

A more accurate measurement of blood pressure can be obtained using a catheter placed in an artery which is then connected to a manometer.

Heart rate

The heart rate is the number of heart beats per minute. Normal resting heart rate is 70–120 beats per minute in the dog and 140–200 beats per minute in the cat. An excessively fast heart rate is called **tachycardia** while an excessively slow heart rate is called **bradycardia.**

Heart rhythm

The heart rhythm is the spacing between beats. It is normal for the heart rate to increase slightly during inspiration and slow during expiration. This variation is called respiratory **sinus arrhythmia**. Abnormal alterations in rhythm are called **dysrhythmias** (or arrhythmias).

Stroke volume

The stroke volume is the volume ejected from the heart with each heart beat.

Cardiac output

This is the amount of blood ejected by the heart every minute. It can be calculated by:

• Cardiac output = stroke volume × heart rate

Pulse

The peripheral arteries expand slightly as the pressure wave from a heart beat passes. This can be felt with the fingertips. Palpating the pulse can help assess heart rate and rhythm and gives a guide to stroke volume. If the heart is ejecting less blood (eg a diseased heart) the pulse will feel weak.

Mucous membranes

The mucous membranes are normally pink. A reduction in the cardiac output results in pallor of the mucous membranes. The normal capillary refill time is 1–2 seconds. In animals with reduced cardiac output the capillary refill time is prolonged.

Cyanosis (blue-tinge) of the mucous membranes indicates that the blood is poorly oxygenated. This can occur when there is pulmonary oedema as a result of congestive heart failure.

The electrical activity of the heart

The rhythmic beating of the heart is controlled by a pacemaker – the **sino-atrial node**, which is located in the wall of the right atrium. Impulses from this node cause the atria to contract together. The impulse then passes to another pacemaker node – the **atrioventricuar (AV) node**.

Excitation spreads from the AV node through the **bundle of His** fibres and through the **Purkinje fibres** in the walls of the ventricles. In this way muscular contraction of both ventricles is co-ordinated and controlled.

Electrical activity in the heart can be measured using an **electrocardiogram** (ECG).

- The **P-wave** represents depolarisation of the atria causing atrial contraction.
- The **QRS complex** represents depolarisation of the ventricles causing ventricular contraction (systole).
- The **T-wave** represents repolarisation of the ventricles during relaxation (diastole).

Congenital heart defects

A congenital disease is one which is present at birth. It is not necessarily hereditary. A number of congenital defects affect the heart.

- **Patent ductus arteriosus (PDA)** The ductus arteriosus is a blood vessel which shunts blood from the pulmonary artery to the aorta in the normal fetus. This blood vessel reduces the amount of blood travelling to the lungs (as the lungs are not functional in the fetus). Normally this vessel closes off at birth but in some animals it persists. The persistence of a patent ductus arteriosus eventually results in congestive heart failure. A continuous 'machinery' murmur is audible. The condition can often be treated successfully with surgery to tie off the PDA, or catheter surgery to block it.
- **Aortic stenosis** The aorta is narrowed as it leaves the heart. This results in high pressure in the left ventricle and a reduction in cardiac output. The heart must beat harder to eject the blood. This often results in hypertrophy of the ventricle (increase in size of the muscle wall). The animal may show signs of reduced cardiac output (sometimes called **forward failure**) such as weakness, exercise intolerance, pallor of the mucous membranes and syncope.
- **Pulmonic stenosis** The pulmonary artery is narrowed as it leaves the heart. This results in high pressure in the right ventricle. The ventricle becomes hypertrophied. Clinical signs depend on the severity of the stenosis. The animal may be asymptomatic if the stenosis is mild, or may show exercise intolerance and fainting.
- **Ventricular septal defect** The inter-ventricular septum is malformed so that blood can pass from one ventricle to the other (usually from the left ventricle to the right as there is higher pressure in the left ventricle). The size of the defect varies greatly. Small defects may not cause any clinical signs. Larger defects cause congestive heart failure. A diagonal murmur is audible (loud cranial R and caudel L).
- **Valvular dysplasia** The heart valves are malformed at birth. The

mitral and tricuspid valves are most commonly affected. Congestive heart failure can develop.

- **Persistent right aortic arch (PRAA)** During fetal development the right aortic arch usually degenerates, leaving the left arch to develop into the aorta. If the right aortic arch persists after birth it can form a stricture round the oesophagus at the level of the heart base. Affected animals have difficulty swallowing and regularly regurgitate food. Treatment involves surgery to relieve the constriction.
- **Tetralogy of Fallot** This is actually four abnormalities which occur together. They are:
  - pulmonic stenosis
  - ventricular septal defect
  - overriding aorta
  - right ventricular hypertrophy (this as a consequence of the previous defects).

Treatment is usually palliative. There is increased pressure in the right side of the heart. The animal often has cyanosed mucous membranes, exercise intolerance and a murmur.

Signs of heart failure

Heart failure can occur **acutely** (sudden onset cardiac output failure) or **chronically** (more slowly progressive congestive heart failure).

Acute heart failure is often the result of a rhythm disturbance or myocardial disease. The most common signs of acute heart failure are syncope (fainting) and pallor or cyanosis of the mucous membranes. The fainting episode is usually brought about by excitement or exercise, and the animal often recovers very quickly. Any episode of fainting should be investigated for a possible cardiac cause. If the acute cardiac output failure is prolonged it may result in cardiac arrest and death.

Chronic heart failure is very common in dogs and cats. As the heart starts to fail (from valvular disease, congenital abnormality or myocardial disease) compensatory mechanisms are activated which support the function of the heart. For example the heart rate may increase, the strength of contractions may increase and peripheral blood pressure may be improved by the constriction of peripheral blood vessels. After a while these compensatory mechanisms are no longer able to sustain the function of the heart and the animal is said to have **decompensated heart failure**. The symptoms of chronic heart failure depend upon which side of the heart is failing to function properly.

If the **right** side of the heart is not pumping blood efficiently, blood returning from the body is not able to enter the right atrium normally. Instead it becomes pooled in the veins and organs (the liver in particular). The increased venous volume often results in fluid being pushed out of the veins into the abdomen, resulting in ascites. This combination is known as right-sided heart failure.

If the **left** side of the heart is not pumping blood efficiently the blood from the lungs is not able to enter the left atrium normally. The excessive volume of blood in the pulmonary circulation results in fluid being pushed from the blood vessels into the alveoli and air spaces. This is called **pulmonary oedema**. Animals with pulmonary oedema show signs of a soft moist cough (particularly when recumbent), reduced exercise tolerance and eventually dyspnoea. Severely affected animals may cough up frothy white or blood-stained pulmonary oedema from the lungs. This combination is known as left-sided heart failure.

Diagnosis of cardiac disease

There are a number of tools available in general practice for the diagnosis and monitoring of cardiac disease.

Auscultation is usually the first method used to assess the cardiac function. Auscultation can be used to assess heart rate and rhythm. By palpating a pulse while auscultating the heart any pulse deficits can be noted.

A muffled heart on auscultation may suggest a pericardial effusion, or abnormal soft tissue density within the thorax (neoplasia, diaphragmatic rupture). Heart murmurs are detected by auscultation. The character of the murmur may suggest its origin (for example a continuous 'machinery' is suggestive of a patent ductus arteriosus).

Radiography can be used to assess the shape and the size of the heart. Enlargement of part of the heart on radiographs may aid in diagnosis of a particular cardiac problem (for example an enlarged left atrium causes the trachea to be elevated and is a sign of mitral valve disease). Any fluid in the lungs or pleural cavity can be identified using radiography.

Electrocardiography (ECG) measures the electrical activity of the heart. ECGs are useful to detect rhythm disturbances in the heart. Other information (such as assessing the size of the heart from the size of the QRS complexes) can be obtained from careful reading of an ECG trace obtained in right lateral recumbency.

Echocardiography is the use of ultrasound to assess the structure and function of the heart. The thickness and contractility of the ventricular walls and septum can be assessed. Abnormal soft tissue masses, such as heart-base tumours and valvular lesions, can be visualised using ultrasound. **Doppler** can be used to assess the flow of blood through valves, vessels and septal defects. Pericardial effusions can be confirmed using echocardiography.

Long-term management of animals with congestive heart failure (CHF)

The most important aspect of treatment of animals with CHF is medical treatment to support the function of the heart. Numerous drugs can be used.

- **Diuretics** (frusemide, spironolactone) help to clear fluid from the lungs (in pulmonary oedema) and abdomen (in ascites).
- **ACE inhibitors** (ramipril, enalapril, benazapril) inhibit the actions of angiotensin-converting enzyme (ACE). ACE is released from the kidney when blood pressure has dropped as a result of reduced cardiac output. Its action is to constrict peripheral blood vessels to increase blood pressure. Initially it is a useful compensatory mechanism but in an animal with congestive heart failure it increases the resistance of the blood vessels so that the heart has to beat even harder in order to eject blood. By inhibiting the actions of ACE the heart is able to eject blood more easily.
- **Venodilators** (glyceryl trinitrate) dilate the veins to reduce the pressure of the blood in the venous circulation. They are used in animals with right-sided heart failure.

Animals suffering from chronic heart failure benefit greatly from additional supportive care.

- Overweight animals should be encouraged to lose weight so that the heart has less work to do pumping the blood around the body.
- Any animal in cardiac failure should be fed on a low-salt diet to reduce water reabsorption at the kidney.
- Animals which are being treated with diuretics should have their potassium levels measured and supplemented as necessary.
- Good-quality protein is important as cardiac patients often develop cachexia. Omega 3 fatty acid supplementation (fish oils) may help to reduce cachexia.
- Animals in cardiac failure should be allowed a small amount of gentle exercise. This maintains quality of life and helps to avoid weight gain in prone animals. However, exercise should be controlled as many cardiac patients have exercise intolerance.

3.6.13   Haematopoietic system

What you need to learn

* You need to be able to describe the normal production of components of the haematopoietic system:
  * erythrocytes
  * polymorphonuclear leucocytes
  * lymphocytes
  * platelets.
* Outline and identify the terms associated with gross abnormalities in diagnostic tests:
  * anaemia
  * erythrocytosis
  * leucocytosis
  * thrombocytopenia
  * lymphocytosis
  * neoplastic diseases of the various cell types particularly the leukaemias.
* Describe the causes and recognise the clinical signs of anaemia:
  * dogs
  * cats
  * small mammals and exotics.
* Describe the types of treatment for acute blood loss and chronic blood loss:
  * whole blood
  * colloids
  * pharmacological treatments.
* Recognise the different types of haemorrhage and describe the factors involved in achieving haemostasis:
  * hereditary
  * acquired haemorrhage.

Functions of blood

For functions of blood, red blood cells, white blood cells and platelets, refer to Level 2, 2.3.22.

Haematological abnormalities

See Table 6.4.

Leukaemia is neoplasia of the haematopoietic system. Leukaemias are classified according to which cell lines are affected.

* Abnormal proliferation of the red blood cells is called **polycythaemia vera**. It results in an increased packed cell volume. The blood becomes increasingly viscous. Blood vessel rupture can

Table 6.4

Cell type	Increased numbers	Decreased numbers
Erythrocyte	*Erythrocytosis* – Polycythaemia vera; relative increase caused by dehydration.	*Anaemia* – caused by increased loss; increased destruction, or decreased production of erythrocytes.
Lymphocyte	*Lymphocytosis* – chronic infection, Addison's disease, lymphocytic leukaemia	*Lymphopenia* – Stress, steroid treatment or Cushing's disease, viral infections, immunosuppression, loss of lymph (eg chylothorax).
Monocyte	*Monocytosis* – inflammation, FIV, immune-mediated disease, steroid treatment or Cushing's disease, some malignant tumours, some leukaemias.	*Monocytopenia* – Occasionally occurs following acute inflammation – not clinically important.
Neutrophil	*Neutrophilia* – Stress, inflammation, infection, some tumours, some leukaemias.	*Neutropenia* – Severe infection involving septicaemia or endotoxaemia, bone marrow suppression, acute viral infection (eg parvovirus and FIV).
Eosinophil	*Eosinophilia* – hypersensitivity, immune reactions, parasitism, some leukaemias.	*Eosinopenia* – Stress, steroid treatment or Cushing's disease, acute inflammation and infection.
Basophil	*Basophilia* – Unusual finding, causes similar to causes of eosinophilia, also some leukaemias.	Very low numbers are normal so not recognised as disease condition.
Thrombocyte (platelet)	*Thrombocytosis* – Stress, acute or chronic blood loss, inflammation, some tumours, steroid treatment or Cushing's disease, some leukaemias.	*Thrombocytopenia* – Decreased platelet production, increased platelet destruction or loss.

occur from over distension. Poor blood flow can cause hypoxia in a number of organs.

- Acute leukaemias are aggressive and progress rapidly. The neoplastic change has occurred early in the cell line so that there are high numbers of poorly differentiated white blood cells. Treatment is difficult and the prognosis is often poor.
- Chronic leukaemias are less aggressive and progress more slowly. The neoplastic change has occurred later in the cell line so that there are excessive numbers of well differentiated white blood cells. Treatment is more successful and the prognosis is usually better.

Leukaemias occur in different cell lines:

- **Myeloid Leukaemias** include:
  - Acute Myeloid Leukaemia
  - Chronic myeloid/granulocytic leukaemia
  - Acute myelomonocytic leukaemia

  • **Lymphoid Leukaemias** include:
    • Acute lymphoblastic leukaemia
    • Chronic lymphocytic leukaemia

Anaemia

  • Anaemia is a reduction in the number and/or size of red blood cells in the circulation.
  • Anaemia is described as:
    • **Regenerative** – where the bone marrow responds to the reduction in circulating erythrocytes by releasing immature erythrocytes into the circulation.
    • **Non-regenerative** – where there is no response by the bone marrow to the reduction in circulating erythrocytes.
  • Anaemia can have three primary causes:
    • Increased loss of erythrocytes. This anaemia is usually **regenerative**.
    • Increased destruction of erythrocytes. This anaemia is usually **regenerative**
    • Decreased production of erythrocytes. This anaemia is usually **non-regenerative**

Table 6.5

Type of Anaemia	Examples of Causes
Increased erythrocyte loss	Internal / external haemorrhage – trauma, parasitism, coagulation disorders, ruptured tumours (such as haemangiosarcomas)
Increased erythrocyte destruction	**Intravascular haemolysis:** Immune-mediated haemolytic anaemia (IMHA), cellular parasites (*Babesia, Haemobartonella*), **Extravascular Haemolysis:** Haemolysis of (usually abnormal) RBCs in the liver, spleen or bone marrow.
Decreased erythrocyte production	Bone marrow disorders (FeLV/FIV, irradiation, drugs, toxins, bone marrow tumours), reduced erythropoietin production in chronic renal failure, other hormonal disorders (hypothyroidism, hyperoestrogenism, Addison's disease) chronic liver disease including portosystemic shunts.

Symptoms of anaemia

  • All anaemic animals show symptoms of the reduced oxygen carrying capacity of the blood:
    • Pale mucous membranes
    • Tachycardia
    • Tachypnoea
    • Weak pulses

- Weakness
- Reduced exercise tolerance
- Collapse and death.
- Other symptoms of anaemia depend on the actual cause:
  - Haemorrhagic anaemia – external bleeding, internal bleeding, petechiae or echymoses.
  - Haemolytic disorders – icterus (jaundice), enlargement of the spleen, liver or lymph nodes.
  - These symptoms are similar in dogs, cats and exotic species.

Treatment of acute blood loss

Also see 3.6.33 – 3.6.36.

- Treatment of blood loss relies on supporting the circulation, improving its oxygen carrying capacity, and aggressive treatment of the underlying cause of the anaemia.
- Fluid therapy is the cornerstone of treatment of anaemia. The use of colloids, whole blood or blood product transfusions or the use of artificial oxygen carrying fluids such as oxyglobin are very important in stabilising the animal while determining the cause of the anaemia.
- Treatment of the cause of anaemia can include:
  - Stopping external or internal haemorrhage. This may involve surgery (for example to remove the spleen where a bleeding splenic haemangiosarcoma is detected); treatment of a coagulation disorder (for example vitamin K for treatment of anticoagulant rodenticide (warfarin) toxicity) or parasite treatment where necessary.
  - Preventing further destruction of erythrocytes. This often involves the use of immunosuppressive drugs such as glucocorticoids or azathioprine.
  - Correcting hormone disorders. This may include injection of erythropoietin for animals with chronic renal failure; supplementation with thyroxine for hypothyroid animals; or castration of dogs with oestrogen-producing testicular tumours.
  - Chemotherapy for the treatment of neoplastic disorders such as the leukaemias.

Haemorrhage

- Haemorrhage is most commonly caused by blood vessel injury. This may be due to trauma, or due to erosion of a blood vessel by infection or neoplasia. Where the damage is not too severe clotting mechanisms will eventually stop the bleeding. Where damage is severe or there are multiple injuries the animal may bleed to death if the haemorrhage is not stopped artificially.

- Haemorrhage can also be caused by disorders in the clotting cascade. This is usually an acquired condition caused by poisoning with anticoagulants such as warfarin (anticoagulant rodenticide).
- Clotting disorders can also be hereditary. Examples are Von Willebrand's disease (seen in Dobermann's) and haemophilia. Animals affected by these conditions should not be allowed to breed. Great care must be taken if these animals require surgery.

3.6.14   Alimentary system – general

What you need to learn

- You need to be able to describe the normal functions of the gastrointestinal tract:
  - see Level 2, 2.3.36.
- Describe terms and clinical signs related to the abnormalities of digestive system:
  - dysphagia
  - anorexia
  - pica
  - inappetence
  - polyphagia
  - megaoesophagus
  - regurgitation
  - vomiting
  - diarrhoea
  - constipation
  - tenesmus
  - melaena.
- Outline the principles associated with nursing animals with diseases of gastrointestinal organs to include nutritional requirements/management:
  - stomach
  - intestines
  - colon
  - liver
  - pancreas.

See NVQ Level 2, 2.3.36

- The digestive system breaks down ingesta into its component molecules so that they can be absorbed and utilised by the body.
- The digestive system is basically a tubular tract extending from the mouth to the anus. It also include a number of glands which open into the tract.
- The digestive system and its contents are continuous with the outside of the body.

- The tract is divided into parts, each of which has a particular function.
- Cats and dogs eat meat (they are **carnivores**). Meat is digested by **chemical digestion** (action of **enzymes**).

The oral cavity

For the oral cavity, tongue, salivary glands, swallowing, the oesophagus and stomach, chemical digestion, the small intestine, digestion, protein digestion, carbohydrate digestion, and the large intestine, see Level 2, 2.3.36.

Glossary of terms relating to digestive abnormalities

Dysphagia – Difficulty eating. Can be due to problems in the mouth, throat or oesophagus. The animal is often very hungry. Examples are dental disease; neurological disorders affecting the swallowing mechanism; foreign body in the throat or oesophagus.

Anorexia – Lack of desire to eat. Often caused by systemic illness. Often occurs in nauseous animals.

Pica – Depraved appetite. Often show signs of eating peculiar substances such as soil or stone, or licking surfaces such as carpet, wallpaper and concrete. Usually associated with a deficiency in a particular dietary component. Can be behavioural.

Coprophagia – Eating faeces. Can occur in polyphagic animals. Often a behavioural problem – often seen in kennelled dogs. Normal maternal behaviour.

Inappetance – Reduced appetite, can be completely anorexic or just eating less than usual. Can be a symptom of many disorders.

Polyphagia – Greatly increased appetite. Can be associated with Diabetes mellitus, steroid therapy or Cushing's disease, hyperthyroidism and maldigestive disorders such as Exocrine Pancreatic Insufficiency (EPI)

Megaoesophagus – Dilation of part of the oesophagus. Can be caused by a number of diseases such as hypothyroidism or the muscle disease **myasthenia gravis**. Can be caused by sedation. Often results in dysphagia or regurgitation.

Ptyalism – Drooling. Can be caused by dysphagia or nausea. Often occurs in animals which are travel sick. Regularly caused by administration of oral medication to cats.

Regurgitation – Food and fluid pass back up through the oesophagus and out of the mouth **before they have entered the stomach**. Regurgitation is a passive process (doesn't involve any abdominal contractions). The food is undigested and is often in a tubular shape. The pH of the regurgitated ingesta is usually neutral.

NB regurgitation can occur many hours after eating. Regurgitation can be caused by the animal simply bolting its food, or can be a result of failure of the peristaltic mechanisms which move food into the stomach. Most owners will describe this as vomiting so careful questioning should be used to distinguish vomiting from regurgitation. If there is any doubt the pH of the material should be checked.

Vomiting – Food and fluid pass out of the stomach, back up the oesophagus and out of the mouth. Vomiting is an active process involving abdominal contractions and a complicated set of co-ordinated movements. The vomited material is usually partly digested and may be stained with bile. It has an acidic pH.

Haematemesis – vomiting material which contains blood, fresh or digested.

Diarrhoea – Passing faeces which are unformed and more liquid than normal faeces. Can range from soft stools to brown watery faeces. Can be caused by disease of the small or large intestine. Can be acute (usually infectious or inflammatory cause) or chronic (often associated with malabsorption or maldigestion).

Constipation – Condition where faeces becomes impacted in the rectum and colon. Can be caused by dehydration, sedentary lifestyle, reduced diameter of pelvic canal (eg following pelvic fracture), pain on defaecation and other causes of dyschezia: enlarged prostate gland, rectal strictures or tumours or perineal hernias.

Tenesmus or **Dyschezia** – Difficulty passing faeces, usually involving excessive straining. Can be associated with constipation, an enlarged prostate gland, rectal strictures or tumours or perineal hernias.

Faecal Occult Blood – **Hidden** blood on the faeces, detected using laboratory tests. Usually caused by small bleeds caused by gut parasites or ulceration.

Melaena – Presence of visible **partially digested** blood in the faeces. Faeces appear dark and tarry. Origin of digested blood is the proximal digestive tract – oesophagus, stomach and small intestine.

Haematochezia – Presence of visible **fresh blood** in the faeces. Origin of fresh blood is usually the distal digestive tract – caecum, colon, rectum, anal glands.

Nursing animals with gastrointestinal disease

The major problems associated with gastrointestinal disorders are:

• reduction of food and fluid intake
• increased loss of fluid and nutrients

These two factors can leave the patient with dehydration, malnutrition and metabolic disturbances. Nursing of these patients involves addressing these problems, and depends on the underlying problem.

- Anorexic animals **which are not vomiting** should be encouraged to eat and drink. Hand-feeding food with a strong flavour and smell is often very useful. The food should be easily digestible and preferably concentrated so that a small amount provides plenty of nutrition. The owner should be consulted so that the patient's preferred diet is available.
- Animals which are regurgitating should be fed from head height so that gravity assists the passage of food from the oesophagus into the stomach. Small moist meals should be provided regularly, and the animal shouldn't be allowed to bolt the food.
- Animals which are vomiting should not be fed until the cause of the vomiting has been determined and treated. Fluid therapy is usually necessary to support these patients until the vomiting has stopped. Animals which are vomiting blood should be treated with appropriate medication to prevent further damage to the stomach lining.
- In many cases of acute vomiting, 24 hours of starvation along with supportive and symptomatic treatment is sufficient to allow repair to damaged gastric mucosa and a return to normal gastric function.
- Animals with diarrhoea are likely to need fluid therapy. Initially this can be oral rehydration fluids but in more severe cases intravenous fluid therapy may be necessary to restore circulating volume and correct electrolyte abnormalities. Haemorrhagic diarrhoea can lead to anaemia so colloid plasma expanders may be used in the fluid therapy.
- Animals with liver disorders should be fed on a prescription diet which supports the function of the liver while appropriate medical treatment is provided.
- Animals with pancreatic disorders such as exocrine pancreatic insufficiency (EPI) will need in-feed supplements to replace the missing pancreatic digestive enzymes.
- Animals suffering from pancreatitis (inflammation of the pancreas) must not eat food until the disorder has been treated. Even the sight or smell of food can stimulate release of pancreatic enzymes which exacerbates the pancreatitis. These patients require fluid therapy to support them until feeding can recommence.
- The veterinary nurses should be responsible for recording and describing all vomiting and diarrhoea incidents. They are also responsible for keeping the animal and its environment clean following vomiting or diarrhoea.
- For further information relating to nutrition of animals during disease see 3.6.08.

3.6.15 Stomach

What you need to learn

❧ You need to be able to describe the causes and patterns of vomiting in relation to medical diseases:
  ❧ acute and chronic vomiting.

Vomiting (emesis)

Vomiting can be acute and chronic:

Acute vomiting involves sudden onset, frequent vomiting. The animal is usually lethargic and depressed and can quickly begin to suffer from dehydration and metabolic imbalances. It can be caused by:

• gastritis
• foreign body ingestion
• gastric ulceration
• some drugs (such as steroids and aspirin)
• some chemicals (such as detergents and pesticides)
• acute systemic disease (acute renal failure, pyometra, sepsis etc)
• If the vomiting continues there may be damage to the gastric mucosa resulting in haematemesis, or there may be vomiting of bile.
• Acute vomiting may be associated with acute diarrhoea. This can help with diagnosing the cause of the problem.
• Acute **non-productive** vomiting and retching is a classic indicator of gastric dilatation and volvulus syndrome (GDV).

Chronic vomiting is regular intermittent vomiting which may continue for days, weeks or even months. The animal is often well in itself in between bouts of vomiting. There is often weight loss and a reduced appetite. Other than this physical examination is often unremarkable. There may be a pattern in the occurrence of the vomiting such as early morning. Causes of chronic vomiting include:

• dietary intolerance
• chronic gastritis
• gastric foreign body
• gastric ulceration
• gastric neoplasia
• non-gastric neoplasia (such as mast cell tumours which release histamine and stimulate increased production of gastric acid)
• gastric retention disorders (gastric outflow obstruction or gastric motility disorders). In these patients there may be food in the vomit more than 12 hours after a meal.

Diagnostic tests which are used to find the cause of the vomiting include:

- Blood samples to check for systemic disease and to assess hydration status and electrolyte imbalances.
- Plain abdominal radiography for radio-opaque foreign bodies, pyometra, GDV, peritonitis and others.
- Contrast radiography to assess gastric outflow obstruction, radio-lucent foreign bodies, motility disorders.
- Ultrasonography to detect presence of neoplasms, pyometra, changes to the structure of the gastrointestinal tract.
- Endoscopy to visualise and biopsy the gastric and small intestinal mucosa.
- Exploratory laparotomy to directly visualise and biopsy the gastrointestinal tract.

3.6.16 Intestines

What you need to learn

☙ You need to be able to describe the causes of enteritis, and/or its association with systemic disease:
- ☙ acute and chronic enteritis
- ☙ obstructive
- ☙ dietary
- ☙ maldigestion
- ☙ malabsorption
- ☙ infectious non-infectious
- ☙ parasitic.

- Small intestinal disorders are very common in small animal practice.
- Careful questioning of the owner should allow small intestinal disease to be distinguished from large intestinal (colon) disorders. This is important for investigation and treatment of the underlying cause.
- Clinical signs of small intestinal disorders include:
  - **Diarrhoea** – in small intestinal disorders the diarrhoea is usually watery and voluminous. There tends to be only a mild increase in the frequency or urgency of defaecation in contrast with large intestinal diarrhoea where there is a marked increase in frequency and urgency of defaecation.
  - **Vomiting** – primary vomiting, can be acute or chronic depending on the cause.
  - **Inappetance**
  - **Borborygmi** – rumbling sounds from the intestines.
  - **Flatulence**

- **Melaena** – Blood from the small intestine is usually partly digested by the time it is passed in the faeces. With large intestinal disorders the blood in the faeces tends to be fresh (haematochezia).
- **Weight loss** – This is particularly marked in disorders involving malabsorption or maldigestion. These animals are usually also polyphagic. Reduced plasma proteins levels in these animals may result in oedema and ascites.
- **Abdominal discomfort** – particularly where there is pancreatitis, foreign body or ulceration.
- Inflammation of the small intestine is called **enteritis**.
- Enteritis can be acute or chronic (lasting for more than 2–3 weeks).
- Causes of enteritis include:
  - Bacterial overgrowth
  - Bacterial infection – *Campylobacter, Salmonella, E.coli*
  - Viral infection – Canine *coronavirus, parvovirus, rotavirus*; Feline enteric *coronavirus, panleucopaenia.*
  - Helminth parasite burdens – roundworms and tapeworms.
  - Protozoal parasite burdens – *Coccidia, Giardia, Trichomonas.*
  - Toxin ingestion – drugs, organophosphates, heavy metals
  - Metabolic disorders – Addison's disease, renal failure, liver disease, hyperthyroidism (cats)
  - Diet – food intolerance (sudden change in diet, rapid eating, intolerance of certain foodstuff.) **NB** food allergy is very difficult to prove.
  - Haemorrhagic gastroenteritis – several haemorrhagic diarrhoea requiring prompt aggressive treatment with fluid therapy and antibiosis.
  - Intestinal obstruction – foreign bodies, intussusception, volvulus, strictures, neoplasia.
- Causes of chronic non-inflammatory small-intestinal diarrhoea include disorders of maldigestion or malabsorption of nutrients. These include:
  - Exocrine Pancreatic Insufficiency – deficiency in pancreatic digestive enzymes such as amylase, lipase and proteolytic enzymes. This results in **maldigestion**. Treatment involves supplementing the enzymes in an in-feed supplement.
  - Small Intestinal Bacterial Overgrowth (SIBO) – caused by motility disorders, foreign body, inflammatory bowel disease, tumour. Damage to the intestinal mucosa and villi results in **malabsorption** of the products of digestion.
  - Dietary sensitivity or intolerance.
  - Lymphangiectasia (dilation of mucosal lymphatics which causes a protein losing enteropathy).
  - Lymphosarcoma infiltrating the gut.

3.6.17 Colonic disease

What you need to learn

❧ You need to be able to describe the causes of colitis, and /or its association with systemic disease:
  ❧ acute and chronic colitis.

- The large intestine or colon is responsible for absorbing water and electrolytes from the material in its lumen, as well as for the storage of the resulting faecal matter.
- The two main symptoms of colonic disease are constipation and diarrhoea. Vomiting occurs occasionally in colonic disease and tenesmus is a frequent feature of both constipation and colonic diarrhoea.
- Inflammation of the colon is called **colitis**.
- Colitis diarrhoea is often associated with markedly increased frequency and urgency of defaecation. The volume of stool is usually no more than normal.
- There is usually mucus and often fresh blood in the stools. There may be vomiting in severe colitis.
- Colitis can be:
  - **Acute** – dietary indiscretion leading to bacterial invasion, infection (*Salmonella*, *Campylobacter*), parasitic colitis (whipworms, hookworms and some protozoa such as *Giardia*).
  - **Chronic** – inflammatory bowel disease, colonic neoplasia, caecal inversion, ileocolic intussusception.
  - Treatment of acute colitis involves withholding food for 24 h while providing fluid therapy (oral or parenteral). If an underlying cause has been detected appropriate treatment should be provided. This may include anti-parasite treatments, antibiotics, exclusion diet, anti-inflammatory treatment.
- Further investigation of colitis may involve endoscopy, biopsy, contrast studies, ultrasonography and blood tests.

3.6.18 Hepatic disease

What you need to learn

❧ You need to be able to outline the causes and clinical signs of hepatic disease, with particular reference to hepatitis:
  ❧ acute and chronic hepatitis
  ❧ jaundice
  ❧ cirrhosis.
❧ Describe the principles of nursing and long-term management of animals with hepatic diseases.

See Level 2, 2.3.46.

The gall bladder:

- Bile made in the liver is stored in the **gall bladder**.
- After a meal the gall bladder contracts, expelling the bile through the **bile duct** and into the gut. Contraction of the gall bladder is stimulated by a hormone called **cholecystokinin**.
- Bile contains bile salts, haem pigments, and sometimes cholesterol.
- The liver has a huge functional reserve. Before symptoms develop there must be damage to approximately three quarters of the liver.
- Liver disease can be acute or chronic and can be primary, or secondary to other systemic conditions.
- The liver has numerous functions, so that impairment of liver function results in a wide variety of symptoms. These symptoms may include:
  - Anorexia
  - Vomiting and diarrhoea
  - Weight loss with poor condition and stunted growth
  - PU/PD
  - Drug Intolerance
  - Ascites (from reduced blood protein levels)
  - Icterus (jaundice) – results from obstruction to the normal flow of bile. Bile enters the circulation causing yellow discoloration of the mucous membranes and skin. The urine also contains large amounts of bilirubin. Reduced flow of bile into the gut results in pale (acholic) faeces.
  - Neurological signs (due to excess ammonia in the blood causing hepatic encephalopathy)
  - Pale (acholic) stools
  - Orange urine (from excess bilirubin)
- Inflammation of the liver is called **hepatitis**. Some of the causes include:
  - Bacterial infection – leptospirosis, septicaemia
  - Viral infection – Infectious canine hepatitis (canine adenovirus) or feline infectious peritonitis (FIP).
  - Toxins – drugs, copper, bacterial endotoxins
- Other conditions which may affect the liver include:
  - Hepatic lipidosis – overload of the liver with fat, occurs particularly following sudden anorexia in overweight cats, or in animals with diabetes mellitus.
  - Neoplasia
  - Cholangiohepatitis (inflammation of both the liver and biliary system)
  - One consequence of liver damage is **cirrhosis**. This is the replacement of functional hepatic tissue with fibrous scar tissue. It

often follows severe or chronic liver damage. The functional capacity of the liver is reduced. The flow of bile becomes obstructed so that the animal becomes icteric. Liver failure eventually follows as the condition is slowly progressive. Cirrhosis is therefore the end stage of many liver diseases.

- Treatment of animals with hepatic disease is based on eliminating the cause, treating the symptoms and providing optimum conditions for hepatic regeneration.
- A major tool in treatment of these patients is management of the diet. Protein should be reduced but of high quality. Most of the calories should be provided in the form of carbohydrates. Essential fatty acids and fat soluble vitamins should be supplemented but the amount of fat in the diet should be moderate. Vitamin B should be supplemented. Copper should be restricted. A number of commercial diets which contain these components are available.
- Animals with hepatic disease should be rested and confined as this improves blood supply to the liver (parasympathetic nervous system) and reduce any abdominal pain.
- Anorexic animals or those with vomiting and diarrhoea often require fluid therapy.
- Corticosteroids are often used in inflammatory hepatic conditions.
- Animals suffering from hepatic encephalopathy should be kept in a darkened quiet room. They are treated with intravenous fluids and oral or rectal lactulose which binds ammonia.

3.6.19   Exocrine pancreatic disease

What you need to learn

- ❦ You need to be able to describe the causes and clinical signs of pancreatic disease:
  - ❦ acute and chronic pancreatitis
  - ❦ exocrine pancreatic insufficiency.
- ❦ Describe the principles of nursing and long-term management of animals with pancreatic disease.

- The pancreas is a mixed gland which lies between the greater curvature of the stomach and the duodenum.
- The exocrine part of the pancreas produces pancreatic juice consisting of digestive enzymes (including amylase, trypsin, chymotrypsin, and lipases) and bicarbonate ions.
- Pancreatic juice is released into the duodenum through two pancreatic ducts.
- The release of pancreatic juice is stimulated by cholecystokinin.
- Inflammation of the pancreas is called pancreatitis. It can be acute or chronic. Chronic pancreatitis often results from repeated bouts of acute pancreatitis.

- Both acute and chronic pancreatitis can result in permanent damage to the pancreas with scar tissue replacing the normal tissue.
- Pancreatitis is often caused by damage to pancreatic cells which then leak digestive enzymes, causing further damage to adjacent tissues.
- Some factors which may initiate damage to the pancreatic cells may include:
  - high fat diet or obesity
  - some drugs (such as steroids)
  - pancreatic ischaemia (when pancreatic cells are starved of oxygen, for example during an episode of hypovolaemia)
  - obstruction of the pancreatic duct
  - trauma
- Clinical signs of pancreatitis are variable and may include:
  - Acute vomiting
  - Depression
  - Anorexia
  - Pyrexia
  - Cranial abdominal pain
  - Possibly weakness and shock.
- Treatment of pancreatitis involves withholding food and providing aggressive fluid therapy. Even the sight or smell of food can stimulate release of pancreatic enzymes which exacerbates the pancreatitis.
- Treatment of the underlying cause and any symptoms should also be provided. This may include antibiotics, anti-emetics, anti-inflammatories and pain relief.
- Once the animal is recovering from the acute stage of pancreatitis food can be offered. This should be low fat and high carbohydrate.
- The owners of obese animals should be counselled about their pet's diet. The owners should be advised to put the animal on a low fat diet and slowly reduce the animal's weight.
- One consequence of chronic pancreatitis is exocrine pancreatic insufficiency (EPI). In this condition the chronic damage to the pancreas results in a loss of functional cells. The pancreas is unable to produce sufficient digestive enzyme to allow the animal to digest its food. The digestive enzymes which are deficient are amylase, lipase and proteolytic enzymes.
- Symptoms of EPI are:
  - diarrhoea – voluminous, pasty (containing ++ fat) loose stools.
  - weight loss
  - polyphagia
  - the animals are bright and well in themselves.
- Treatment involves supplementing the deficient enzymes using an in-feed supplement. This supplementation must continue life-long.
- The patient should be weighed regularly.

- The owner should be counselled that the treatment can be expensive and is life-long. These patients usually respond well to treatment but tend to remain relatively thin.
- Occasionally severe damage to the pancreas can result in damage to the endocrine function, and diabetes mellitus may result. This may be temporary or permanent.

3.6.20   Renal system

What you need to learn

- You need to be able to describe the function of the kidney and the production of glomerular filtrate and subsequently urine.
- Describe the terms, and associated clinical signs, related to the disease of the kidney:
  - nephritis
  - glomerulonephritis
  - pyelonephritis
  - interstitial nephritis.
- Outline the causes for the major abnormal renal conditions:
  - acute renal failure
  - chronic renal failure.
- Describe the principles of nursing animals with acute, chronic renal failure and nephrotic syndrome:
  - medical management
  - provision of water
  - appropriate dietary control.

See Level 2, 2.3.50 for functions of the kidney and the production of glomerular filtrate and urine.

Terms relating to renal disease

Nephritis – Inflammation of the kidney. This term is a general term and does not indicate which parts of the kidney are affected.

Nephrosis – Non-inflammatory damage to the renal tubules – often caused by ischaemia (lack of oxygen) or toxicity (drugs, antifreeze, some antibiotics and heavy metals, non-steroidal anti-inflammatories).

Glomerulonephritis – Inflammation of the glomeruli and associated capillary beds. It is usually due to deposits of immune complexes (clumps of antibody and antigens). It may be associated with FeLV or FIP infections in cats, or chronic infections in dogs. The deposited immune complexes lead to a change in the permeability of the nephrons so that protein is able to leak out into the urine. Chronic

proteinuria can result in a state of hypoproteinaemia and the condition is described as **nephrotic syndrome**. Clinical signs include:
- Signs of hypoproteinaemia (weight loss, oedema, ascites).
- Chronic renal failure and uraemia if a significant amount of tissue has been damaged
- Sudden death/respiratory compromise due to pulmonary thromboembolism.

Pyelonephritis – Inflammation of the renal pelvis, usually associated with bacterial infection. Pyelonephritis is usually due to ascending infection from the lower urinary tract. Animals with a depressed immune system are predisposed, as are animals with a glucose in the urine (diabetic animals). Symptoms include:
- pyrexia
- vomiting
- anorexia
- renal pain

Pyelonephritis can result in acute or chronic renal failure if not treated promptly.

Interstitial Nephritis – Inflammation of the interstitial renal tissue. This term is rarely used.

Renal failure

Renal failure has occurred when the kidney is not able to excrete non-protein nitrogenous waste (urea and creatinine) effectively, due to reduced functional renal capacity. There is also a change in water and electrolyte balance in the body.

- **Azotaemia** is an increase in non-protein nitrogenous waste (urea and creatinine) in the blood. In renal failure azotaemia occurs when three-quarters of the nephrons are not functioning. There are also pre-renal causes of azotaemia (such as dehydration) and **post-renal** causes (such as an obstruction to the flow of urine out of the body). In these cases the function of the kidneys may be normal. Azotaemia is therefore not always associated with renal failure.
- **Uraemia** is the combination of clinical signs and biochemical abnormalities associated with loss of functional nephrons. Uraemia is always associated with azotaemia and renal failure.
- **Acute Renal Failure** (ARF) is characterised by:
  - sudden deterioration in renal function
  - sudden development of azotaemia
  - sudden loss of ability to regulate water and electrolyte balance
  - ARF may be reversible if diagnosed promptly and treated aggressively.
- It may be caused by **nephritis** (bacterial pyelonephritis,

leptospirosis, acute glomerulonephritis, and some viruses) or by **nephrosis** (due to renal ischaemia from dehydration, hypovolaemia, anaesthesia or sepsis; or toxicity).

- In the early stages of ARF urine output is reduced (**oliguria**) or absent (**anuria**). This is later followed by an increased urine output (**polyuria**).
- Symptoms of ARF are the non-specific signs of uraemia (depression, anorexia, vomiting, diarrhoea) and either oliguria or polyuria.
- Treatment of ARF involves eliminating the cause and maintaining the animal while repair and regeneration of renal function takes place.
- Fluid therapy is vital for patients in renal failure.
- Electrolyte abnormalities must be identified and corrected.
- Treatment of vomiting may be necessary.
- Monitoring of the patient must include: urine output, hydration status and electrolyte levels.
- Animals which are not vomiting should be fed on a low protein, low phosphorous and high carbohydrate diet. A number of commercial diets are available for feeding to animals in renal failure.
- **Chronic Renal Failure** (CRF) is characterised by:
  - Gradual loss of renal tissue (months to years) so that the kidneys lose the ability to function normally.
  - Irreversible structural damage to the kidneys. The disease will eventually progress to end-stage even when the inciting cause has been removed.
  - Poor long-term prognosis but reasonable quality of life while on treatment.
- The main cause of CRF is acquired disease in older animals (chronic interstitial nephritis, pyelonephritis or gomerulonephritis; leptospirosis, tumour). It is also caused by inherited disease in younger animals.
- Animals with CRF usually present with chronic symptoms of uraemia. These include non-regenerative anaemia (from reduced erythropoietin production), weight loss, uraemic stomatitis and hypertension. There is also usually pu/pd, anorexia, lethargy and weight loss.
- Treatment of CRF involves eliminating the cause where possible and reducing the clinical signs of uraemia.
- Fresh water should be freely available and the patient should be allowed outside regularly to prevent soiling of bedding as these patients are polyuric.
- Dietary treatment is the most important tool in the treatment of CRF. There should be restricted, but good quality protein; reduced phosphorous and sodium. The food should be warmed to increase palatability. Some animals may need appetite-stimulating medication to encourage eating.

- Fluid therapy may be necessary to 'rescue' animals when they are first presented, and to support the remaining renal function while other treatments commence.
- Synthetic erythropoietin can be given by injection to improve the PCV in anaemic patients.
- The owners of patients with CRF should be kept informed of their pet's progress. They should be informed honestly but sensitively that the prognosis for these patients is guarded, and that reasonable quality of life is the goal of treatment. Euthanasia should be considered when the animal is in end-stage renal failure and is no longer responding to treatment as quality of life is seriously compromised at this point.
- Animals with nephrotic syndrome have clinical signs of hypoproteinaemia. Treatment of these patients involves minimising protein loss in the urine by feeding a low protein prescription diet. Oedema should only be treated (with careful use of diuretics) if it is involving the pleura or causing abdominal discomfort.

3.6.21   Urinary tract

What you need to learn

- You need to be able to describe clinical problems and terms related to the lower urinary tract and urination:
  - cystitis
  - stranguria
  - haematuria
  - polyuria
  - dysuria
  - oliguria
  - anuria
  - pollakurea.
- Outline the importance of urinalysis in the diagnosis and management of renal and urinary tract disease.
- Describe the causes, signs and treatments for disorders of the lower urinary tract:
  - cystitis
  - urinary calculi
  - urinary obstruction
  - incontinence
  - feline lower urinary tract disease
  - prostatitis.
- Outline nursing principles associated with animals suffering with urinary disorders to include dietary management.

The functions of the ureters, bladder and urethra can be found in Level 2, 2.3.51, 2.3.52, and 2.3.53.

Terms relating to disorders of the lower urinary tract

Cystitis – Inflammation of the bladder. Animals with cystitis feel discomfort when urine comes into contact with the inflamed bladder lining. Because of this they tend to show pollakiuria. There is often haematuria and the animal spends a lot of time licking at the perineum.

Haematuria – The presence of blood in the urine.

Pollakiuria – Increased frequency and urgency of urination, usually passing small amounts of urine each time.

Dysuria – Difficulty or pain when passing urine.

Stranguria or *tenesmus* – Straining to pass urine – must be differentiated from faecal tenesmus.

Polyuria – Formation and excretion of increased amounts of urine. Often associated with polydipsia (increased drinking).

Oliguria – Passing reduced amounts of urine.

Anuria – Cessation of urine production and excretion. Usually associated with urinary tract obstruction or acute renal failure.

• **Urinalysis** is an extremely useful tool in the diagnosis and treatment of diseases of the lower urinary tract.
• See 3.5.14–3.5.18

Specific conditions affecting the lower urinary tract

Cystitis – Inflammation of the bladder
• **Causes:** Bacterial infection, trauma, urine crystals or calculi, neoplasia. Animals with glucosuria (such as diabetic animals) are predisposed to bacterial cystitis because the glucose supports bacterial growth. Animals with suppressed immunity (such as animals on steroid treatment or with Cushing's disease) are also predisposed to cystitis.
• **Symptoms:** Animals with cystitis feel discomfort when urine comes into contact with the inflamed bladder lining. Because of this they tend to show pollakiuria and dysuria. There is often haematuria and the animal spends a lot of time licking at the perineum. Some animals appear to become incontinent when they have cystitis.
• **Treatment:** Treatment of underlying cause. Antibiotics. Increase water intake to produce dilute urine which flushes material out of the bladder and makes crystal formation more difficult. If crystals are detected these may be dissolved using prescription diets or treatments which alter the pH of the urine. Encourage exercise to allow regular urination. If the animal is incontinent care should be taken to avoid urine scalds (regular washing and application of barrier cream).

Urinary Calculi – Presence of crystals or mineralised stones in the

renal pelvis, ureters, bladder or urethra.
- **Causes:** Concentrated urine, urine pH, diet, infectious agents, inactivity and obesity, increased urine transit time.
- **Symptoms:** Vary in severity. Range from mild pollakiuria and haematuria, to stranguria, vocalisation and general malaise. Can lead to complete urinary tract obstruction.
- **Treatment:** Identification of the type of crystal/stone. Some can be dissolved by manipulating the pH of the urine (for example struvite crystals can be dissolved by acidifying the urine). Some stones cannot be dissolved and must be removed by flushing or cystotomy. Urinary tract infections should be treated appropriately. Increase water intake to produce dilute urine which flushes material out of the bladder and makes crystal formation more difficult. Urine samples should be monitored following treatment to ensure all crystals have disappeared.

Urinary Obstruction
- **Causes:** Urolithiasis, FLUTD, neoplasia, trauma.
- **Symptoms:** Severe stranguria, vocalisation, anuria, excessive attention to perineum. Progresses to post renal azotaemia and acute renal failure. Can lead to bladder rupture and death if left untreated. Males are more likely to obstruct than females as they have a longer narrower urethra.
- **Treatment:** Urine should be removed immediately. This is usually achieved by catheterising the urethra, often under general anaesthesia. If this is not possible because the urethra is blocked it may be necessary to perform a urethrotomy. Cystocentesis should be avoided as the bladder is under pressure and may tear upon introduction of a needle. Treatment of the underlying condition should be addressed once the obstruction has been relieved.

Incontinence – Inability to completely control urination. May be mild (with dribbling of urine when animal recumbent) or complete (no control of urination at all).
- **Causes:** Sphincter mechanism incontinence (SMI) (mainly in older spayed bitches), ectopic ureters (congenital condition where ureters attach to the urethra rather than the bladder), neurological impairment (usually following spinal or pelvic trauma), urinary tract infection.
- **Symptoms:** Animal passing urine without being aware of it. Urine scalding of perineum and hind limbs. Licking at perineum. Soiling of coat.
- **Treatment:** Identification and treatment of underlying cause. Phenylpropanolamine or oestrogen treatment can be very useful in management of SMI. Surgical correction of ectopic ureters.
NB urine scalding should be avoided by the application of barrier creams to the perineal skin where necessary. Incontinent animals

should be allowed many opportunities to urinate through the day. Owners should be counselled not to punish their pet if it soils its bedding through incontinence.

Feline Lower Urinary Tract Disease (FLUTD) – Common condition affecting cats.

- **Cause:** Combination of cystitis, bacterial infection, struvite crystals, and production of waxy or cellular urethral plugs. Neutered, obese, sedentary animals are predisposed.
- **Symptoms:** Signs of cystitis and sometimes urinary tract obstruction.
- **Treatment:** Catheterisation if obstructed. Antibiotics to treat infection. Increase water intake. Manipulation of diet to dissolve struvite crystals. Commercial diets are available which contain urinary acidifiers; and with low magnesium and phosphate content to prevent struvite formation. Male animals are more likely to obstruct than females as they have a longer narrower urethra. Animals which repeatedly block may need a perineal urethrostomy procedure.

Prostatitis – Inflammation of the prostate gland in entire male animals.

- **Cause:** Prostatic hyperplasia (effect of testosterone), bacterial infection, cysts, abscesses, neoplasia, trauma.
- **Symptoms:** Caudal abdominal pain, stranguria, haematuria, constipation (from enlarged prostate gland obstructing the rectum), pyrexia, altered hind limb gait, general malaise.
- **Treatment:** Treatment of underlying cause; antibiotics, anti-testosterone treatment (eg delmadione) or castration to reduce hyperplasia, surgical treatment of prostatic cysts. Prostatic neoplasia carries a very poor prognosis.

3.6.22 Nervous system

What you need to learn

- ❧ You need to be able to outline the function of the central and peripheral nervous system and describe clinical signs associated with abnormal neurological function.
- ❧ Describe the terms related to abnormalities of the central nervous system:
  - ❧ epilepsy
  - ❧ convulsions
  - ❧ status epilepticus.
- ❧ Describe the causes, signs, and first aid treatment for seizures.
- ❧ Understand the principles of nursing and monitoring an animal with seizures

❧ immediate and long-term nursing care.
❧ Describe the causes and nursing priorities appropriate to an unconscious patient.

For functions of the nervous system, see Level 2, 2.3.15.

• Disorders of the nervous system can have numerous symptoms.
• In general:
• Disorders of the brain cause symptoms such as seizures, depressed mental processes, weakness and inco-ordination, paralysis central blindness, cranial pain
• Disorders of the spine cause severe pain; weakness or paralysis caudal to the lesion. (This may include loss of continence).
• Disorders of the peripheral nerves cause neurological deficits in the parts of the body supplied by those nerves.

Disorders of the central nervous system

Seizures (also called convulsions or fits) – Unco-ordinated, unconscious, vigorous contractions of all the body muscles. Seizures result from disruption of the electrical activity in the brain.
Epilepsy – Medical condition where the patient suffers from recurrent seizures.
Status Epilepticus – This is when the seizure is prolonged, or when one seizure is directly followed by another without recovery in between. Status epilepticus is potentially life-threatening.

Causes of seizures can be divided into:
1 Seizures in the normal brain as a response to metabolic or toxic abnormalities. The disease is **extracranial** (outside of the brain). Examples are hypoglycaemia, and circulating toxins due to liver or kidney failure.
2 Seizures caused by disease of the structure of the brain. The disease is **intracranial** (within the brain). Examples are brain tumours, trauma, inflammation of the brain (**encephalitis**), and **hydrocephalus** (build-up of CSF in the ventricles).
3 Idiopathic epilepsy. In this case the seizures result from a chemical imbalance in the brain. It is not associated with intra or extracranial disease.

• Idiopathic epilepsy is not uncommon in dogs but very rare in the cat.
• The first seizure is usually seen when the animal is 1–4 years old.
• Seizures can be triggered by stress.

An epileptiform seizure can be divided into three phases:
• During the **pre-ictal phase** (a few minutes before the fit starts) the animal is often restless or excitable.

- During the **seizure** the animal usually loses consciousness for a variable period of time.
- There is often loss of continence.
- Paddling of the legs while recumbent and jerky movements usually occur.
- During the **post-ictal phase** (after the seizure) the animal is often disorientated and restless. The post-ictal phase usually lasts for a few hours but can be as long as a week.

- Partial seizures can occur where the animal is unaware of its surroundings but does not lose consciousness. Twitching of part of the body may occur.
- Animals are completely normal in between seizures.
- Seizures often occur in **clusters** with an animal suffering a number of brief seizures of a period of a few hours.
- A thorough history should be obtained to identify possible causes of the seizure.
- First aid involves preventing injury to the dog and handlers during the fit.
- The owner is often distraught because it is very upsetting to see an animal having a fit. They must be calmed and if necessary moved into a different room while their pet is treated.
- Medical treatment (anti-convulsants such as phenobarbitone and diazepam) will be given if the fit is prolonged (status epilepticus), or during a cluster of fits.
- The animal should be carefully moved away from objects which may cause injury.
- The room should be darkened and noise kept to a minimum.
- Owners should be made aware that a dog may bite during a seizure so should be handled with great care.
- If the fit is single or very infrequent, long-term treatment may not be necessary.
- Animals which are suffering from frequent fits, severe fits or cluster fits should be treated with an anti-convulsant such as phenobarbitone. This treatment is usually lifelong.
- Anti-convulsant medication can cause hepatic toxicity. Owners should be aware that regular blood testing to assess blood levels of the drug, and hepatic function will be necessary.
- Owners should be trained to detect signs of cluster fits and status epilepticus so that they can seek veterinary attention when necessary.
- Epileptic animals should not be allowed to be in situations which may prove dangerous should a seizure occur (eg they should not be allowed unsupervised access to water).

Treatment of the unconscious patient

Loss of consciousness is manifested as:

- Collapse with flaccid muscles (although muscular spasm and movement occurs during seizures).
- The animal is unaware of its surroundings.
- Loss of continence is common (urination and defaecation).
- The reflexes are usually still intact.
- Pulse and respiration are present although they may be altered.

Collapse can occur without loss of consciousness (locomotor collapse):

- Weakness due to pain (for example arthritic old dogs which are unable to stand)
- Neurological disorders

Collapse with or without unconsciousness can occur due to:

- Weakness due to circulatory compromise (heart failure, anaemia, haemorrhage)
- Severe disease such as metabolic or endocrine disorders (uncontrolled diabetes mellitus, Addison's disease, etc).
- Toxicity or poisoning.
- Electric shock.
- Shock.

Basic first aid principles should be applied to the unconscious patient:

- A clear airway should be obtained and maintained.
- The animal should be kept warm and treated for any pain.
- Treatment of the underlying condition should start (control haemorrhage, fluid therapy, etc.)
- If respiration and heartbeat ceases, resuscitation can be attempted. This is often called cardiopulmonary resuscitation (CPR) or cardiopulmonary-cerebral resuscitation (CPCR).

All staff should be aware of CPR procedures as prompt treatment is vital:

- The **airway** is cleared and intubation is performed (The tube should be cuffed to prevent inhalation of foreign material.) Tracheotomy may be performed where necessary.
- **Breathing**: Ventilation should begin as soon as possible to provide oxygen.
- **Circulation**: Compression of the chest wall should be performed. The aim is to push blood through the heart and therefore provide cardiac output.
- In cats and small dogs the chest wall can be compressed from side to

side. In larger dogs the chest is compressed from one side with the animal in lateral recumbency.

- Drugs (such as adrenaline, atropine or lignocaine) may be administered once airway, breathing and circulation have been established.
- CPR should only be performed if the animal has a disease which is treatable.
- If possible the owner's consent should have previously been sought.

CPR should not be attempted if:

- The animal is in the terminal stages of disease such as kidney or liver failure.
- The animal has severe head injuries which make recovery of mental function unlikely.
- The owner has asked that CPR should not be attempted.

Once the first aid treatment has been provided the veterinary surgeon will investigate the cause of the unconsciousness, using relevant ancillary tests.

3.6.23 Spinal injuries

What you need to learn

- 🐾 You need to be able to outline the conditions related to spinal injuries and their causes:
  - 🐾 tetraplegia/tetraparesis
  - 🐾 paraplegia/paraparesis
  - 🐾 hemiplegia/hemiparesis.
- 🐾 Identify the neurological tests/examination commonly performed on animals:
  - 🐾 muscle tone
  - 🐾 the ability to stand
  - 🐾 radiography
  - 🐾 myelography
  - 🐾 examination of peripheral and spinal nerve reflexes
  - 🐾 MRI.
- 🐾 Describe the nursing and long-term management and prognosis of animals with spinal injuries.

- If a spinal injury is suspected immediate veterinary attention is required as prompt treatment can limit damage to the spinal cord.
- It is vital that there is no movement of the fracture site during transportation.
- A number of assistants may be required to move the patient, taking care to maintain the alignment of the spine.
- The animal should be moved onto a stretcher or board. Cats can be placed in a rigid box.

- Blankets can be used to envelop the patient and restrict movement.
- If the animal is amenable it is possible to further restrict movement with the use of restraining ties.
- Spinal injuries can result in weakness or paralysis caudal to the injury.
- **Tetraparesis** is weakness of all four limbs.
- **Tetraplegia** is paralysis of all four limbs.
- **Paraparesis** is weakness of both hind limbs.
- **Paraplegia** is paralysis of both hind limbs.
- **Hemiparesis** is weakness of the fore and hind limb on one side.
- **Hemiplegia** is paralysis of the fore and hind limb on one side.
- To assess if any neurological deficit has occurred following a spinal injury a number of neurological tests or examinations are performed.
- The animal should be observed both standing and walking. Any alteration in gait should be noted. Dragging of the limbs is a sign of neurological injury. The nails should be checked for signs of scuffing.
- The sensation in the limbs should be checked. Normal animals will withdraw the limb when a painful stimulus is applied (eg pinching the nailbed using forceps).
- The anal reflex should be checked by inserting a thermometer into the rectum. Normally the anal sphincter muscle contracts round the thermometer.

Local reflexes (such as the patellar reflex) can be checked by the vet. Further diagnostic tests are necessary to localise and characterise the spinal lesion:

- Plain radiographs are used to check for fractures and dislocations. Lysis of the vertebra (from infection or tumour) can also be seen. In some animals the intervertebral discs become mineralised and displaced discs can be seen on plain radiographs.
- Myelography (injection of radio-opaque dye into the space surrounding the spinal cord) is usually necessary to detect spinal lesions (disc protrusions, bony lesions pressing on the spinal cord, tumours). These lesions show up as a deviation or narrowing in the column of dye.
- Magnetic Resonance Imaging (MRI) may be necessary to detect lesions which can't be visualised using these other methods. Brain lesions can be seen using MRI as can any other spinal lesion, whether it is a bony lesion or a soft tissue lesion.
- Nursing of patients with spinal injuries depends on the extent of the injury.
- Animals which are recumbent should be provided with a deep clean bed to avoid development of pressure sores. The animals should be

turned frequently and with great care.

- The animal should be cage rested to avoid movement which may cause pain or a worsening of the condition.
- The animal may need hand feeding, particularly if it is recumbent.
- Special attention must be given to urination and defaecation. Incontinent animals must be kept clean. Barrier cream should be applied if there is a risk of urine scalding. Some animals may need assistance in passing urine or faeces. Some animals may require an indwelling urinary catheter.
- Many recumbent patients benefit from physiotherapy to limit stiffness and muscle wastage.
- The owner should be kept informed of their pet's condition.
- Animals which have no deep pain sensation in their hind limbs following treatment of their injuries have an extremely poor prognosis and euthanasia should be offered.
- Some animals with paraplegia will tolerate a mobility device such as a cart to replace the function of their hind limbs. Care must be taken when selecting patients for this as some highly strung animals will not adapt to the loss of use of their limbs.
- Euthanasia should be offered for animals which are permanently incontinent.

3.6.24   Endocrine system

What you need to learn

- You need to be able to outline the function of the endocrine system.
- Outline the organs and hormones related to pathology of endocrine glands.
- Describe the conditions/diseases associated with endocrine system and outline diagnostic tests:
  - diabetes mellitus
  - diabetes insipidus
  - Cushing's disease
  - Addison's disease
  - hyperthyroidism
  - hypothyroidism
  - juvenile hyperparathyroidism
  - sertoli cell tumours
  - renal hyperparathyroidism.
- Describe the causes and signs of diabetes mellitus.
- Describe the treatment, stabilisation and long-term management of diabetes mellitus:
  - monitoring of urine glucose
  - administration of insulin

* regular feeding and exercise
* blood glucose/sugar.
* Describe the causes and signs and First Aid treatment of insulin overdose and other possible complications:
  * medical and management
  * Insulin resistance and ketoacidosis
  * Hypoglycaemia.
* Describe the clinical signs and treatment of diabetes insipidus and the associated required laboratory tests:
  * routine renal function
  * water deprivation
  * partial water deprivation.
* Describe the clinical signs, diagnostic test and treatment of other common endocrine conditions:
  * hyperadrenocorticism and hypothyroidism in the dog
  * hyperthyroidism in the cat.

* The endocrine system co-ordinates and controls many functions of the body.
* Endocrine glands synthesise and secrete *hormones* directly into the blood stream (compare with exocrine glands).
* Hormones are chemical messengers which travel in the blood stream to *target organs*. At the target organ the hormone binds to receptors and causes a response.
* In some places the cells of the endocrine cells are not organised into glands, but act as individual cells – eg gastrin secretion in the gastrointestinal tract.

The pituitary gland

* The pituitary gland lies on the ventral surface of the midbrain. It is connected to the hypothalamus.
* The hypothalamus receives information from the body and organises the appropriate response from the endocrine system. The hypothalamus secretes a number of *releasing hormones* which all act on target cells in the pituitary gland.
* The pituitary gland is separated into two lobes called the *anterior hypophysis* (or *adenohypophysis*) and the *posterior hypophysis* (or *neurohypophysis*).
* The two lobes secrete different hormones (see Table 6.9).
* FSH and LH are known as the *gonadotrophins*.
* The *pineal gland* is a small gland between the cerebral hemispheres and the cerebellum. It produces the hormone *melatonin*. The pineal gland functions as a biological clock, affecting the gonadotrophins. It regulates gonadal activity throughout the day and also through the seasons.

Table 6.6

Hormone	Hypophysis:	Target Cells:	Action:
Adrenocorticotrophic hormone (ACTH)	Anterior	Adrenal cortex	Cortisol synthesis
Growth hormone (GH) (sometimes called somatotrophin)	Anterior	All tissues	Stimulates growth and repair of tissues, and speeds the breakdown of fat stores.
Follicle stimulating hormone (FSH)	Anterior	Ovary, testes	Maturation and growth of ovarian follicles and spermatozoa.
Luteal hormone (LH) (sometimes called lutenising hormone)	Anterior	Ovary, testes	Induces ovulation, stimulates formation of oestrogen and testosterone.
Prolactin	Anterior	Mammary glands	Increased milk synthesis
Thyroid stimulating hormone (TSH)	Anterior	Thyroid glands	Stimulates thyroid function
Oxytocin	Posterior	Mammary glands, uterus	Milk release, uterine contraction, prostaglandin secretion
Anti diuretic hormone (ADH) (sometimes called vasopressin)	Posterior	Kidney (collecting ducts)	Increased water reabsorption.

The thyroid gland

- The paired thyroid glands lie on either side of the trachea (see Figure 6.6).
- It is composed of *follicles* of cuboidal epithelial cells which secrete the thyroid hormones.
- The thyroid hormones are called *tri-iodothyronine* (T3) and *tetra-iodothyronine* (T4) which is better known as *thyroxine*. T3 is the active form of the hormone.
- Synthesis of the thyroid hormones requires iodine.
- TSH released from the pituitary gland causes an increase in the production of thyroid hormones.
- Control of the plasma levels of thyroid hormones is through *negative feedback*:
  - Hypothalamus detects a decrease in plasma T3 and T4 levels
  - The pituitary gland is instructed to release TRH into the blood
  - TRH acts on the thyroid gland to stimulate production of T3 and T4
  - The hypothalamus detects the increase in plasma T3 and T4, and suppresses the release of TRH from the pituitary.
- The thyroid hormones affect all the body tissues and have two main actions as follows.

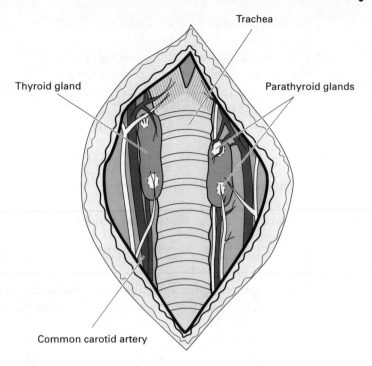

Figure 6.1 The thyroid glands, ventral view.

- **Metabolic:** Thyroid hormones control the *basal metabolic rate (BMR)*. This is the rate at which energy must be used to maintain vital functions such as respiration, heartbeat, peristalsis and biosynthesis (construction of proteins and other molecules). The BMR is high in young animals to allow for growth. BMR levels off in mature animals and then declines with old age.
- **Growth and Development:** Thyroid hormones are involved with the growth and development of tissues such as the skeleton, central nervous system, reproductive system and hair cycle.
- A group of cells called *C-cells* within the thyroid gland secrete the hormone *calcitonin*. This hormone causes calcium to be deposited in the bones. Calcitonin therefore has a role in calcium homeostasis.

The parathyroid glands

- The parathyroid glands are closely associated with the thyroid gland.
- They synthesise and secrete the *parathyroid hormone (PTH)*.
- PTH is involved in controlling calcium distribution in the body.
- Calcium (Ca^{2+}) is a very important ion. It is involved in muscle contraction, blood clotting and nerve conduction; as well as

providing teeth and bone structure. Calcium levels are very tightly controlled.
- The main actions of parathyroid hormone are:
  - Increasing absorption of Ca^{2+} from the gut.
  - Stimulating reabsorption of Ca^{2+} through the proximal convoluted tubule in the kidney.
  - Promoting movement of Ca^{2+} from the skeleton into the plasma

The pancreas

- The anatomy and exocrine function of the pancreas has already been discussed.
- Within the pancreas are islands of endocrine tissue called the *Islets of Langerhans.*
- These areas contain three types of cells; *alpha* (α), *beta* (β) and *delta* (δ) cells.
- Beta cells secrete **insulin**. Insulin is secreted when blood glucose levels rise, for example after a meal. It performs two functions both of which lower blood glucose levels:
  - Insulin stimulates synthesis of *glycogen* which is a polymer of glucose. Glycogen can be stored in the liver and skeletal muscle cells.
  - Insulin aids the transport of glucose *from* the blood *into* respiring cells.
- Alpha cells secrete **glucagon**. Glucagon is secreted when blood glucose levels decrease.
- Glucagon has the opposite effect to insulin. It stimulates the conversion of glycogen back to glucose, thereby raising blood glucose levels.
- Delta cells produce **somatostatin**. Somatostatin reduces gut motility and inhibits secretion of pancreatic and gastric secretions.

The adrenal glands

- The adrenal glands lie just cranial to the kidneys. They are retroperitoneal (see Figure 6.10).
- Each adrenal gland is divided into two independent parts; the outer **cortex** and the **medulla**.

The adrenal cortex

- The adrenal cortex produces *steroid* hormones. The release of these hormones is controlled by ACTH from the pituitary gland and is regulated by negative feedback mechanisms.
- The three main groups of hormones produced are:
  - The **Glucocorticoids** (eg cortisol, cortisone.)
  - The **Mineralocorticoids** (aldosterone.)

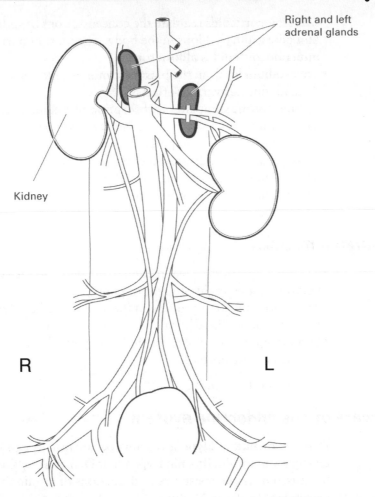

Right and left adrenal glands

Kidney

R   L

Figure 6.2 Diagram showing the position of the adrenal glands.

- The **Sex Hormones** (progesterone, testosterone, oestrogen.)
- Glucocorticoids are very important in allowing animals to cope with physical and mental stress. Glucocorticoid levels are much higher in stressed animals.
- They have numerous functions:
- Carbohydrate metabolism: Glucocorticoids raise blood glucose levels and stimulate the release of glucose from glycogen stores. (These effects are opposite to those of insulin). They also stimulate mobilisation of fats from adipose tissue.
- Protein metabolism: Glucocorticoids promote conversion amino acids into glucose (this process is called *gluconeogenesis*).
- Immune suppression: Glucocorticoids cause eosinopenia and lymphopenia.
- Anti-inflammatory effect: Glucocorticoids can delay wound healing.

- Mineralocorticoids regulate the concentrations of sodium (Na^+) and potassium (K^+) ions in the body. The most important mineralocorticoid is **aldosterone.**
- Low sodium levels in the plasma stimulate aldosterone release. Aldosterone has various effects:
  1. Aldosterone stimulates reabsorption of sodium in the kidney. This in turn causes water retention at the kidney.
  2. Uptake of sodium suppresses potassium reabsorption at the kidney resulting in decreased potassium levels.
- The sodium: potassium ratio is tightly controlled.
- The production of sex hormones in the adrenal cortex is of minor importance.

The adrenal medulla

- The functions of the renal medulla are related to the sympathetic nervous system (fight or flight response).
- Two hormones are produced in the medulla; *adrenaline* and *noradrenaline*. These hormones have similar effects.
- Stimulation of the adrenal medulla by sympathetic nerves causes release of these hormones.

See also Level 2, 2.3.59.

Disorders of the endocrine system

Diabetes mellitus – Hyperglycaemia occurs usually caused by deficiency in insulin (Insulin Dependant Diabetes Mellitus). Can also be caused by tissue resistance to the actions of insulin (Non Insulin Dependant Diabetes Mellitus).

Diabetes insipidus – Deficiency in anti-diuretic hormone (ADH) production or failure of the kidneys to respond to ADH. Results in inability to concentrate urine properly.

Cushing's Disease (Hyperadrenocorticism) – Excessive secretion of cortisol from the adrenal cortex. Can be pituitary dependant (from excessive secretion of ACTH from the pituitary gland) or adrenal dependant (unilateral tumour of the adrenal gland which secretes excess cortisol). Can also be caused by prolonged treatment with gucocorticoids.

Addison's Disease (Hypoadrenocorticism) – Deficiency in glucocorticoids and mineralocorticoids due to failure in the function of the adrenal cortex.

Feline Hyperthyroidism – Presence of a benign but functional tumour of the thyroid gland which secretes excess thyroid hormones into the circulation. Occurs in middle aged to old cats.

Canine Hypothyroidism – Deficiency in production and release of thyroid hormones, usually caused by damage to the thyroid glands. Usually occurs in middle aged dogs. Extremely rare in cats.

Juvenile or Nutritional (secondary) **Hyperparathyroidism** – Excessive parathyroid hormone (PTH) in circulation, usually caused by low dietary calcium and high dietary phosphate such as an all meat diet in juvenile animals.

Renal (secondary) **Hyperparathyroidism** – Excessive parathyroid hormone in circulation, caused by retention of phosphorous at the kidney in animals with renal failure. This alters the Ca:P ratio and stimulates the release of excessive PTH.

Sertoli Cell Tumour – Production of excessive oestrogen from a (usually benign) functional tumour of the Sertoli cells in the testicle. The affected testicle is enlarged. The effects of oestrogen are seen in the male animals. These include atrophy of the opposite testicle, bilateral alopecia, mammary development and attractiveness to other male dogs. Treatment is castration which is curative.

Diabetes mellitus

- Insulin Dependent Diabetes Mellitus (IDDM) is usually caused by hypoplasia of the islet cells in the pancreas. Loss of islet cells can also be caused by pancreatitis, auto-immune disease, toxicity or neoplasia.
- Non-Insulin Dependent Diabetes Mellitus (NIDDM) is caused by decreased sensitivity of tissues to the actions of insulin. This can occur in obese animals or under the effects of some hormones (progesterone, glucocorticoids and catecholamines (adrenaline and norarenaline)).
- The function of insulin is to assist in the transport of glucose from the blood into the tissue cells. In Diabetes mellitus the blood glucose levels are markedly elevated, while the tissues are starved of glucose.
- Symptoms of Diabetes Mellitus include:
- **Polyuria and polydipsia** – when glucose exceeds a certain threshold it is excreted at the kidneys and takes water with it by osmosis. This causes polyuria. The polydipsia compensates for the loss of water and prevents dehydration.
- **Polyphagia** – the tissue cells are starved of glucose so the animal is driven to take in even more carbohydrate.
- **Weight loss** – the animals is unable to use glucose as an energy source so it starts to break down fat, and then muscle (although animals with NIDDM may be obese.)
- **Recurrent urinary tract infections** – the presence of glucose in the

urine encourages bacterial growth.

- **Cataracts** – caused by alteration of water balance in the lens of the eye.
- If untreated the diabetic animal may develop **diabetic ketoacidosis (DKA)**. This is a result of excessive breakdown of fats within the body. Ketones (energy source derived from fat breakdown) are produced in the liver. These cause metabolic acidosis and exacerbate the existing condition.
- Symptoms of DKA include the symptoms of diabetes mellitus along with:
- Anorexia
- Vomiting and diarrhoea
- Lethargy
- Strong smelling breath (ketotic breath smells like pear drop sweets.)
- Weakness progressing to collapse and death
- DKA is a life-threatening condition and must be treated promptly and aggressively with fluid therapy and insulin therapy.
- **Diagnosis of Diabetes Mellitus involves**:
- Blood sampling to confirm marked hyperglycaemia. In uncomplicated cases the rest of the biochemistry and haematology profile is normal.
- Urinalysis shows glucosuria and possible ketonuria. The specific gravity is high (>1.040). There may be signs of urinary tract infection. There is sometimes enlargement of the liver due to hepatic lipidosis (from mobilisation of fat stores).
- **Treatment of Diabetes Mellitus**:
- In IDDM the loss of beta-cell function is usually permanent and insulin therapy is necessary. In NIDDM the animal is not sensitive to the actions of insulin and so insulin therapy is usually not helpful. In these animals careful weight loss and control of diet is useful.
- **Insulin Therapy**:
- Daily injection of insulin is the cornerstone of treatment, and is necessary for the rest of the animal's life.
- The insulin is administered by subcutaneous injections once or twice daily (depending on the type of insulin used).
- Just before giving the insulin injection the animals should be offered a small amount of its meal. The insulin should only be given if the animal eats this food (this avoids causing hypoglycaemia by giving insulin to an inappetant animals). The rest of the animal's food should be given when the insulin is having its peak activity (usually eight hour after injection).
- **Urine Sampling**:
- Urine sampling 2–3 times daily is useful in monitoring glucosuria.
- It can also be used to observe trends in glucosuria. Care should be taken however as urine levels of glucose do not always reflect blood

glucose levels.

- **Diet:**
- The animal should be placed on a diet which is high in complex carbohydrates (starch and dietary fibre). This provides a slow-release source of glucose. The diet should also be restricted in fat. Animals which are obese should have this corrected using a low fat diet. The diet should be fed at the same times each day. The animals should also be exercised should be regular but controlled. Excessive exercise can lead to hypoglycaemic episodes.
- **Neutering:**
- Female animals should be spayed to avoid the effects of progesterone on insulin production.
- **Monitoring animals with diabetes mellitus:**
- Blood glucose measurement is the most accurate method of monitoring response to insulin therapy.
- For the first few days of treatment a glucose curve can be performed. This involves taking blood samples every few hours to observe the effect, and the duration of action, of the insulin.
- Urine sampling 2–3 times daily is useful in monitoring ketonuria in the initial stages of treatment. It can also be used to observe trends in glucosuria. Care should be taken however as urine levels of glucose do not always reflect blood glucose levels.
- The simplest way of monitoring diabetic animals which are stable on insulin treatment is through the resolution of the clinical signs of diabetes. This includes measuring thirst, appetite and weight of the animal.
- **Insulin overdose:**
- This can occur if:
- Too much insulin is injected
- The animal is inappetant
- The peak effect of the insulin occurs before the animal eats its main meal.
- Insulin overdose causes profound hypoglycaemia.
- Symptoms of hypoglycaemia include:
- Weakness and lethargy
- Tremors
- Ataxia
- Collapse and death.
- Owners should be warned of these symptoms and should be told that if the animal is still conscious it should be given plenty sugary food (honey, sugar, syrup etc.) and then taken or veterinary attention. If the animal is unconscious it should be taken for immediate veterinary attention.
- **Failure of Insulin Therapy:**
- This can occur for many reasons including:

- Underlying disease (Diabetes mellitus often occurs with Cushing's disease, and will be refractory to treatment until the Cushing's disease is treated).
- Improper injection technique
- Improper storage and handling of insulin
- Concurrent infection (urinary, respiratory and skin infections in particular)
- Oestrus
- Change in diet or exercise levels
- Short action of insulin (these animals often need slow acting insulin and twice daily injection)
- Non insulin dependant diabetes mellitus.

Diabetes insipidus

- Anti-diuretic Hormone (ADH) is produced by the pituitary gland in response to hypovolaemia or dehydration.
- ADH reduces the rate of urine production by promoting reabsorption of water in the distal and collecting tubules in the kidney.
- Diabetes insipidus is caused by failure of synthesis or release of ADH (**central Diabetes Insipidus**) or by failure of the renal tubules to respond to the ADH (**nephrogenic Diabetes Insipidus**).
- Symptoms of Diabetes insipidus include:
- Severe polyuria, possibly with incontinence.
- Severe polydipsia (compensatory – avoids dehydration due to the polyuria).
- Patients generally fit and well in themselves.
- Diagnosis of Diabetes insipidus
- This involves ruling out the many other causes of PU/PD
- Water intake should be measured to confirm that the animal is genuinely pu/pd.
- Blood samples should be performed – these will usually be normal in an animal with diabetes Insipidus.
- Urinalysis will show an extremely low specific gravity (always less than 1.010). The presence of glucose, ketones or signs of infection suggest some other cause of pu/pd.
- Once other causes of pu/pd have been eliminated, specific tests for DI can be performed.
- The **water deprivation test** should be performed with great care (and must never be used in animals with renal dysfunction):
- Food is withheld for 12h. The animal should have an empty bladder and be weighed in the morning. Urine specific gravity is measured.
- Food and water is withheld during the test.

- The bladder is re-emptied and the animal re-weighed every 1–4 hours. Hydration status and urine specific gravity should be re-tested.
- The test finishes when the animal has lost 5% body weight, or when it appears clinically dehydrated or unwell. The test should also finish if urine specific gravity exceeds 1.025.
- Dogs with Diabetes insipidus fail to concentrate their urine over 1.012. The urine of normal animals becomes more concentrated as the animal becomes more dehydrated.
- Once the test is completed the animal should be allowed free access to water.
- **Treatment of Diabetes Insipidus:**
- Dogs with confirmed Diabetes insipidus can be treated with exogenous ADH (called vasopressin) usually by nasal or eye drop.
- If the DI is nephrogenic the animal will not respond to treatment with vasopressin. These animals are difficult to treat. Thiazide diuretics may decrease urine volume by increasing reabsorption of salt.

Canine hyperadrenocorticism (Cushing's disease):

- Hyperadrenocorticism (HAC) is excessive secretion of cortisol from the adrenal cortex.
- It can be:
- **pituitary dependent** – from excessive secretion of ACTH from the pituitary gland. This type accounts for 85–90% of cases.
- **adrenal dependent** – unilateral tumour of the adrenal gland which secretes excess cortisol. This type accounts for about 10% of cases.
- It can also be caused by prolonged treatment with gucocorticoids. This is called *iatrogenic* hyperadrenocorticism.
- **Symptoms** of HAC include:
- Polyuria and polydipsia – due to cortisol inhibiting the action of ADH at the collecting duct.
- Polyphagia
- Pot bellied appearance – due to hepatomegaly and weak abdominal muscles.
- Lethargy
- Muscular weakness and atrophy
- Alopecia mainly affecting the flank, thighs and abdomen – due to effect of cortisol on the hair cycle.
- Excessive panting
- Reproductive failure
- Calcinosis cutis – deposition of calcium in the skin.
- Persistent infections – due to suppression of the immune system
- Diabetes mellitus – due to cortisol-induced insulin resistance.

- **Laboratory Findings**
- Haematology shows neutrophilia, eosinopenia and lymphopenia (sometimes called a stress leucogram).
- Biochemistry shows elevated ALKP (steroid induced isoenzyme). There is often elevated ALT, cholesterol and glucose.
- Urinalysis often shows dilute urine, often with signs of urinary tract infection.
- **Diagnostic Tests:**
- ACTH Stimulation test:
- Baseline plasma sample is taken for cortisol measurement.
- The animal is given and intravenous injection of synthetic ACTH.
- One hour later another plasma sample is taken for measurement of cortisol.
- In normal animals the ACTH stimulates the adrenal gland to release cortisol so that levels rise to 2–3 times the baseline value.
- Animals with HAC show an exaggerated response, or start with an extremely high baseline cortisol level which does not show significant increase on stimulation.
- Low Dose Dexamethasone Test:
- Baseline plasma sample is taken for cortisol measurement.
- A low dose (0.01mg/kg) of dexamethasone is injected intravenously.
- At four and eight hours after injection repeat plasma samples are obtained for cortisol measurement.
- The test is based on the negative feedback mechanism which controls ACTH and cortisol release.
- In normal animals the dexamethasone suppresses further release of ACTH and hence cortisol. This effect is seen by four hours post injection and levels continue to be suppressed after eight hours.
- In animals with HAC the dexamethasone injection fails to suppress the release of cortisol so that cortisol levels remain high or only reduce by a small amount.
- High Dose dexamethasone test
- This can be used to distinguish pituitary dependant HAC from adrenal-dependant HAC.
- **Treatment of HAC:**
- Surgical removal of adrenal tumour – technically difficult.
- Medical treatment with trilostane (Vetoryl®).

Canine hypothyroidism

- Deficiency in production and release of thyroid hormones.
- It is usually caused by damage to the thyroid glands. The damage is most commonly caused by the immune mediated condition lymphocytic thyroiditis, but can also be through neoplastic destruction.

- Usually occurs in middle aged dogs. Extremely rare in cats.
- **Symptoms** of hypothyroidism include
- Alopecia – mainly of the flanks and tail. This is due to the effect of the thyroid hormones on the hair cycle. Clipped hair fails to regrow,
- Dry scaly skin, often thickened and hyperpigmented
- Weight gain
- Bradycardia
- Subnormal temperature
- Infertility and anoestrus
- Weakness and exercise intolerance
- Puffy face with 'tragic' expression
- Neuropathies – particularly laryngeal paralysis and megaoesophagus.
- **Laboratory Findings**
- Haematology – mild non-regenerative anaemia
- Biochemistry – Elevated cholesterol
- **Diagnostic Tests**
- Measurement of basal thyroid levels – not very reliable
- Measure T4/TSH ratio
- TRH stimulation test –
  - A baseline serum sample is taken for measurement of T4
  - An intravenous injection of TRH is given
  - Repeat serum samples are taken six hours post injection for measurement of T4.
  - Most normal animals show at least a 50% increase in T4 levels.
  - Animals with hypothyroidism do not show a marked increase in T4.
  - This test is sometimes difficult to interpret as it can be affected by non-thyroidal illness, and normal animals may not show an elevation in T4 after TRH injection.
- A number of thyroid panels are available which measure various values. These are currently the most accurate tests but must still be interpreted with caution.
- Trial treatment with thyroxine supplementation is a reasonable option if there has been difficulty obtaining a clear result and if suspicion of hypothyroidism is high.
- **Treatment of Hypothyroidism:**
- Oral thyroid hormone replacement with synthetic thyroxine.
- Response to treatment can be monitored with repeat blood sampling, or simply with resolution of clinical signs.

Feline hyperthyroidism

- Feline hyperthyroidism is almost always caused by the presence of a benign but functional tumour of the thyroid gland which secretes excess thyroid hormones into the circulation.

- Occurs in middle aged to old cats.
- **Symptoms** of hyperthyroidism include:
- Weight loss
- Hyperactivity – may become more aggressive or over-friendly
- Polyphagia
- Poor quality staring coat
- Diarrhoea
- Tachycardia, often with a systolic murmur – due to hypertrophic cardiomyopathy
- Palpable enlargement of thyroid gland, usually unilateral. This is called a *goitre*.
- **Laboratory Findings**
- Biochemistry – elevated ALKP and ALT
- **Diagnostic Tests**
- Measurement of T4 from serum sample
- In early hyperthyroidism the T4 level may remain normal
- **Treatment of Hyperthyroidism**
- Anti-thyroid drugs. Methimazole is currently the only licensed drug in cats. Carbimazole is unlicensed but has been used successfully in the past. Treatment is lifelong if surgery is not performed.
- Surgical removal of the thyroid tumour. Usually only attempted once condition has been stabilised using anti-thyroid drugs.
- Use of radioactive Iodine – some specialist centres have the facilities to administer radioactive iodine which is concentrated in the thyroid gland and destroys only the abnormal tissue. This is the optimum treatment but suitable facilities for handling the radioactive material are only found at a handful of specialist centres.

3.6.25 Skeletal system

What you need to learn

❧ You need to be able to describe the function of the skeletal system.

For functions of the skeletal system and development of bones, see Level 2, 2.3.04.

3.6.26 Bones

What you need to learn

❧ Identify importance of a suitable diet for growing animals in order to avoid nutritional induced problems:
  ❧ relevance of level and balance of calcium
  ❧ phosphorous
  ❧ vitamin D

* hypervitaminosis A.
* Describe the impact of metabolic diseases on bone with respect to clinical and radiological signs of bone disease:
    * secondary nutritional hyperparathyroidism
    * rickets
    * metaphyseal osteopathy.
* Identify the major non-metabolic pathological changes of bone:
    * pulmonary osteopathy
    * osteopathy
    * osteomyelitis.
* Describe the site and types of commonly encountered bone tumours:
    * osteoma
    * osteosarcoma.

During growth there is a great demand for skeletal growth. For this reason nutritional problems in young animals can have severe adverse effects on skeletal growth and development.

As well as nutritional deficiencies and excesses, overfeeding is a major cause of orthopaedic (bone-related) problems in young animals. This is because the immature skeleton is unable to cope with the excessive stresses applied through carrying too much weight. This can result in disorders such as hip dysplasia and osteochondrosis dissecans (OCD).

* **Calcium** and **phosphorous** are vitally important in the growth of bone, as well as for nerve and muscle function and blood clotting.
* Almost all of the body's calcium and phosphorous is in the teeth and bones.
* A suitable diet for growing animals should contain an adequate but not excessive amount of these minerals at the correct ratio. Extra calcium should not be given as an in-feed supplement to young animals as this can result in excessively swift bone growth.
* A source of **vitamin D** is necessary to aid in the absorption of calcium through the gut and decrease the excretion of these minerals from the kidney.
* Care should be taken to avoid excessive intake of **Vitamin A** in young animals (such as may occur with feeding liver) as hypervitaminosis A can cause degenerative changes in the physes leading to abnormal bone growth in young animals. Hypervitaminosis A is rarely seen nowadays but tends to affect more cats than dogs.

Secondary nutritional hyperparathyroidism

* Parathyroid hormone (PTH) controls the levels of calcium and phosphorous in the blood.

- If an animal is fed a diet which is low in calcium, particularly if Vitamin D has been added, it will develop hypocalcaemia.
- This causes the parathyroid glands to release PTH which causes breakdown of bones and release of calcium from the skeleton.
- This results in a poorly mineralised, weak skeleton. This can be seen on radiography.
- Clinical signs include:
  - Skeletal pain
  - Lameness
  - Deformity
  - Pathological fractures
  - Abnormal posture
- Large breed dogs are most commonly affected.
- Treatment involves correcting the diet and supplementing calcium.

Rickets

Fortunately this is now a very rare condition. It is caused by dietary deficiency of vitamin D and calcium/phosphorous.
- The condition is often accompanied by nutritional hyperparathyroidism because of the hypocalcaemia.
- The skeleton is weak and poorly mineralised. This can be seen on radiography as with nutritional hyperparathyroidism. Thickened growth plates may also be visible on radiography.
- Treatment involves improving the diet and supplementing Vitamin D.

Metaphyseal osteopathy (also called hypertrophic osteodystrophy)

- Idiopathic disease (unknown cause) which affects young growing dogs. Giant breeds are more commonly affected.
- Over-supplementation of minerals and vitamins causing fast growth is a possible factor in the development of this disease. It has also been suggested that persistent infection of osteocytes with the canine distemper virus following vaccination with a live virus may be another potential cause.
- The clinical signs are lameness and often pyrexia.
- Radiography shows abnormalities in the metaphyses. These may be areas of lucencies or extra bone growth.
- Treatment includes improving the diet but lowering the plane of nutrition to reduce the animal's growth rate. Pain relief and fluid therapy may be necessary in the acute phase of the disease.

Pulmonary osteopathy (also called Marie's disease or hypertrophic osteoarthropathy)

- This disease is usually associated with a space-occupying lesion in the thorax (or rarely the abdomen).
- There is proliferation of new one in the distal forelimbs. Swelling of the overlying soft tissues also occurs.
- The animal is often lame and stiff on the affected leg. The presenting complaint may be associated with the thoracic lesion.
- The cause of the bony lesions is not fully understood.
- Occasionally removal of the thoracic lesion can result in reversal of the bony changes, but often the thoracic lesion is a malignant neoplasm.

Osteomyelitis

- Osteomyelitis is inflammation of the bone including the bone marrow.
- It is almost always caused by an infectious agent. Bacteria are the most common cause but fungi and viruses occasionally can cause bony infection.
- The infection can be caused by direct contamination of the bone, during fracture or repair of a bone. Infection may spread locally for example from surrounding soft tissues or periodontal disease. Occasionally bony infection can be caused by haematogenous spread.
- Clinical signs of osteomyelitis include:
  - Pyrexia
  - Lethargy
  - Inappetance
  - Heat, pain and possibly discolouration over the site of the affected bone.
  - Exudation of purulent material may occur particularly if there is a wound.
  - In more chronic cases there may be lameness and pain without acute systemic signs.
  - Pathological fracture may occur occasionally
- Diagnosis is made using haematology, biochemisty, bacteriological sampling of any exudates and radiography.
- Osteomyelitis can be seen on radiography as an irregular periosteal reaction. There are often areas of lysis.
- Treatment involves long term antibiotic therapy. Pain relief and fluid therapy may be necessary in the acute stage of the disease. In chronic cases surgical debridement may be necessary.
- Owners should be warned that treatment of osteomyelitis is

difficult and time-consuming. In severe cases amputation may be necessary.

Bone tumours

- Bone tumours are either **primary** (originating in the bone) or **secondary** (invasion of bony tissue from another source, usually local invasion, occasionally metastasis).
- Primary bone tumours include:
  - Osteoma (benign bony tumour)
  - Osteosarcoma (by far the commonest bone tumour)
  - Chondrosarcoma
  - Fibrosarcoma
  - Haemangiosarcoma
  - Multiple myeloma
  - Secondary bone tumours include:
  - Fibrosarcoma
  - Synovial sarcoma
  - Numerous tumours which invade the mandible (squamous cell carcinoma, melanoma, acanthomatous epulis)

Osteosarcoma

- Extremely aggressive primary bone tumour.
- Predilection sites are proximal humerus, distal radius, distal femur and proximal and distal tibia.
- Clinical signs include:
  - Swelling
  - Severe pain
  - Lameness
  - Muscle atrophy
  - Pathological fracture
  - Depression, lethargy and inappetance.
- Diagnosis is by radiography and bone biopsy.
- Radiography show both destruction of bone (lysis) and new bone formation. There is often elevation of the periosteum (called Codman's triangle). Osteosarcomas may invade a joint but rarely cross a joint to affect the adjacent bone.
- Osteosarcomas are highly metastatic and have usually already spread haematogenously by the time diagnosis is made.
- Treatment involves removing the primary tumour (amputation or possibly limb-sparing techniques), and treatment of the metastases using chemotherapy.
- The prognosis is very guarded. With aggressive prompt treatment the animal's life expectancy may be extended to 12–18 months.
- Euthanasia should be offered if the owner declines treatment.

3.6.27   Joints

What you need to learn

🐾 You need to be able to explain the major forms of joint disease:
   🐾 acute and chronic arthritis osteochondritis (degenerative joint disease)
   🐾 hip/elbow dysplasia.

Synovial joints

- Fluid-filled space, the **synovial cavity**, separates the articulating bones.
- Freely movable joints.
- The synovial cavity is lined with a **synovial membrane** which produces the lubricating **synovial fluid**. The outside of the synovial membrane is protected by a tough fibrous joint capsule. Often parts of the joint capsule are strengthened by ligaments.
- The articular surfaces of the bones in a synovial joint are covered with articular cartilage (usually hyaline cartilage).
- A few synovial joints (eg the stifle) possess fibrocartilage discs or **menisci** which sit between the bones which aid in smooth movement of the joint.

Diseases of the joints

- Inflammation of the joint is called **arthritis.**
- Arthritis is the consequence of any damage to the joint.
- **Traumatic arthritis (sprain) usually affects a single joint.** There is pain and swelling of the affected joint, usually with associated lameness. Treatment is usually rest and external support of the joint. Surgical repair is sometimes necessary
- **Osteoarthritis** is arthritis with some degree of bony involvement. It is characterised by degenerative changes to the cartilage as well as the formation of bony spurs called **osteophytes** at the joint margins. The synovial membrane is often inflamed and the joint capsule is thickened. There may be damage, such as tearing, to the menisci.
- Multiple joints may be affected.
- Clinical signs of osteoarthritis include:
   - Lameness and stiffness
   - Joint swelling
   - Crepitus
   - Reduced range of movement of the affected joint(s)
- Acute osteoarthritis can be caused by:
   - Infection – usually bacterial, rarely mycoplasmal, fungal or protozoal.

- immune mediated conditions (idiopathic polyarthritis, rheumatoid arthritis, vaccine reactions)
- trauma

Chronic osteoarthritis can have numerous causes:

- Primary osteoarthritis – uncommon
- Secondary to:
  - Osteochondrosis (common disorder in young dogs caused by disturbance to endochondral ossification during growth, often related to over feeding and excessive growth rates particularly in large breed animals)
  - Elbow or hip dysplasia
  - Trauma (such as cranial cruciate ligament damage)

Treatment of osteoarthritis

- This involves relieving the pain and discomfort of the condition and allowing joint repair to occur. If possible the primary cause of the disease should also be addressed.
- Exercise should be controlled. The animal should be allowed some exercise to keep the joints mobile but this should not be excessive.
- Overweight animals should be put onto a reduced plane of nutrition to reduce the amount of weight being carried by the diseased joints.
- Medical therapy such as non-steroidal anti-inflammatories or corticosteroids reduces the pain and inflammation.
- Medication which promotes the repair of the joints can also be used. Examples are chondroitin and glucosamine supplements.
- Surgery and joint flushing can be used in severe or unresponsive cases.
- In acute arthritis any causative agents should be identified and appropriate treatment provided. For infectious or septic arthritis antibiotic therapy is necessary. For immune mediated arthritis medication to suppress the immune reaction is necessary (often corticosteroids).

Hip and elbow dysplasia

- This disease is caused by a combination of environmental, dietary and genetic factors.
- Hip dysplasia is the most common cause of osteoarthritis in young dogs.
- It is more common in large breed dogs but can be seen in all types of dogs and cats.
- The dysplastic joint develops abnormally. The condition is then exacerbated by laxity and sub-luxation or luxation of the joint.
- Clinical signs of hip or elbow dysplasia include pain and lameness

in the affected joint. There is often history of an episode such as a fall which has exacerbated the condition.

- Diagnosis is based on palpable laxity of the affected joint along with radiographic features consistent with dysplasia.
- Management of these patients involves:
  - Restricting the animal's growth rate
  - Reducing the weight of overweight animals
  - Controlling the amount of exercise allowed
  - Pain relief may be required intermittently.
  - Severely affected animals may need surgery such as femoral head excision, hip replacement, or triple pelvic osteotomy.
- These conditions are partly inherited so animals which are affected should not be allowed to breed.
- There is a BVA/KC (British Veterinary Association/Kennel Club) scheme for giving dogs a **hip score**. This score indicates the degree of anatomical dysplasia. The higher the score, the more dysplastic changes have been seen on the radiograph. An average breed score is provided and only animals with a hip score which is significantly lower than the breed average should be used for breeding.

3.6.28   Muscle

What you need to learn

- You need to be able to describe common conditions associated with muscle disease/condition:
  - myositis
  - tendonitis.

Muscular disorders

- Inflammation of a muscle is called **myositis**.
- An example is masticatory myositis (inflammation of the muscles of mastication usually affecting West Highland White Terriers).
- Generalised inflammation of the skeletal muscles is called **polymyositis**.
- Polymyositis is often caused by infectious agents such as *Toxoplasma* or *Neospora*.
- Non-inflammatory disease of the muscle is called **myopathy**.
- Examples include inherited conditions such as Scottie cramps and myotonia.
- There are also acquired myopathies such as metabolic myopathies associated with:
- Cushing's disease or long term steroid therapy
- Hypothyroidism

- Hypokalaemic polymyopathy which occurs in renal failure and is inherited in Burmese cats.
- **Muscular dystrophy** is a rare progressive degenerative disease of the skeletal muscles. It is seen most commonly in Golden Retrievers and carries a guarded prognosis.
- **Myasthenia gravis** (MG) is a disorder which affects the neuromuscular junction and prevents nerve transmission. It manifests as generalised weakness and exercise intolerance. Megaoesophagus is one of the possible complications of MG.
- **Tendonitis** is the inflammation of a tendon.
- It is most commonly caused by trauma or over exercise but can also result from infection.
- Treatment involves pain relief and rest.

3.6.29 Cutaneous system

What you need to learn

- You need to be able to describe the function of the cutaneous system and recognise clinical signs associated with skin disease.
- Identify terms related to the diseases of the cutaneous system:
  - pruritus
  - seborrhoea
  - pyoderma.
- Describe the causes, signs and symptoms of parasitic skin disease:
  - fleas
  - lice
  - mange mites
  - harvest mites
  - *Cheyletiella*
  - *Demodex*
  - hookworm (see 3.5.20/21)
  - *Malassezia*.
- Describe advantages/disadvantages of various antiparasitic preparations and advise owners of the zoonotic aspects of ringworm and other parasitic conditions.
- Describe the causes, signs, tests and treatment, including long-term management, for allergic skin conditions:
  - intradermal skin testing
  - patch testing
  - exclusion diets for food hyper-sensitivity.

Disorders of the cutaneous system

See Level 2, 2.3.14 for functions of the skin, structure of the skin and hair cycle.

Clinical signs associated with skin disease

- Full clinical examination of an animal with skin disease allows the nature and distribution of the skin lesions to be identified.
- **Primary skin lesions** are those which have developed as a direct result of the disease process.
- **Secondary lesions** are those which follow on from the original lesions by extension or as a result of attention from the patient.
- Clinical signs often seen in skin disease include:
  - **Alopecia** – hair loss in an are which is normally hair-covered,
  - **Dermatitis** – inflammation of the skin
  - **Erosions** – superficial ulcerated areas of skin
  - **Erythema** – reddening of the skin caused by inflammation.
  - **Excoriation** – erosions and ulcers caused by self inflicted trauma
  - **Furunculosis** – rupture of hair follicles as a results of severe inflammation
  - **Hyperkeratosis** – increased thickness of the stratum corneum
  - **Intertrigo** – frictional damage in areas of folded, poorly-ventilated skin such as the axillae and inguinal areas.
  - **Lichenification** – Thickening of the superficial layers of the skin.
  - **Plaques** – swellings with a flat surface more than 1cm in diameter
  - **Pruritus** – intense, persistent itching (**NB** note spelling, prur*itis* is *incorrect*)
  - **Pustule** – small pus-filled lesion
  - **Pyoderma** – Infection of the skin involving the formation of pus.
  - **Seborrhoea** – excessive secretion of sebum causing a greasy skin and coat.

Parasitic skin disease

- Ectoparasites are involved with most of the skin disease seen in general practice.
- A summary of the organisms involved and the symptoms of infestation can be seen in Table 6.7.

Also see 3.5.20-21.

Skin disease caused by Malassezia pachydermatis

- *Malassezia pachydermatis* is a yeast which is found on the skin of healthy animals. It has only fairly recently been recognised as causing skin disease in dogs (and rarely, cats).
- In affected animals the population of yeast becomes overwhelming and causes clinical signs such as:
- Erythema (reddening of the skin) with alopecia and scaling.
- Greasy exudate which matts the coat

Table 6.7

Ectoparasite	Symptoms	Distribution of Lesions
Lice	Biting lice cause pruritus and self trauma, sucking lice can cause anaemia in large numbers.	Can be found anywhere but often pinnae, axillae, inguinal areas
Fleas	Skin disease usually only seen in hypersensitive or heavily infested animals. Pruritus, erythema, anaemia if heavy burden. Can cause symmetrical ventral alopecia in cats.	Flea allergy dermatitis (FAD) usually affects rump, thighs, abdomen and flanks.
Ticks	Seldom cause skin problems, bites occasionally become infected.	Can attach anywhere, often seen on head and face.
Dipteran larvae (myiasis)	Moist soft skin, maceration, deep ulcers filled with maggots, strong smell. Animal usually debilitated.	Pressure points, perineum, under matted coat or any wounds.
Hookworm Uncinaria	Dermatitis caused by presence of larvae which can penetrate skin.	Usually interdigital dermatitis.
Mites: Sarcoptes scabei	Severe pruritus, small papules/pustules. Self trauma causing hair loss. If untreated leads to weight loss, lymphadenopathy, depression and secondary infections.	Edge of pinnae, elbows, hocks and ventral thorax. Prefers lightly haired areas.
Mites: Notoedres cati	Pruritus, crusting, skin thickening. Very rare in UK	Lesions worst on head.
Mites: Demodex	Usually non-pruritic, alopecia, thickening of skin, scaling. Pruritus occurs with secondary infections.	Localised often forelimb or head (usually benign and resolves without treatment) or Generalised affecting various parts of body, usually including the feet (this form of the disease is very serious and difficult to treat).
Mites: Trixacarus caviae	Severe pruritus, erythema and alopecia in guinea-pigs.	Mainly affects dorsum and pinnae
Mites: Cnemidocoptes pilae	Affects parakeets such as budgies and cockatiels. Scaling on beak and cere, beak can become distorted. Mild pruritus only.	Beak and cere mainly affected. Other lightly feathered areas such as neck, legs and feet can be affected.k
Mites: Otodectes cynotis	Mild to severe pruritus; head shaking; canal filled with thick brown wax. Often inflammation and secondary changes in ear canal.	Almost always external ear but occasionally found at different sites (especially in cats).
Mites: Cheyletiella spp.	Heavy scaling of skin, 'walking dandruff', variable pruritus.	Mainly dorsum in dogs and rabbits, can be localised or generalised in cats.
Mites: (Larvae) Trombicula autumnalis	Moderate pruritus, occasionally patches of red larvae can be seen.	Feet, face, ears and ventrum

- Hyperpigmentation and lichenification of the skin in chronic cases.
- Otitis externa
- Commonly affected sites include ventral neck, interdigital skin , axillae and inguinal areas.
- It is thought that *Malassezia* is often a secondary invader when other skin disease is present such as atopy and keratinisation defects.
- There is usually concurrent infection with bacteria such as *Staphylococcus aureus*.
- Diagnosis of *Malassezia* infection can be achieved by:
- **Microscopy**: This is the most useful method. Examination of tape strips, and direct smears from affected areas show increased numbers of *Malassezia* yeasts.
- **Culture**
- **Biopsy** (not a sensitive test)

Anthelmintic and parasiticide treatment

Table 6.8 Ectoparasites

Product	Treats	Comments
Fipronil	Fleas, ticks, lice, some mites (cheyletiella,	Spot-on and spray formulations
Selamectin	Fleas, ticks, lice, some mites (otodectes, cheyletiella, sarcoptes)	Spot-on formulation, sarcoptes requires repeat treatment after 30 days
Ivermectin	Most endo/ecto parasites	Not licensed, MUST NOT be used in collie or part collie dogs. Toxic in chelonians.
Lufenuron	Fleas	Insect growth inhibitor, doesn't kill adult fleas but renders them infertile.
Imidacloprid	Fleas	Spot-on formulation
Amitraz	Sarcoptes, Demodex	Weekly baths. Organophosphate so must be handles with great care.

- Owners will regularly request information about parasite control (See Table 6.8).
- It is important to be familiar with the parasiticide treatments used by the practice, and to be aware of the indications and contraindications for use.

When giving advice about ectoparasiticides it is important to know the following:

- How old must the animal be before the treatment can be used.
- What dose should be used.

- How the product should be administered (usually sprays or spot-ons, occasionally orally or in baths)
- How often the treatment should be used.
- Which parasites are killed using the product.
- What the possible side-effects are.
- Any handling precautions (eg Amitraz is an organophosphate and must be handed with care; some spot-ons and sprays contain flammable liquids etc.)
- Whether any environmental treatment is necessary (it is usually necessary to treat the environment if a flea infestation is suspected).
- How long the product will take to work.
- It is extremely important to make owners aware that dermatophytosis (ringworm) is a potential zoonosis (ie it can be passed on to humans, causing similar lesions to those seen in cats and dogs).
- For this reason owners should be advise to take care when handling an animal with suspicious lesions, and to wash their hands carefully using a suitable product afterwards.

Allergic skin disease

- Allergic skin disease is one of the most common diseases seen in small animals practice.
- The two main allergic diseases seen are **flea allergy** and **atopy**.
- The main symptom of allergic skin disease is marked pruritus and erythema. This is followed by scratching and self-inflicted trauma leading to secondary lesions, usually infected with bacteria and *Malassezia*.
- Clinical signs persist until the allergen (the substance which is causing the allergic reaction) is removed. This means that many cases of allergic skin diseases become chronic if the allergen can't be identified.

Flea allergy

- Pruritic dermatitis caused by allergy to flea saliva.
- In dogs the pruritus is mainly distributed over the rump. In the cat the distribution varies more and can be on the face, distal limbs and ventral abdomen.
- Diagnosis is based on the clinical signs and evidence of flea infestation.
- It is wise to rule out flea allergy before launching an in-depth investigation of allergic skin disease. This involves treatment of all the animals in the household and treatment of the environment.
- The patient may also require treatment of the pruritus and secondary lesions.

Atopy

- An inherited tendency to develop allergic reaction to environmental allergens.
- Most common allergens which are involved in atopy include:
  - House dust mites (*Dermatophagoides*)
  - Pollens (grass, trees and some weeds)
  - Some moulds
- Some breeds are predisposed to developing atopy. These include West Highland White Terriers, Shar-peis, Cairn terriers, Jack Russell Terriers, Alsatians, Boxers and many others.
- Clinical signs of atopy are:
  - Pruritus, particularly affecting the ventrum, feet, ears, hocks and carpi, usually in a symmetrical pattern.
  - Erythema, alopecia, progressing to hyperpigmentation and lichenification of the skin
  - Secondary infections, most commonly with *Staphylococcus* and *Malassezia*.
  - Sebborhoea.
- Diagnosis involves:
  - Treating secondary infections and parasites.
  - Excluding dietary sensitivity by offering an exclusion diet (diet which contains only novel proteins (those which the animal will not have been exposed to before) so that the animals cannot have developed allergy to those proteins).
  - Intradermal allergy tests (injecting a selection of allergens into the skin and monitoring the sites for allergic reaction)
  - Serological allergy tests (detection of antibodies to selected allergens from a serum sample).
- Treatment involves:
  - Allergen avoidance – this is the most useful part of treatment if it is possible. Animals with pollen allergies should be exercised away from obvious sources of pollen and should have their feet and ventrum rinsed with water after each walk. Placing a regularly washed cotton sheet or hypoallergenic cover over the animal's bed helps reduce exposure to allergen in the house. Regular vacuum cleaning of the house also helps reduce the amount of pollen and house dust mites present.
  - Controlling concurrent (bacterial and fungal) infections
- Glucocorticoids stop the allergic reactions but should be used with great care especially if they are to be used long term.
- Antihistamines reduce the pruritus in some but not all dogs. They have fewer side-effects than steroids so should be tried.
- Essential Fatty Acid (EFA) supplementation can be helpful in about half of the cases of atopy. Beneficial effects may not be obvious for

three months so owners must be advised of this before attempting treatment.

3.6.30 Medical conditions of the eyes

What you need to learn

* You need to be able to describe the common conditions which affect the eyelids and conjunctivae, the clinical signs and treatment:
    * conjunctivitis
    * blepharospasm
    * increased lacrimation
    * uveitis
    * iritis.
* Describe the major causes of eyelid and conjunctival disease including ulceration:
    * allergic
    * infective
    * degenerative
    * entropion
    * ectropion
    * distichiasis
    * keratoconjunctivitis sicca (KCS)
    * cataracts.
* Recognise the common causes of defective vision due to increased intraocular pressure and retinal problems:
    * PRA
    * collie eye anomaly
    * glaucoma.
* Recognise the common causes of defective vision due to retinal problems.

Symptoms of ocular disease

* **Conjunctivitis** – Inflammation of the conjunctiva
* **Hyperaemia** – (engorgement of the blood vessels causing reddening) of the conjunctiva
* **Chemosis** – oedema of the conjunctiva
* **Ocular discharge** – (ranging from mucoid to purulent)
* **Blepharospasm** – excessive blinking and holding the eyelids closed – sign of ocular discomfort
* **Epiphora** – excessive lacrimation (tear production)
* **Keratitis** – Inflammation of the cornea
* **Corneal oedema** – corneal swelling leading to blue appearance to cornea

- **Iritis** – Inflammation of the iris only
- **Uveitis** – Inflammation of the uveal tract (iris, ciliary body and choroid)
- **Hyphaemia** – Blood in the anterior chamber
- **Hypopyon** – Pus in the anterior chamber
- **Glaucoma** – Increase in the pressure within the eye

Conditions affecting the eyelids and conjunctiva

Conjunctivitis

Symptoms include:

- Hyperaemia of the conjunctiva
- Chemosis
- Epiphora and ocular discharge (ranging from mucoid to purulent)
- Blepharospasm.

Causes include:

- Bacteria (often *Staphylococcus*, *Streptococcus* and *Chlamydia*)
- Viruses (Feline herpes virus)
- Physical irritation – foreign bodies, dust and smoke particles, abnormal eyelashes
- Chemical irritation – cleaning products, ectoparasiticides
- Immune mediated disorders – atopy, follicular conjunctivitis
- Tear film abnormalities – dry eye (keratoconjunctivitis sicca)
- Corneal ulceration.

Treatment depends on the cause and may involve:

- Removing cause if known
- Topical antibiotic
- Topical anti-viral treatment (such as trifluorothymidine)
- Topical anti-inflammatory treatment.

Entropion

- Inversion of the eyelid with in-rolling of the eyelashes so that they cause corneal irritation.
- Symptoms include:
- Blepharospasm
- Epiphora
- Keratitis, corneal oedema and corneal ulceration
- Commonly affects breeds with lots of facial skin folds such as Shar-peis, Chows, Clumber spaniels, Rottweilers, Golden retrievers and numerous other breeds.
- Entropion is sometimes secondary to painful ocular conditions which cause blepharospasm. Correcting the primary condition

results in resolution of the entropion.
- Treatment of primary entropion is usually a surgical procedure during which a small strip of skin is excised to return the eyelid to its normal position.

Ectropion

- Eversion of the eyelid, often related to the conformation of the breed.
- Breeds which are commonly affected include St Bernards, Bloodhounds, Bassett Hounds, Mastiffs and other similar breeds.
- Causes fewer problems than entropion as the eyelashes are not in contact with the cornea.
- Can result in keratitis and chronic conjunctivitis in severe cases as the animal is unable to closes its eyelids properly.
- In severe cases surgery may be necessary to correct the condition.

Distichiasis

- Common congenital abnormality in dogs
- Extra cilia (eyelashes) emerge from the meibomian glands on the eyelid margin.
- Symptoms include:
  - Epiphora
  - Keratitis, corneal oedema and corneal ulceration
  - Blepharospasm.
  - Treatment may involve:
- Plucking the cilia – temporary measure as these will regrow.
- Electrolysis
- Surgical excision of the affected strip of meibomian glands.
- A similar but less common condition occurs where *ectopic cilia* grow from the palpebral conjunctiva. This condition is treated with surgery to remove the haired area of conjunctiva.

Prolapse of the nictitans gland

- Prolapse of the nititans gland so that it appears as a smooth red swelling at the medial canthus.
- Also known as '**Cherry Eye**'
- Commonly affects breeds including Bulldogs, Mastiffs, Rottweilers, American Cocker Spaniels.
- Treatment involves suturing the gland back into place. **NB** the gland should not be removed as it contributes to the tear film.

Keratoconjunctivitis sicca (KCS) (also known as dry eye)

- Deficiency of tears causing drying of the corneal surface.

- The most common cause is immune-mediated destruction of the lacrimal gland. It can also be caused by chronic conjunctivitis in cats.
- Symptoms include:
- Conjunctivitis
- Thick mucopurulent ocular discharge which is often adherent to cornea
- Dull appearance to cornea
- Keratitis
- Corneal pigmentation.
- Diagnosis is through measurement of tear production using a marked strip of paper called a **Schirmer Tear Test**.
- Normal tear production causes dye from the base of the strip to travel 15–25 mm along the strip in 1 minute.
- Values of 10–15 mm/min are suspicious of KCS
- Values of < 5mm/min confirm KCS.

Conditions affecting the lens

Cataracts

A cataract is an opacity of the lens.
Causes include:
- Age-related changes in the lenses of older animals
- Congenital cataracts
- Secondary to ocular conditions such as uveitis or neoplaisa
- Secondary to metabolic conditions such as Diabetes mellitus
- Trauma – if the lens capsule is damaged.
  In many older animals the opacity of the lens causes impaired vision but the animal is able to cope using the remaining vision and other senses.
- In more complete cataracts the vision may be severely affected or lost altogether.
- Treatment may be necessary in these more severely affected animals. Treatment is surgical breakdown and extraction of the affected part of the lens.
- Care must be taken that only animals which have still got normal retinal function and which are not suffering from uveitis are selected for this surgery.
- Medical treatment is ineffective.

Conditions affecting intra-ocular pressure

Glaucoma

- Glaucoma is increased pressure of the fluid within the eye (aqueous humour).

It can be caused by:

- Primary glaucoma – anatomical interference with drainage of aqueous humour, inherited in numerous breeds.
- Secondary glaucoma – closure of the irido-corneal angle (where aqueous humour drains away) due to other disease process.
- Commonest causes of secondary glaucoma are:
- Lens luxation – movement of the lens from where it is anchored. The lens can move forwards into the anterior chamber causing increased pressure behind the iris.
- Uveitis – can cause adhesions which block aqueous drainage.
- Intra-ocular neoplasia – can cause swellings or adhesions which block aqueous drainage.
- Trauma – can cause adhesions which block aqueous drainage.
- Treatment involves:
- Medically constricting the pupil (causing miosis) so that the angle of drainage is opened. Topical treatments such as pilocarpine can be used to do this.
- Using carbonic anhydrase inhibitors such as dichlorphenamide reduces the production of aqueous humour.
- Surgery may be necessary in unresponsive cases but these cases should be referred to an experienced ophthalmologist.
- Enucleation may be necessary in painful, unresponsive cases.

Conditions affecting the retina

Collie Eye Anomaly (CEA)

- Failure in the development of the retina during foetal development.
- Results in undeveloped defects on the retina.
- Affects mainly rough collies, smooth collies, Shetland sheepdogs and occasionally border collies.
- The condition can result in retinal detachment and intra-ocular haemorrhage.
- CEA is an inherited condition and there are a number of schemes which assess the eyes of potential breeding animal.

Progressive Retinal Atrophy (PRA)

- Degeneration of the photoreceptor unit in the retina.
- Symptoms start as night blindness and progress to total blindness.
- There may be secondary cataract formation.
- Irish Setters, Rough Collies, Poodles, Dachshunds and Cocker Spaniels are most frequently affected.
- The condition is inherited and affected animals should not be allowed to breed.

3.6.31   Medical conditions of the ears

What you need to learn

❧ You need to be able to describe common conditions which affect the external ear canal, including common causes, clinical signs and treatment:
- ❧ otitis externa
- ❧ otitis media
- ❧ otitis interna
- ❧ infective
- ❧ parasitic
- ❧ degenerative.

❧ Recognise the common conditions which affect the middle and internal ear canal, the common causes, the clinical signs and treatment:
- ❧ Otitis media
- ❧ inner ear disease.

❧ Describe the method for collecting samples from ears and examine to recognise the causes of ear disease.

Terms relating to ear (aural) disease:

- **Otitis Externa** – Inflammation of the external ear canal as far as the ear drum.
- **Otitis Media** – Inflammation of the middle ear.
- **Otitis Interna** – Inlfammation of the inner ear affecting both auditory and vestibular systems.
- **Aural Haematoma** – Development of a blood filled pocket within the pinna.

Otitis externa

This condition can have a number of causes such as:
- Parasites – almost always infestation with *Otodectes cynotis*. Can be caused by *Psoroptes cuniculi* in rabbits.
- Foreign body – often grass seeds lodged in canal.
- Allergic skin disease such as atopy.
- Bacterial infection – often secondary to another condition
- Fungal infection – usually *Malassezia*, often secondary to another condition.
- Breeds with narrow, haired ear canals, and those with floppy ears are predisposed to otitis because wax and cellular debris tends to accumulate within the canal

Symptoms may include

- head shaking.
- erythema progressing to ulceration of canal and pinna.
- pain.
- discharge – ranging from thick black wax (parasitic) to purulent (infections).
- aural haematoma – usually secondary to head-shaking.

Treatment depends on the cause and may include:

- Oral antimicrobial and anti-inflammatory treatment (useful if condition is very painful initially). **NB** Swabs should be taken for laboratory analysis in any complicated cases to ensure that the correct antimicrobial therapy is being used.
- Topical antimicrobial and anti-inflammatory treatment (if animal not too painful and if ear drum not damaged)

Treatment of underlying allergic conditions

- Anti-parasite treatment where necessary.
- Removal of foreign body or flushing of material from the ear under general anaesthetic.
- Surgery – indicated only for recurrent non-responsive cases. Can involve lateral wall resection (LWR), Vertical Canal Ablation (VCA) or Total Ear Canal Ablation (TECA).

Otitis media

- Usually caused by an extension of otitis externa when the tympanic membrane has been damaged.
- Occasionally caused by ascending infection through the auditory tubes.
- Symptoms are similar to those of otitis externa.
- Treatment is similar to that used for otitis externa, but most topical preparations should be avoided when the tympanic membrane is damaged.

Otitis Interna

- Usually caused by an extension of otitis externa and otitis media.
- Usually accompanied by vestibular symptoms such as nystagmus, circling and loss of balance due to effects of infection and inflammation on the vestibular apparatus.
- May be accompanied by Horner's syndrome (3rd eyelid protrusion, constricted pupil etc on affected side) from damage to the sympathetic nerve supply to the head where it passes close to the tympanic bulla.
- Cats with otitis interna occasionally show peculiar symptoms such as hypersensitivity and tail-chasing.

- Radiography of the tympanic bulla may be necessary to confirm the presence of otitis interna.
- Treatment is difficult and may involve medical treatment (antibiotic and anti-inflammatory treatment) or surgical management.

Collecting samples from the ear

- If an ear infection is severe or failing to respond to initial treatment samples of material should be taken for laboratory analysis.
- This allows identification of which bacteria or yeasts are causing the infection, as well as what medication is most suitable for the elimination of those micro-organisms.
- A sample of the ear wax is collected using a sterile swab. This may need to be performed under general anaesthesia.
- The swab is placed into transport material and despatched to the laboratory.
- Some of the sample is can be transferred onto a clean microscope slide for in-house microscopy.
- Yeasts such as *Malassezia*, and parasites such as *Otodectes* or *Psoroptes* can easily be identified using the practice microscope.

3.6.32   Poisons

What you need to learn

- You need to be able to recognise clinical signs of a poisoned animal.
- Describe the general principles of collection and storage of samples from possible poisoning cases and appreciate difficulties involved with forensic examination:
  - see Level 2, 2.4.39.
- Identify poisons encountered in small animal practice with signs and treatment or antidotes where possible:
  - rodentocides
  - carbon monoxide
  - acrolein
  - ethylene glycol
  - lead
  - phenolic compounds
  - acids/alkalis
  - herbicides
  - insecticides
  - molluscocides.
- Describe how different poisons affect the body and their route of entry:
  - convulsants
  - irritants

- corrosives
- anticoagulants
- inhaled
- ingested
- skin absorbed.
- Itemise the commonly used drugs with toxic effects, state their signs and treatment:
  - organophosphorus compounds
  - corticosteroids
  - NSAIDs.
- Describe the general methods of treatment for poisoning including when emetics can and cannot be used:
  - emesis
  - gastric lavage
  - emollients
  - washing agents
  - antidotes.
- Explain the conditions often confused with poisoning.
- Describe the principles of nursing animals suffering from poisoning to include long-term management.

A **poison** is a substance which when inhaled, ingested, or absorbed into the body will cause adverse effects.

Poisoning can occur through accident, overdose (eg flea spray), allergic reactions, carelessness (leaving medication where a pet can find it), or ignorance (treating animals with human medication such as paracetamol). Malicious poisoning is extremely rare.

The clinical signs of poisoning are dependent on the toxin involved. Common symptoms are:

- drooling (often seen with overdose of organophosphates)
- vomiting (a common symptom caused by irritation of the gastrointestinal tract)
- lack of co-ordination and seizures (metaldehyde, lead)
- depression and weakness
- abdominal pain
- dilated pupils (organophosphates)
- bleeding (following ingestion of anti-coagulant poisons such as the rodenticide warfarin)
- organ failure – renal failure often follows ingestion of ethylene glycol (antifreeze) or toxic amounts of raisins; liver failure can be caused by ingestion of theobromine (in chocolate) or metaldehyde (slug pellets)
- collapse and death (carbon monoxide poisoning, some venomous stings/bites).

Obtaining an accurate history is vital in suspected cases of poisoning.

Important questions are:

- What poison has been ingested?
- How much of the poison has been ingested?
- How long ago was the poison ingested?

When investigating the cause of a suspected poisoning, various samples can be collected and sent for laboratory analysis. Samples should always be collected aseptically to prevent contamination and erroneous results. Suspected poisons can also be toxic to the handler so precautions, such as the wearing of plastic gloves, should be taken when obtaining samples.

Samples can be taken pre- or post-mortem (see also 2.4.39).

- Whole blood should be sent in an EDTA or heparin tube (eg heavy metal toxicity).
- Serum should be sent in a clotting tube (eg chocolate toxicity).
- Brain, kidney and liver samples from a post-mortem should be frozen before transport to the laboratory.
- Stomach contents (or gastric lavage fluid) can be collected in a waterproof bag or vial. This can be frozen if necessary.
- Foodstuffs and water can be sent in a watertight container. These should be refrigerated or frozen.
- Environmental samples (bedding or soil samples) should also be collected if they are indicated in a poisoning case.

Many different substances can be poisons.

- **Medicines**
  - Almost any medication taken at a high dose is toxic. Poisoning with ibuprofen and aspirin is commonly seen. Toxicity from illegal drugs, such as marijuana (cannabis), is occasionally seen.
- **Pesticides**
  - weed killers (including chlorates and paraquat)
  - insecticides (including flea products, mange treatments and sheep dips)
  - slug pellets (metaldehyde)
  - rodenticides (baits containing warfarin, strychnine).
- **Foodstuffs**
  - raisins
  - chocolate (contains the toxin theobromine)
  - acrolein (a poison released when cooking fat is allowed to overheat)
  - alcohol.
- **Household chemicals**
  - antifreeze (ethylene glycol)

- petrol and oil
- cleaning fluids
- lead (from paint, plumbing materials, lead weights and shot)
  NB lead toxicity is common in birds such as swans and geese as a
  result of ingestion of lead fishing weights
- wood treatments
- phenolic compounds
- acids (limescale removers such as hydrochloric or formic acid)
- alkalis (drain cleaners such as sodium hydroxide; fertilisers
  containing ammonia).
- **Gases**
  - carbon monoxide from poorly ventilated boilers.
- **Plants**
  - laburnum
  - foxglove
  - deadly nightshade
  - oak
  - ragwort
  - yew.
- **Bites**
  - Bites from adders are occasionally seen.
  - Bites can be inflicted by exotic species.
- **Stings**
  - Multiple wasp and bee stings can have toxic effects.

Poisons can be **inhaled** (eg carbon monoxide, acrolein), **ingested**
(taken in through the mouth, the commonest route), or **absorbed**
across the skin and mucous membranes (stings, insecticides such as
organophosphates).

Almost any medication taken at a high dose is toxic. Drugs which
commonly cause problems include the following.

- **Corticosteroids** – examples are prednisolone, dexamethasone,
  betamethasone. High doses cause immunosuppression and can
  cause ulceration of the gut. Treatment of overdose involves
  prevention of gut damage using antacids, adsorbents such as
  sucralfate or anti-ulcer drugs such as ranitidine and cimetidine.
- **Non-steroidal anti-inflammatories (NSAIDS)** – examples are
  carprofen, meloxicam, phenylbutazone and ketoprofen. NSAIDs
  used in human medicine include paracetamol and aspirin. High
  doses cause liver or kidney failure. Gastric ulceration can also be
  caused by NSAID ingestion. Treatment of overdose involves
  prevention of gut damage using antacids, adsorbents such as
  sucralfate or anti-ulcer drugs such as ranitidine and cimetidine.
  Supportive treatment such as fluid therapy is usually necessary.
  Overdose is fatal when organ failure occurs.

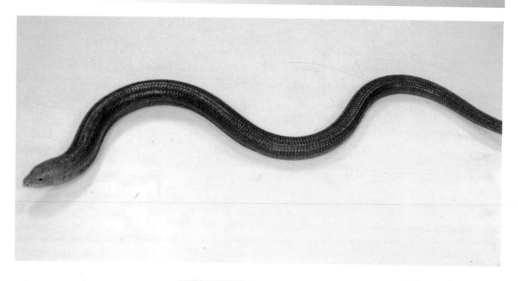

Plate 1 (Above)
Glass lizard (legless).

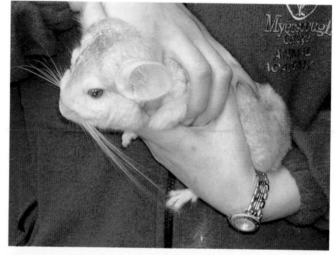

Plate 2 (Right)
How to hold a chinchilla.

Plate 3 (Below)
Axolotl.

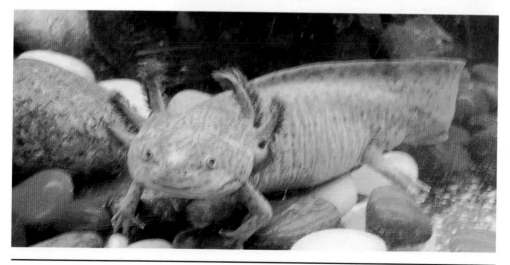

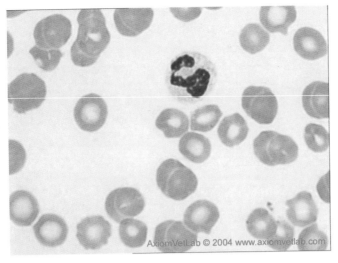

Plate 4 A mature canine neutrophil.

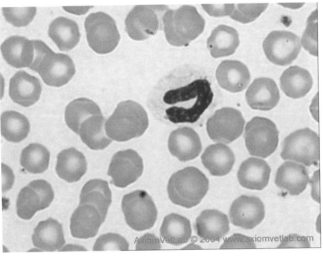

Plate 5 A canine band neutrophil with dohle body.

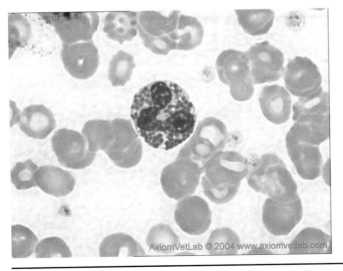

Plate 6 A canine eosinophil.

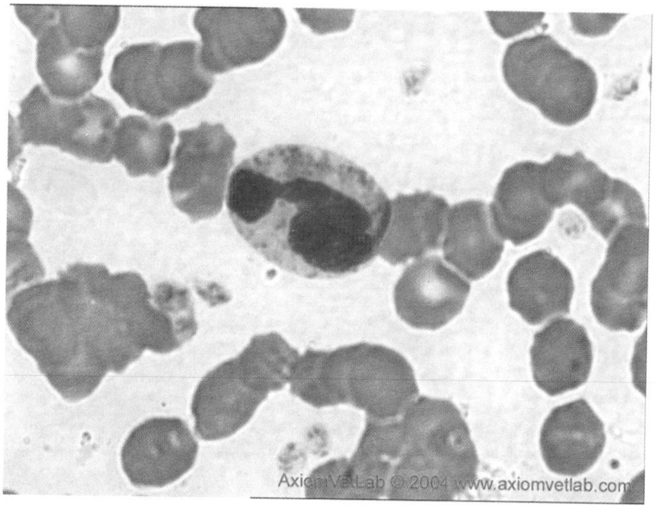

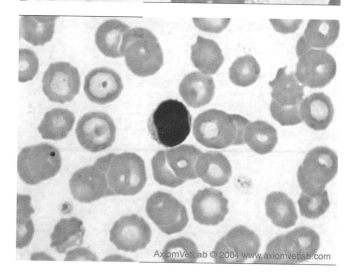

Plate 7   A canine basophil.

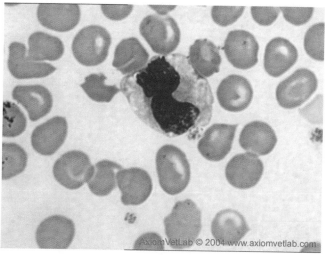

Plate 8   A canine lymphocyte.

Plate 9   A canine monocyte.

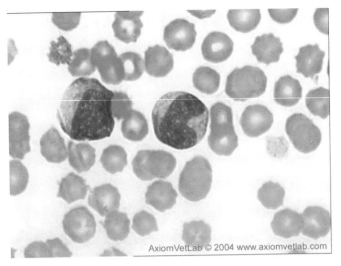

Plate 10 A canine myelocyte and metamyelocyte.

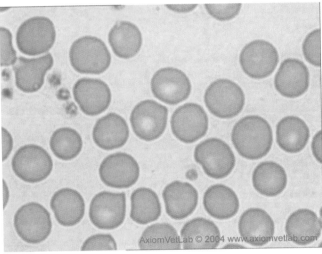

Plate 11 Mature erythrocytes.

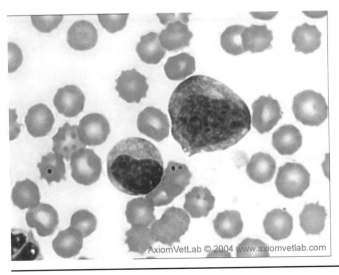

Plate 12 A canine myelocyte and myeloblast.

• **Organophosphorous compounds** – are usually a component of insecticides such as flea sprays, mange treatment and sheep dips; examples are dichlorvos, cypromethrin and amitraz.

First aid in poisoning

Remove the source of toxicity

Poisons can be adherent to the coat so a collar which prevents licking should be applied, then the coat should be cleaned as soon as possible once the animal is stable. Clipping the coat will remove a great deal of contaminating material.

If the coat is contaminated with oily material, such as oil or creosote, detergents should be avoided in the first instance as they may increase the absorption of toxins through the skin. Instead the coat should be cleaned with Swarfega to remove as much oil as possible, and only then should a detergent be used to remove the contaminant.

Prevent further absorption of ingested poison

This often involves stimulating **emesis** (vomiting). Emetic substances (those used to induce emesis) include xylazine, apomorphine, washing soda crystals and ipecachuana syrup. **NB** Salt should not be used as an emetic as it is ineffective and may be absorbed, causing electrolyte imbalances.

Vomiting should **not** be induced if:

• the poison is corrosive as further damage to the upper gastrointestinal tract will occur
• the patient is unconscious, fitting, or too weak to hold its head up as these animals are at risk of inhaling the vomit.

Gastric contents remain in the stomach for approximately four hours so there is no point inducing emesis more than four hours after ingestion.

Gastric lavage involves anaesthetising the patient and flushing the stomach with tepid water to remove all of the gastric contents.

Adsorbents such as activated charcoal are used to bind to the toxin, preventing absorption through the gut wall.

Cathartics speed the elimination of unabsorbed poisons in the faeces. Examples are sorbitol and magnesium sulphate. These can cause dehydration and should be used with care.

Treat with an antidote if one is available

Examples of suitable antidotes for use in poisoning include

- vitamin K (used to treat warfarin toxicity)
- naloxone (treats opiate toxicity)
- atropine (used to treat organophosphate toxicity)
- ethanol (used to treat ethylene glycol toxicity)
- sodium calcium edetate (used to treat lead toxicity)
- antivenins (treat bites from poisonous snakes, spiders and fish).

Treatment of symptoms

This depends on the poison but usually involves supportive treatment such as fluid therapy. If convulsions occur these should be treated with anticonvulsant agents such as phenobarbitone and diazepam.

Oxygen therapy may be necessary for animals with respiratory compromise.

Close monitoring is very important to assess deterioration or recovery.

The Veterinary Poisons Information Service (VPIS) provides 24-hour information for veterinary surgeons. It can:

- supply data on the clinical effect of most poisons
- advise on antidotes
- advise on treatment methods.

The symptoms of poisoning are variable and often non-specific. Many other conditions can be mistaken for poisoning, particularly where a number of animals are involved. When investigating poisoning it is important to eliminate other possible causes such as:

- trauma
- drowning
- starvation
- endo- and ectoparasites
- bacterial, viral, or fungal infections
- metabolic disease
- nutritional disease such as mineral or vitamin deficiency
- electric shock/lightning strike.

Once emergency treatment has been administered the animal must be closely monitored.

Animals which have been bathed will need to be dried off with a towel and then allowed to undergo recovery with a heat source to prevent hypothermia.

Some effects of poisoning take time to become clinically apparent. Blood samples must be taken to assess organ function and monitor the progression of any anaemia. It may be necessary to take repeated samples over a few weeks following the poisoning. The effects of poisoning with substances such as ragwort, organophosphates or paraquat may be delayed for weeks or even months.

The animal should be assessed for any permanent damage such as brain damage from strychnine or lead toxicity.

Euthanasia may have to be considered for animals which are in severe pain; have permanent organ failure, brain damage or which fail to respond to treatment.

3.6.33 Fluid therapy (definition of terms)

What you need to learn

* You need to be able to describe terminology relating to fluid therapy:
  * ion
  * cation
  * anion
  * electrolyte
  * osmosis and osmotic pressure
  * isotonic solution
  * hypotonic solution
  * hypertonic solution.
* Describe different types of fluid within the compartments of the body:
  * intracellular fluid
  * extracellular fluid
  * intravascular fluid
  * interstitial fluid
  * transcellular fluid.
* Identify the common cations and anions found in the intracellular and extracellular fluids.
* Describe the principles of water balance in the body and relevance of pH in respect of body fluids.
* Identify the sources of water to the body.

The following are terms used in describing fluid therapy:

* **Ion** – a charged atom or particle
* **Cation** – a positively charged ion
* **Anion** – a negatively charged ion
* **Electrolyte** – a liquid or solution that is capable of conducting electricity because it dissociates into ions, eg salt (or sodium chloride, NaCl) dissociates into chloride ions (Cl^-) and sodium ions (Na^+)

- **Osmosis** – the passage of water through a semi-permeable membrane
- **Osmotic pressure** – the pressure with which the water molecules are drawn across the semi-permeable membrane
- **Isotonic solution** – has the same osmotic pressure as blood
- **Hypotonic solution** – has a lower osmotic pressure than blood
- **Hypertonic solution** – has a greater osmotic pressure than blood.

Different types of fluid within the body

Approximately 60% of the body weight is fluid (this is lower in the elderly and higher in the young).

This fluid comprises the following:

- **Intracellular fluid** (ICF) – is the fluid found within the cells and it makes up 60% of body fluids.
- **Extracellular fluid** (ECF) – is the fluid found outside the cells and it makes up 35% of the body fluid.
- **Plasma** makes up the remaining 5%.

Extracellular fluid is further divided into:

- **intravascular fluid** – which is found within the vascular compartment
- **interstitial fluid** – which is the fluid found in the spaces between cells.
- **Transcellular fluid** – comprises the special fluids formed by secretory mechanisms, eg cerebrospinal fluid (CSF).

The distribution of electrolytes (in descending order) within the intra- and extracellular fluids are as follows:

- **ICF** – potassium, magnesium, sodium and chloride, calcium
- **ECF** – sodium, chloride, calcium, bicarbonate, potassium.

Water balance

To maintain a normal water balance the patient needs to take in approximately 50 ml/kg/day fluid.

When there is reduced intake of water or increased loss of water the following starts to occur:

- The osmotic concentration within the animal increases and fluid is drawn from the intravascular compartment.
- This makes the patient thirsty.
- Osmoreceptors are stimulated and produce anti-diuretic hormone (ADH).
- The ADH aids reabsorption of water and concentrates the urine.

• The renin-angiotensin process starts to stimulate aldosterone to act on the kidney to increase the reabsorption of sodium.

Sources of water

There are various sources of water available to animals:

• drinking water
• water present in food
• water metabolised from fats and carbohydrates.

3.6.34   Water in the body and dehydration

What you need to learn

❧ You need to be able to identify the ways in which water is lost from the body and the volume of water required to replace losses:
  ❧ sensible/insensible losses.
❧ Describe the terms associated with dehydration:
  ❧ pH
  ❧ metabolic acidosis
  ❧ metabolic alkalosis
  ❧ buffer solution respiratory acidosis
  ❧ respiratory alkalosis.
❧ Describe how the body maintains its pH.
❧ Identify clinical signs of dehydration, with reference to percentage of body weight loss:
  ❧ case history
  ❧ skin tenting/condition etc.
❧ Identify the conditions that cause dehydration.
❧ Identify and describe the causes of primary water deficit and sodium and potassium imbalances and how they may occur.
❧ Describe clinical tests for assessing dehydration and identify normal parameters for each test:
  ❧ PCV
  ❧ SG see 3.5.18.
❧ Calculate fluid requirements:
  ❧ normal maintenance
  ❧ fluid deficit correction.
❧ Describe the principles of accurate charting of fluid intake/output.

Water losses

Water losses can be divided into sensible and insensible losses.

• **Insensible loss** – these are losses that cannot be controlled
• breathing/cutaneous loss 20 ml/kg/day

- **Sensible losses:** over which the body has some control
  - faeces – 10–20 ml/kg/day
  - urine – 20 ml/kg/day

Adult animals therefore need to replace 50–60 ml/kg/day approximately to maintain their water balance.

Terms associated with dehydration

- **pH** is a measure used to express the acidity or alkalinity of a substance.
- **Metabolic acidosis** occurs when there is a fall in blood pH with retention of potassium.
- **Metabolic alkalosis** occurs when there is a rise in blood pH with retention of bicarbonate.
- **Buffer solution** is a substance that causes resistance to any change of hydrogen ion concentration (and thus pH) when either acid or alkali is added.
- **Respiratory acidosis** describes a rise in carbon dioxide levels and hence pH.
- **Respiratory alkalosis** describes a decrease in carbon dioxide levels and hence pH.

Maintaining pH

The pH of blood should be 7.35–7.45. It is important that it is maintained within this range to prevent acid-base disturbances. The pH is carefully controlled by:

- buffer systems
- respiration (increasing or decreasing)
- renal function (excretion of bicarbonate).

Clinical signs of dehydration

After taking a case history the patient should be assessed for clinical signs of dehydration as listed in Table 6.9

Conditions causing dehydration

There are various conditions that can lead to dehydration:

- vomiting and diarrhoea
- severe burns
- hyperthermia
- no access to water.

Primary water deficit

In primary water deficit the following series occurs.

Table 6.9 Clinical signs of dehydration

% dehydration	Clinical signs
<5%	No signs detected
5%	Some loss of skin elasticity Mucous membranes and eyes are OK
5–8%	Marked loss of skin elasticity Eyes slightly sunken Capillary refill time is sluggish
10%	Skin tenting Dry ,tacky and pale mucous membranes Eyes are sunken Capillary refill time is slow Early shock
12–15%	Severe skin tenting Very dry and tacky mucous membranes Collapsed Shock Moribund

- The hypothalamus stimulates the animal to drink.
- If there is no intake of water, the blood remains hypertonic and fluids therefore move from inside the cells into the bloodstream by osmosis.
- The pituitary gland releases ADH and this stimulates the kidneys to conserve water by concentrating the urine.
- Skin tenting occurs when the cells start to lose their fluid.

Causes of primary water deficit include:

- prolonged inappetance, eg fractured jaw
- water unavailable
- unconsciousness
- excessive panting
- diabetes insipidus.

Water and electrolyte loss

When the loss of water and electrolytes is equal the blood remains isotonic.

Following a period of this loss, the blood is still isotonic but its volume decreases and hypovolaemia develops. This is followed by collapse.

Poor tissue perfusion and cardiac output lead to acute renal failure.

Vomiting and diarrhoea are the most common causes of water and electrolyte loss.

When electrolyte loss is greater then water loss

If the loss of electrolytes exceeds the loss of water:

• The blood becomes hypotonic as a result of the water and electrolyte loss.
• Fluid moves from the blood into the cells by osmosis.
• There is no stimulus from the hypothalamus to drink.
• The pituitary gland stops producing ADH because the blood is dilute.
• The animal becomes hypovolaemic.

Causes of this type of loss are:

• persistent vomiting
• persistent diarrhoea
• pyometra
• wound drainage.

Tests for dehydration

There are various tests for dehydration to support the use of the clinical signs given above in Table 6.12.

• the **Packed cell volume** (PCV), which has been described in 3.5.18.
• the **Specific gravity of urine**, which has been described in 3.5.18.
• urine output should be 1–2 ml/kg/hour
• total plasma protein should be 55–70 g/l
• central venous pressure (CVP) should be 3–7 cm of water
• daily measurement of body weight.

Fluid calculations

Calculation of the fluid requirements should take into account the size of the animal and the giving set used as follows.

• standard giving set drop rate = 20 drops/ml
• paediatric giving set drop rate = 60 drops/ml

Fluids should be maintained at 50–60 ml/kg/day to replace daily losses.

An example is given here of the maintenance rates for a 5-kg cat using a standard giving set.

• maintenance fluid requirement = 50 ml/kg/day = (50ml × 5 kg)/day = 250 ml/day
• requirement per hour = 250 ml ÷ 24 ~ 10 ml
• requirement per minute = 10 ml ÷ 60 ~ 0.16 ml
• giving set drop rate = 20 × 0.16 ml = 3.2 drops/min
• drip rate = 60 seconds/3.2 drops = 1 drop every 18 seconds

Fluid deficit requirements

The fluid requirement varies with the condition of the animal. The following are examples of the requirements under different circumstances:

- vomiting or diarrhoea episode – 4 ml/kg/episode
- pyrexia – 3 ml/kg/% increase in body temperature
- surgery – 5–10 ml/kg/hour
- PCV – 10 ml/kg/1% increase in PCV
- dehydration deficit – 10 ml/kg/% dehydrated.

Principles of accurate charting of fluid intake-output

All fluid intake should be recorded. This includes:

- the amount of intravenous fluid given
- the amount of water given to drink
- the amount of fluid fed by syringe
- the amount of food given and state if it was moist or dry food.

All fluid loss should also be recorded, including:

- the amount of urine passed
- the amount of faeces/diarrhoea passed
- the amount of vomit
- any excessive panting should also be recorded.

3.6.35   Fluids

What you need to learn

- ☙ You need to be able to describe terms relating to fluids:
  - ☙ hypotonic
  - ☙ hypertonic
  - ☙ isotonic.
- ☙ Identify the common fluids available for fluid therapy:
  - ☙ colloids
  - ☙ plasma
  - ☙ plasma substitutes
  - ☙ blood
  - ☙ crystalloids, eg Hartmanns, Ringers, dextrose, saline, normal saline.
- ☙ Describe fluids' ionic content and concentration.
- ☙ For each common fluid, state whether hypotonic, hypertonic or isotonic.
- ☙ Identify their use for specific conditions.
- ☙ Identify the routes available for fluid therapy:

- intravenous
- subcutaneous
- intra-peritoneal
- oral
- intraosseous.
- Identify the veins used for intravenous therapy and describe their locations:
  - cephalic
  - saphenous
  - jugular
  - marginal ear vein (rabbit).
- Describe the equipment necessary for intravenous fluid therapy and the necessary precautions for preventing infection:
  - giving sets
  - I/V catheters
  - infusion pumps.
- Describe the principles of calculating a transfusion/infusion rate and managing an intravenous drip.
- Identify and describe procedures for monitoring during administration of fluids:
  - central venous pressure monitoring systems
  - blood pressure monitoring equipment.
- Mucous membrane, pulse etc.
- Describe the principles of providing parenteral nutrition.

Common fluids available for fluid therapy

- **colloids** – plasma substitutes (eg Gelofusine®, Haemaccel®)
- **blood** and **plasma**
- **crystalloids** – Hartmann's, Ringer's, dextrose, saline (sodium chloride), normal saline (0.9% sodium chloride).

Hartmann's solution

The ionic content of Hartmann's solution is:

- sodium 131
- potassium 5
- calcium 2
- chloride 111
- bicarbonate (as lactate) 29.

It is an isotonic solution.

Hartmann's solution is used for vomiting and diarrhoea, pyometra, water and electrolyte loss.

Sodium chloride 0.9% and glucose 5%

The ionic content of this solution is:

- sodium 154
- chloride 154.

and it has an energy value of 785 kilojoules (ie 188 calories)

It is an isotonic solution. Sodium chloride 0.9%/glucose 5% solution is used for maintenance and for primary water deficits.

Sodium chloride 0.9% (normal saline)

The ionic content of this solution is:

- sodium 150
- chloride 150.

It is an isotonic solution. Normal saline is used for vomiting and for water and electrolyte loss.

Dextrose 5%

The ionic content of dextrose 5% is:

- 5% dextrose.

It is an isotonic solution. Dextrose 5% is used for primary water loss and for hypoglaecemia.

Ringer's solution

The ionic content of Ringer's is:

- sodium 147
- potassium 4
- calcium 2.5
- chloride 156.

It is an isotonic solution. Ringer's solution is used for primary water loss and for vomiting.

Haemaccel®

The ionic content of Haemaccel® is:

- sodium 143
- potassium 5
- calcium 3
- chloride 154
- it also contains gelatins.

It is an isotonic solution. Haemaccel is used for blood loss, to restore the circulating volume.

Routes available for fluid therapy

A variety of routes exist by which fluid therapy can be administered.

- intravenous
- subcutaneous
- intraperitoneal
- oral
- intraosseous.

Veins used for fluid therapy

The veins used for the administration of fluid therapy include:

- **Cephalic veins** are located on the dorsal aspect of the distal forelimbs.
- **Saphenous veins** are located on the lateral aspect of the proximal hindlimbs.
- **Jugular vein** is found on the lateral aspect of the neck.
- **Marginal ear vein** is found on the dorsal aspect of the ear and is used in rabbits.

Equipment for fluid therapy

The following equipment is required when initiating fluid therapy:

- giving set
- intravenous catheters, eg butterfly, over the needle
- infusion pumps
- bag of intravenous fluids
- electric clippers
- antiseptic solution and swabs
- spirit (with or without cotton wool)
- tape, eg micropore, zinc oxide
- blade (optional)
- bandage.

To prevent infection the area should be aseptically prepared using antiseptic solution and spirit before insertion of the catheter. The catheters and giving sets used should be sterile.

Calculating an infusion rate

Calculation of an infusion rate is described in 3.6.34.

Managing an intravenous drip

The management of an intravenous drip requires the following:

- Protection -the dressing on the leg (protecting the catheter and attached giving set) should be changed if it becomes soiled/wet.
- Observation – if the catheter is not in the vein then the following will be seen – a wet bandage and swelling of the limb above the catheter site. The catheter may be visible if the patient has pulled it out completely.
- Check – the drip should be checked to see that it is running and not occluded by kinks in the giving set or by the patient pulling their leg back
- Pulse
- Respiration
- Urine output – can only accurately be measured if it is collected into a collection bag, alternatively the urine could be collected in a kidney dish and measured. Urine output should be 1–2 ml/kg/hour.
- Mucous membrane colour and CRT.
- Any signs of noisy breathing or coughing

How to change a drip bag

- Close off the giving set.
- Remove the tag from the new bag by twisting it.
- Remove the giving set from the old bag.
- Place the giving set into the new bag with a rotating movement, be careful not to twist it in as this will in turn twist the giving set tubing.
- Open the giving set to the appropriate level.
- Place the old bag in the clinical waste bin.

Monitoring administration of fluids

When monitoring the administration of fluids the following check s should be made.

- **Mucous membranes** should be pink in colour with a capillary refill time of less then two seconds.
- **Pulse** should be within the normal range with an adequate pulsation.
- **Central venous pressure**, which is the measurement of the venous

blood return to the heart, should be between 3 and 7 cm of water.
- **Blood pressure** monitoring by sphygmomanometry, ultrasonic Doppler, or oscillometric devices, directly into an artery, should be 120 mmHg/80 mmHg, mean blood pressure = 94 mm/Hg
- **Urine ouput** should be between 1 and 2 ml/kg/hour.

Parenteral nutrition

Parenteral nutrition involves feeding intravenously, this method is used when enteral methods are not possible or when starvation has exceeded 5 days.

A central vein must be used, eg jugular. If a peripheral vein is used, eg cephalic, then thrombophlebitis can occur.

Energy is provided as a mixture containing:

- dextrose
- lipid emulsions
- protein.

The aseptic management of catheters, feeding solutions and giving sets is paramount as any infection can be fatal.

Monitoring of parenteral nutrition

The following must be monitored on a daily basis sometimes up to four times a day.

- vital parameters
- urine glucose
- body weight
- PCV
- TP
- electrolytes.

3.6.36   Blood transfusions

What you need to learn

- You need to be able to describe the collection and storage of blood for transfusion:
  - storage times
  - conditions for blood/plasma.
- Describe the reasons for transfusion reactions to blood or blood products and identify clinical signs.
- Identify and describe the consequences of over transfusion of intravenous fluids.

🐾 Explain the significance of transfusion rates.
🐾 Outline central venous pressure and describe its measurement.
🐾 Describe the considerations for the management of patients undergoing fluid infusions:
    🐾 self mutilation
    🐾 infection
    🐾 patency etc.

Collection of blood

- Blood should be collected from healthy, vaccinated patients (dogs 30 kg and over, cats 4 kg and over, cats should be tested for FELV, FIV and FIP prior to collection).
- Sedation may be required.
- Blood should be collected from a jugular vein.
- Blood should be collected into a prepared blood collection bag, either acid citrate dextrose (ACD), citrate phosphate dextrose (CPD), or should be syringe-treated with an anticoagulant (eg heparin).
- Only 1% body weight may be collected from dogs.
- Only 30 ml maybe collected from cats.

Storage of blood

- If heparin was used (within a syringe) as anticoagulant then the blood must be used within 48 hours.
- Blood collected in CPD collection bags may be stored at 1–6 °C for 28 days.
- Blood collected in ACD collection bags may be stored at 1–6 °C for 21 days.

Collection of plasma

- Collected in the same manor as blood.
- The blood is then centrifuged immediately.
- The plasma is decanted off.

Storage of plasma

- Plasma can be frozen at –20 °C for up to 3 months.
- Plasma can be frozen at –70 °C for up to 6 months.

Transfusion reactions

Reactions to transfusion can be either immediate or delayed.

Immediate reactions

Immediate reactions can occur as a result of:

- histamine release
- differences between recipient and donor red cells (cross-matching should be performed)
- prior sensitisation of the donor by a previous transfusion.

Delayed reactions

These occur up to two weeks following the transfusion and are the result of the recipient having an immune response to the donor's red cells.

Clinical signs of a transfusion reaction

The following clinical signs are seen in a transfusion reaction:

- hypotension
- muscle tremors
- pyrexia
- panting
- tachycardia
- jaundice
- anaemia.

Overtransfusion of fluids

If the volume of fluid administered intravenously greatly exceeds the recommended amount then the following will become evident:

- oedema of soft tissues
- fluid within in the lungs – lung noises (crackling) will be heard
- coughing
- excessive urination.

It is important that the fluid volumes and rates are calculated for each patient and monitored accordingly to prevent volume overload and its consequences.

Central venous pressure

CVP is a measurement of the venous blood return to the heart. It is measured using the following technique.

- Position the patient in lateral recumbency with the head and neck extending over towels or a pillow.
- A long jugular catheter is inserted into a jugular vein.

- The catheter is advanced towards the anterior vena cava so that the tip of the catheter is sitting by the right atrium.
- A three-way tap is attached to the catheter.
- Tubing is attached to the opposite end of the three-way tap and a second three-way tap is attached at the opposite end of the tubing.
- Infusion fluid and a giving set are then attached to one side of the three-way tap and a open-ended manometer is attached to another side of the three-way tap.
- Fluid must be run through the manometer before connecting to the catheter.
- The reading on the manometer should be zero. This indicates that it is level with the right atrium (approximately the level of the sternum).
- The fluid in the manometer will rise and fall with respiration.

Normal values of CVP are 3–7 cm of water. Trends in the results are more useful than one-off readings with this type of monitoring.

- High values indicate right-sided heart failure, pericardial disease, or over infusion of fluids.
- Low values indicate dehydration, venous pooling, or reduced plasma concentration.

Management of patients undergoing fluid infusions

- **Prevent patient interference** – This can be done by using Elizabethan collars, placing a bandage over the catheter, and bandaging the remaining feet.
- **Prevent infection** – Use of aseptic technique when applying the catheter, swabbing of the injection site with spirit before injection of any drugs, changing the giving sets carefully and aseptically, and changing the dressings if soiled will all help to prevent infection.
- **Patency** – The catheter must remain 'open' so it should be flushed twice daily with a heparin flush, this can done through an injection port or directly into the catheter (remembering to be as aseptic as possible). Splints may also be used to prevent the patients pulling their limbs back and therefore occluding the catheter.

3.6.37 Shock

What you need to learn
- You need to be able to describe shock.
- Describe the various types of shock, including:
  - hypovolaemic
  - endotoxic
  - neurogenic

- cardiogenic.
- Identify the clinical signs relating to shock and the appropriate First Aid treatment:
  - TPR
  - mucous membrane
  - colour/capillary refill
  - PCV
  - urine production
  - degree of consciousness.
- State the important factors in the treatment of hypovolaemic shock.
- State the types of intravenous fluid suitable for treating shock:
  - colloids
  - crystalloids.
- Recognise the use of other drugs in the management of shock:
  - steroids
  - analgesics
  - antibacterials.

Shock is a group of symptoms resulting from a severe deterioration in the animal's clinical signs. It occurs when there is inadequate perfusion of all the body tissues with blood resulting in widespread cell damage.

Shock manifests as circulatory compromise (reduced capillary refill time, pallor of mucous membranes, tachycardia, weak/irregular pulses, cold extremities, decreased urine output as a result of decreased renal perfusion), and alteration in the level of consciousness.

There are different types of shock:

- **Hypovolaemic shock** – The loss of circulating blood volume causes a change in perfusion of the tissues. Hypovolaemic shock can be caused by blood loss or severe dehydration. After trauma extensive tissue damage and severe pain can further exacerbate the compromise to tissue perfusion.
- **Cardiogenic shock** – The failure of the heart to pump blood causes a decrease in tissue perfusion.
- **Anaphylactic shock** – This is the immediate response of the body to the entry of an antigen to which the animal is sensitised (allergic). Large amounts of antibodies are produced which have wide-ranging effects. Hypovolaemia is caused by loss plasma into the tissues from leaking blood vessels.
- **Endotoxic shock** – This is caused by an inflammatory response to severe infection. It is usually caused by bacteria.
- **Neurogenic shock** – This occurs when there is serious damage to the central nervous system, for example spinal or brain injury.

Treatment of shock involves using supportive therapy to improve the animal's circulation and the treatment of the underlying problem.

Fluid therapy is vital in restoring circulating blood volume, and improving tissue perfusion. If hypovolaemic shock is diagnosed then colloid fluid therapy can be used to increase the circulating blood volume and to improve the osmotic pressure of the blood.

If the haemorrhage has been severe and acute, whole blood can be used to replace plasma proteins, red blood cells, clotting factors and platelets.

When the circulating blood volume is greatly reduced the placement of an intravenous catheter is more difficult. It may be necessary to use a jugular catheter.

If shock is **endotoxic** or **anaphylactic** crystalloid fluid therapy should be used to correct electrolyte imbalances and correct any dehydration. Care should be taken with fluid therapy in animals with heart failure as there is a danger of increasing the blood pressure and further compromising cardiac output.

Treatment of the underlying condition may include appropriate antibacterial treatment (for example in endotoxic shock), analgesia, and medication with drugs which improve cardiac function such as ACE inhibitors and diuretics. Steroids are potent inhibitors of inflammatory mediators. They are useful in the treatment of anaphylactic, neurogenic and endotoxic shock where the widespread release of inflammatory mediators greatly worsens the animal's condition.

Oxygen therapy may be necessary and should be provided using a tent, mask, or nasal catheter.

Hypothermia is a risk, so shocked animals must be kept warm. Intravenous fluids should also be warmed if possible.

A quiet, comfortable environment aids recovery.

3.6.38   Urinary catheterisation

What you need to learn

* You need to be able to describe types of catheters commonly used in veterinary practice:
  * Tieman's
  * Foley bitch
  * Jackson's
  * dog.

🐾 Identify the reasons for catheterisation.
🐾 Describe the process of cleaning and sterilising catheters:
  🐾 means of cleaning
  🐾 sterilising gas
  🐾 autoclave
  🐾 liquid.
🐾 Describe safety checks on catheters before use.
🐾 Describe catheterisation:
  🐾 dogs male, female
  🐾 cats male, female.

See also Unit 2, 2.4.17

Types of catheters

Types of catheters are shown in the photos (Figures 6.11 and 6.12):
• Tieman's catheter
• Foley catheter
• Jackson's cat catheter
• Portex dog catheter (nylon disposable)
• Metal bitch catheter
• Dowse's catheter
• Conventional cat catheters.

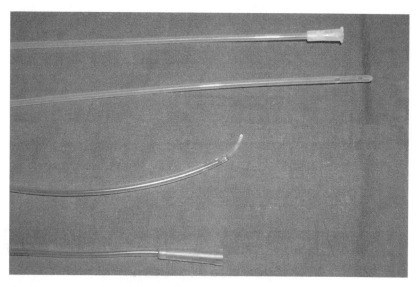

Figure 6.3   Dog catheter (top), Tieman's bitch catheter (bottom).

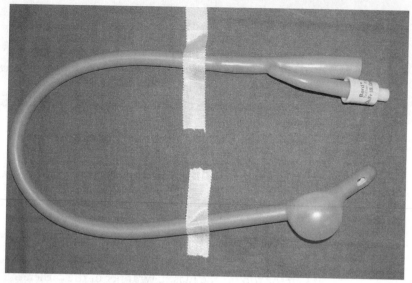

Figure 6.4 Foley catheter.

Indications for placing a urinary catheter

These include:

- urinary retention
- urinary incontinence
- diagnostic procedures, eg to introduce radiographic contrast media
- to monitor urine output
- before and during abdominal surgery – to prevent contamination of the surgical field
- following surgery – when the patient cannot move or it is inadvisable for the patient to move
- urinary calculi and obstruction
- to prevent urinary scalding
- to obtain a sterile urine sample.

Cleaning and sterilising urinary catheters

- Clean the catheter using an antiseptic solution, flush the inside using a syringe. The inside must always be flushed with water following flushing with antiseptic solution.
- The catheter can be chemically sterilised using ethylene oxide, the catheter must be fully dry (including the inside) for sterilising by this method.
- Catheters can be sterilised using moist heat (in an autoclave) although they may melt at high temperatures.
- Catheters can be cold-sterilised using cold sterilization fluid. This method is not as effective as the other two methods given above.

Safety checks

- Ensure sterility – if pre-packed you should check that they are sterile, that the packing has not been damaged or opened and that they are not past their use by date.
- Check the catheters for any damage and check that they are fully patent.
- Ensure the correct catheter type and size are chosen.

Principles of urinary catheterisation

Male dog

- General anaesthesia may be needed.
- Restrain the patient in lateral recumbency or in the standing position.
- Cut the top off the plastic wrapper of the catheter.
- Extrude the penis.
- Gently insert the catheter by feeding from the remaining plastic wrapper.
- Stop when urine is seen.

Female dog

Catheterisation can be done either in the standing position or in dorsal recumbency and requires two people. The technique that follows is used in dorsal recumbency using a Foley catheter.

- General anaesthesia is usually needed.
- Restrain the patient in dorsal recumbency.
- Draw the hind legs in a cranial direction.
- Lubricate the speculum and insert it into the vagina.
- Insert the catheter and on advancement of the catheter slowly release the hind legs caudally.
- Inflate the balloon – resistance will be felt if the catheter is not in the bladder.
- Remove the stylet and urine will be seen.

Male cat

- General anaesthesia is usually needed.
- Restrain the patient in lateral recumbency.
- Extrude the penis.
- Insert the catheter using slight rotation.
- Advance the catheter until urine is seen.
- Suture the catheter in place if it is being used as an indwelling catheter.

Female cat
- General anaesthesia is usually needed.
- Restrain the patient in lateral recumbency.
- Cut the top off the plastic wrapper.
- Insert and advance the catheter along the floor of the vagina. Stop when urine is seen.

Multiple choice questions

1. The causal agent of Infectious Canine hepatitis is:
   - ☐ A   a morbillivirus
   - ☐ B   a spirochaete bacteria
   - ☐ C   a rhabdovirus
   - ☐ D   Adenovirus 1

2. Leptospira icterohaemorrhagia is mainly spread by:
   - ☐ A   direct contact with infected urine
   - ☐ B   a tick bite
   - ☐ C   direct contact with fomites
   - ☐ D   inhalation

3. Which of the following feline diseases is the most likely to result in anaemia:
   - ☐ A   Feline Infectious Peritonitis
   - ☐ B   Chlamydiosis
   - ☐ C   Feline Calici Virus
   - ☐ D   Feline Immunodeficiency Virus

4. Which of the following is untrue:
   - ☐ A   viruses contain both RNA and DNA
   - ☐ B   toxoplasma gondii is a protozoa
   - ☐ C   bacteria do not have a nucleus
   - ☐ D   the minimum incubation period of canine distemper is 7 days

5. A mechanical host which transmits a disease but no life cycle development occurs during the transmission, is known as:
   - ☐ A   definitive
   - ☐ B   paratenic
   - ☐ C   intermediate
   - ☐ D   biological

6. A patient which has been exposed to an organism, has not shown symptoms but continues to shed the organism into the environment at times of stress is known as:
   - ☐ A a healthy open carrier
   - ☐ B a convalescent closed carrier
   - ☐ C a latent closed carrier
   - ☐ D an open symptomatic carrier

7. An excessive long term intake of vitamin A (retinol) in a cat may result in:
   - ☐ A central retinal degeneration
   - ☐ B dilated cardiomyopathy
   - ☐ C ankylosis of cervical vertebra
   - ☐ D nutritional secondary hyperparathyroidism

8. The BER of a 3 kg cat with severe burns would be:
   - ☐ A 160 kcals
   - ☐ B 180 kcals
   - ☐ C 360 kcals
   - ☐ D 720 kcals

9. Which of the following is untrue:
   - ☐ A extracellular fluid can be interstitial
   - ☐ B synovial fluid is transcellular
   - ☐ C a cation is a negatively charged ion
   - ☐ D 60% of body fluid is intracellular

10. Extracellular fluid contains the highest amount of which of the following:
    - ☐ A sodium
    - ☐ B potassium
    - ☐ C chloride
    - ☐ D magnesium

11. A 10% dehydrated dog would most likely exhibit which one of the following clinical parameters:
    - ☐ A a low PCV
    - ☐ B low plasma protein levels
    - ☐ C a urine output of 20 mls/kg
    - ☐ D a slow capillary refill time

12. A 10kg dog has been anorexic for 2 days following orthopaedic surgery which lasted for 2 hours. Its fluid requirement would be approximately:
    - ☐ A 500 ml
    - ☐ B 750 ml
    - ☐ C 1 litre
    - ☐ D 1.10 litres

13. An iosotonic crystalloid fluid with a high barcarbonate content would be:
    - ☐ A sodium chloride 0.9%
    - ☐ B Haemacell
    - ☐ C Ringers
    - ☐ D Hartmanns

14. A patient requires 2 litres of fluid to be administered over 12 hours. What would the drip rate be per minute if a standard giving set was used.
    - ☐ A 3 ml per minute
    - ☐ B 7 drops per minute
    - ☐ C 55 ml per minute
    - ☐ D 166.66 drops per minute

15. In a feline patient parenteral nutrition should be administered:
    - ☐ A via a jugular vein
    - ☐ B subcutaneously
    - ☐ C via a naso gastric feeding tube
    - ☐ D via a PEG tube

16. A canine blood transfusion collected into a collection bag containing acid citrate dextrose should be used within:
    - ☐ A 48 hours
    - ☐ B 3 weeks
    - ☐ C 28 days
    - ☐ D 3 months

17. Two days following a blood transfusion a patient has a reaction due to an immune response to the donor's red cells. Clinical signs may consist of:
    - ☐ A hypertension and oedema of soft tissues
    - ☐ B pulmonary oedema and coughing
    - ☐ C muscular tremors and bradycardia
    - ☐ D pyrexia and tachycardia

18. During the monitoring of a fluid infusion, which of the following should have the highest priority:
    - ☐ A measurement of CVP
    - ☐ B change giving set daily
    - ☐ C flush catheter twice daily with heparin
    - ☐ D monitor temperature, pulse, respiration

19. The general term for a micro organism which has the ability to cause disease is known as a:
    - ☐ A   prion
    - ☐ B   phagocyte
    - ☐ C   pathogen
    - ☐ D   antibody

20. Immunity provided by a vaccine is known as:
    - ☐ A   passive immunity
    - ☐ B   cell mediated immunity
    - ☐ C   active immunity
    - ☐ D   innate immunity

21. Humoral immunity is dependent on the body's production of:
    - ☐ A   T Lymphocytes
    - ☐ B   Immunoglobulins
    - ☐ C   Colostrum
    - ☐ D   Antigens

22. Inactivated vaccines:
    - ☐ A   contain an adjuvant
    - ☐ B   provide a long lasting immune response
    - ☐ C   can be safely stored in a freezer
    - ☐ D   are the freeze dried powder component of a vaccine

23. Paraquat poisoning may be caused if a puppy ate or drank:
    - ☐ A   an insecticide
    - ☐ B   a wood treatment
    - ☐ C   antifreeze
    - ☐ D   a weed killer

24. Acrolein poisoning results because the poison was:
    - ☐ A   ingested
    - ☐ B   inhaled
    - ☐ C   absorbed through the skin
    - ☐ D   absorbed via the mucous membranes

25. Atopy is a/an:
    - ☐ A   nutritional disease
    - ☐ B   anaphylactic shock response
    - ☐ C   allergic disease
    - ☐ D   congenital disease

26. Rupture of the thoracic duct would result in:
    - ☐ A   exudate in the pleural space
    - ☐ B   a haemothorax
    - ☐ C   transudate in the pleural space
    - ☐ D   pulmonary oedema

27. As a result of dental disease a rabbit would be most likely to develop:
   - ☐ A epistaxis
   - ☐ B pharyngitis
   - ☐ C dacryocystitis
   - ☐ D tracheitis

28. Degeneration of the mitral valve in a canine patient would result in:
   - ☐ A chronic endocarditis
   - ☐ B right sided dilated cardiomyopathy
   - ☐ C acquired endocardiosis
   - ☐ D low systolic blood pressure

29. A congenital heart defect which allows blood to be shunted directly from the pulmonary artery to the aorta in the foetus is known as:
   - ☐ A Tetralogy of Fallot
   - ☐ B Patent ductus arteriosus
   - ☐ C Pulmonic stenosis
   - ☐ D Persistent right aortic arch

30. In a cat, regenerative anaemia may develop as a direct result of:
   - ☐ A FIA
   - ☐ B FeLV
   - ☐ C Chronic renal failure
   - ☐ D Carcinogenic drug therapy

31. The presence of fresh blood in the faeces is known as:
   - ☐ A haematemesis
   - ☐ B melaena
   - ☐ C dyschezia
   - ☐ D haematochezia

32. A dog has chronic liver disease, resulting in bile stasis. Which of the following clinical signs would probably NOT be observed?
   - ☐ A icterus
   - ☐ B pale faeces
   - ☐ C anorexia
   - ☐ D pale urine

33. Symptoms of FLUTD in a male cat would most likely NOT include:
   - ☐ A oliguria
   - ☐ B pollakuria
   - ☐ C polyuria
   - ☐ D haematuria

34. Long term treatment of a cat with chronic renal failure should include:
    - ☐ A   diuretics and a reduction of water intake
    - ☐ B   a high protein diet
    - ☐ C   reduced phosphorus in the diet
    - ☐ D   increased taurine

35. A dog suffering from idiopathic epilepsy has status epilepticus whilst in your care. Your highest priory should be to:
    - ☐ A   darken the room/ kennel but observe the dog
    - ☐ B   intubate the patient
    - ☐ C   attempt to rehydrate by offering water by mouth
    - ☐ D   administer I.V. diazepam

36. Diabetes insipidus is:
    - ☐ A   hyperglycaemia
    - ☐ B   deficiency of antidiuretic hormone
    - ☐ C   hypocalcaemia
    - ☐ D   excessive secretion of cortisol

37. Symptoms of chronic hypothyroidism in a dog would include:
    - ☐ A   weight loss
    - ☐ B   muscle paresis
    - ☐ C   calcinosis cutis
    - ☐ D   polyphagia

38. Name the idiopathic bone disease which occurs in adolescent growing breeds where there is lameness, abnormal development of the metaphyses and pyrexia:
    - ☐ A   osteomyelitis
    - ☐ B   pulmonary osteopathy
    - ☐ C   secondary nutritional hyperparathyroidism
    - ☐ D   hypertrophic osteodystrophy

39. Inflammation of the iris, ciliary body and choroid collectively is known as:
    - ☐ A   uveitis
    - ☐ B   keratitis
    - ☐ C   chemosis
    - ☐ D   'cherry eye'

40. Which of the following would NOT result in otitis externa in a cat?
    - ☐ A   Secondary infection with staphylococcus
    - ☐ B   Malassezia pachydermatis
    - ☐ C   Otodectes cyanotis
    - ☐ D   Psoroptes cuniculi

Level 3: Unit 7

Diagnostic imaging

3.7.01   Health and safety

What you need to learn

🐾 You need to be able to describe the important points of legislative Acts and Regulations which apply to radiographic work:
  - 🐾 Ionising Radiation Regulations (1999)
  - 🐾 Code of Practice (1985)
  - 🐾 Guidance notes for the protection of persons against ionising radiations arising from veterinary use ISBN 085951 300 9 HMSO (July 1988)
  - 🐾 Local Radiation Rules and Regulations
  - 🐾 Health & Safety at Work Act (1974)
  - 🐾 Collection and Disposal of Waste Regulations (1988)
  - 🐾 Control of Substances Hazardous to Health (COSHH) Regulations (1999).

There are some important acts and regulations concerned with imaging and health and safety:

- Ionising Radiation Regulations (1999)
- Code of Practice (1985)
- Guidance notes for the protection of persons against ionising radiations arising from veterinary use ISBN 085951 300 9 HMSO (July 1988)
- Local radiation rules and regulations
- Health and Safety at Work Act (1974)
- Collection and Disposal of Waste Regulations (1988)
- Control of Substances Hazardous to Health Regulations (COSHH) (1999)

3.07.02   Dangers of radiation

What you need to learn

🐾 You need to be able to identify the properties of X-rays in respect of health and safety and their dangers:
  - 🐾 burns

- ❧ cataracts
- ❧ teratogenicity
- ❧ induction of leukaemias.
- ❧ Outline the biological effects of radiation:
  - ❧ genetic factors
  - ❧ DNA
  - ❧ carcinogenic
  - ❧ fertility.
- ❧ Identify measures which can be taken to reduce and collimate the primary beam:
  - ❧ cones
  - ❧ light beam diaphragm.
- ❧ Outline ways of controlling the production and effect of scatter:
  - ❧ correct exposure
  - ❧ compression
  - ❧ grids.
- ❧ Recognise and implement safety measures to protect all personnel in accordance with the Code of Practice and Local Rules (See Health and Safety – Introduction to this Unit):
  - ❧ use of radiation monitoring devices
  - ❧ controlled area
  - ❧ designated area
  - ❧ designated persons.
- ❧ Outline the roles of the Radiation Protection Advisor (RPA) and the Radiation Protection Supervisor (RPS).
- ❧ Describe the requirements for equipment maintenance with reference to radiography safety:
  - ❧ X-ray machine
  - ❧ tube head.
- ❧ Outline personnel safety procedures:
  - ❧ staff rotation
  - ❧ monitoring
  - ❧ designated persons.
- ❧ Describe the types and maintenance of protective clothing and their advantages and disadvantages:
  - ❧ gloves
  - ❧ aprons
  - ❧ sleeves
  - ❧ barriers
  - ❧ gonad and thyroid protection.
- ❧ Describe ways of warning personnel and public during exposure:
  - ❧ warning light systems
  - ❧ display radiation symbols
  - ❧ warning notices.
- ❧ Describe ways of restraining or sedating a patient before a radiographic examination

❀ chemical
❀ manual.

In respect of health and safety, X-rays have four properties that increase their danger.

- They are invisible.
- They cannot be felt.
- Their effects are latent – effects will be come evident later rather than immediately.
- Their effects are cumulative.
  There are three types of effects caused by X-rays.
- **Somatic effects** are direct changes and occur soon after exposure, eg burns, cataracts, hair loss, reddening of skin and digestive upsets.
- **Carcinogenic effects** (teratogenicity) occur where damage is caused to tissues through which the X-rays pass. Rapidly dividing cells are most susceptible, eg gastrointestinal tract, skin and haematopoeitic tissue. These changes can be malignant and may develop into such diseases as leukaemia. These effects may not be seen for a long time, eg 20 years after exposure.
- **Genetic effects** occur when the gonads have been exposed to X-rays, causing mutation in the chromosomes of germ cells. This may lead to inherited abnormalities in children, although this has not yet been proven.

Measures to reduce and collimate the primary beam

There are various measures available to reduce and collimate the beam.

- use cones
- use a light beam diaphragm
- keep collimation as tight as possible
- never have any part of the body within the primary beam
- use a vertical beam (horizontal beams should be avoided)
- an aluminium filter should be fitted between the X-ray tube and the collimator
- use lead-lined cassettes and table tops.

Controlling the production and effects of scatter

To control the production of scatter and its effects:

- Use the correct factors. This reduces repeat radiographs and unnecessary exposure. Keep the kilovoltage as low as feasible.
- Use compression. A radiolucent band can be fitted around a large abdomen to reduce the thickness of the tissue; it should be used with caution in patients with abdominal injury or disease.

• Use a grid.

Safety measures to protect personnel

The following provide guidelines for using ionising radiation:

• the Ionising Radiation Regulations 1999
• code of practice for the protection of persons against ionising radiation arising from any work activity (a booklet that explains the regulations with specific references to veterinary radiography)
• guidance notes for the protection of persons against ionising radiations arising from veterinary use 1988 (easy to read guidance notes on veterinary radiography)
• local rules provided by the practice's radiation protection adviser (RPA).

Radiation monitoring devices

• The device should be worn by the person whose name appears on the device.
• The device should be worn on the trunk under protective clothing.
• The device should not be left in the radiography room while not being worn.
• The device should not be exposed to heat or sunlight.

Thermoluminescent dosemeters (TLD) are usually yellow or orange and contain fine crystals sensitive to radiation. The crystals are heated and emit light proportional to the amount of radiation absorbed. They are sent off for readings every 1–3 months, depending on case load.

Film badges are usually blue. They are pieces of radiographic film worn by personnel that are then developed and measured by the degree of blackening.

For equine radiography special **finger badges** can be used that are placed inside the lead gloves. These can also be used in the unlikely event of a patient having to be held.

Controlled area

The controlled area is defined as the area around the primary beam where radiation levels are in excess of the safe level, usually a 2 m radius from the primary beam. The area becomes a controlled area once the X-ray machine is turned on and appropriate warning devices are activated. No-one should have access to the controlled area during exposure.

Designated area

A designated room specially designed for radiography should be accommodated within the practice or hospital.

Designated people

Only designated people are allowed to be involved in radiography. These should be stated on the local rules and each person should have a monitoring device.

- **Radiation protection adviser** (RPA) – These are usually external experts in radiography and are either a veterinary surgeon who hold the veterinary radiography diploma with knowledge on radiation physics or a medical physicist. They advise on protection, the controlled area and draw up the local rules.
- **Radiation protection supervisor** (RPS) – A person appointed within the practice, eg a senior partner. They ensure safety and that the local rules are adhered to.

The X-ray machine and tube head must be serviced annually by professional radiography engineers. If there is a fault this should be reported to the RPS who should then seek advice from the radiography engineers or the RPA.

Personal safety

To ensure personal safety the following guidelines should be followed:

- Rotate staff on a regular basis to ensure the same nurse is not involved with all the radiography.
- Monitoring devices must be worn.
- Only designated people stated by the local rules should be involved with radiography.
- Stand at least 2 m from the primary beam; ideally stand behind a protective screen.
- Wear protective clothing.

Protective clothing

Types of protective clothing available include:

- gloves – should be at least 0.35 mm lead equivalent (LE)
- aprons – should be at least 0.25 mm LE
- sleeves – should be at least 0.35 mm LE
- barriers
- gonad protectors
- thyroid protectors.

Protective clothing should be maintained in good condition by following these rules.

- Always hang aprons up.
- Place gloves, sleeves, gonad and thyroid protectors in their correct storage place after use.
- Do not drop, bend, or roll protective clothing as this can lead to cracking of the material which will then let X-rays through.
- If in doubt, radiograph the piece of clothing; any cracks will be visible on a radiograph.

The **advantage** of protective clothing is that is protects personnel from scatter radiation and its effects.

However, **disadvantages** are:

- It does not protect against the primary beam.
- Clothing is heavy and can be uncomfortable to wear.
- It requires storage space.

Warning personnel and the public

The following warning systems should be set in place:

- **Warning light systems** – red lights or an illuminated sign at any entrance point into the room. These should automatically come on when the X-ray machine is turned on.
- **Radiation symbols and warning notices** – these should be placed at all entrances into the room, see Figure 7.1.

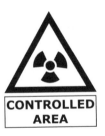

Figure 7.1 Warning notice.

Restraining patients for radiography

Patients can be restrained for radiography in two ways.

- **chemically** – using sedation or general anaesthesia
- **manually** – using sandbags, rope ties, foam wedges and cradles/troughs.

Only in exceptional circumstances should a patient be held for radiography, eg when either of the methods described would be contraindicated or would worsen any existing disease or injury. In this case the veterinary surgeon in charge of the case should hold the patient.

3.7.03   Elementary principles of radiography

What you need to learn

❧ You need to be able to identify terms related to the physics of radiography:
   ❧ electromagnetic radiation
   ❧ primary beam and scattered radiation or atoms etc.
❧ Describe how X-rays are produced.
❧ Identify the main parts of an X-ray machine, describe the structure of an X-ray tube and its housing.
❧ Identify the difference between stationary and rotating anodes and the reasons for their use.
❧ Describe the relative absorption of X-rays by substances of varying density and atomic number.
❧ Describe the effect of applying varying kilovoltages (kV) to the X-ray tube and the influencing factors:
   ❧ species
   ❧ weight of patient
   ❧ density of area to be radiographed.
❧ Describe the effects of varying the milliamperes (mA) to the X-ray tube and the influencing factors and relate to inverse square law:
   ❧ mA
   ❧ time
   ❧ kV
   ❧ film speed
   ❧ Film Focal Distance (FFD).

• **Electromagnetic radiation** – a method of transporting energy, identified by energy, wavelength and frequency
• **Primary beam** – straight lines of X-rays focused into a beam
• **Scatter radiation** (secondary radiation) – produced when the primary beam interacts with tissues or other objects such as the tabletop
• **Atom** – a basic form of matter; a nucleus is present surrounded by electrons
• **Proton** – a positively charged particle found in the nucleus of the atom
• **Neutron** – a particle carrying no charge found in the nucleus of the atom

- **Electron** – a negatively charged particle that surrounds the atom in shells
- **Atomic number** – the number of protons in an atom's nucleus
- **Photon (quanta)** – bundles of energy which make up the primary beam

How X-rays are produced

The production of X-rays needs to take place in a vacuum, therefore avoiding ionisation of air molecules. At either side of the tube head there is an electrode. They are known as the **cathode** (negatively charged) and the **anode** (positively charged).

- Generation of an X-ray beam begins at the cathode. The cathode itself is a coil of wire (referred to as the filament), much like that found in a light bulb. It is usually made of metal called tungsten.
- By heating the filament via the milliamperage (measured in milliamps, mA), a cloud of electrons is produced. This cloud of electrons is then released, by a process known as thermionic emission (boiling off of electrons).
- By altering the milliamperage the amount or quantity of electrons produced at the cathode can be controlled.
- A lot of heat is generated at the filament, which is why the metal tungsten is ideal (it has a high melting point, ~3370°C).
- The filament is heated by the milliamperage via a step-down transformer; this enables the amperage from the mains to be converted into millamperage so that the filament can cope.
- The filament is placed in a focusing cup made of a metal called molybdenum; this also has a high melting point and is a poor conductor of heat. Electrons will repel each other (as they are of all the same charge); the purpose of the cup is to shape the beam and to direct the electrons in one direction only, towards the anode.
- The electrons are negatively charged, therefore they are attracted to the positively charged anode.
- A high electrical potential difference is needed between the filament and anode, so the beam of electrons can be accelerated across to the anode.
- The kilovoltage (measured in kilovolts, kV) supplies this potential difference. The kilovoltage needs to be much higher than the mains, so a step-up transformer is used. This increases the kilovoltage from the mains at 240 volts up to 40,000–100,000 volts (ie 40–100 Kv). The rate at which these electrons travel across to the anode (controlled by the kilovoltage) is the penetrating power of the beam.
- The anode or target is the area at the opposite side of the tube head that the beam of electrons will hit.

- Heat dissipation is very important here as temperatures of 1000°C or more are created. Only 1% of the energy produced by the electrons is X-rays. The other 99% is heat.
- After the beam of electrons has been accelerated across from the cathode to the anode/target, the electrons collide on a specific place on the target known as the focal spot.
- The focal spots range in size between 0.3 mm and 2.5 mm, the smaller sizes producing the sharper image. Some of the larger more modern X-ray machines have two different size focal spots.
- The beam created then leaves the focal spot and travels out of the tube head towards the patient and cassette on the table.
- The time it takes for the beam to reach the patient from the tube head is controlled by a timing device. This is essential so that the duration of X-ray production can be controlled. The device may be clockwork or electronic.

Parts of an X-ray machine

- **Control panel:**
  - on/off switch
  - line voltage compensator
  - kilovoltage control
  - milliamperage control
  - timer
  - exposure button.
- **Tube head:** containing the anode (stationary or rotating)
- **Timer** (measured in seconds, either electronic or mechanical).

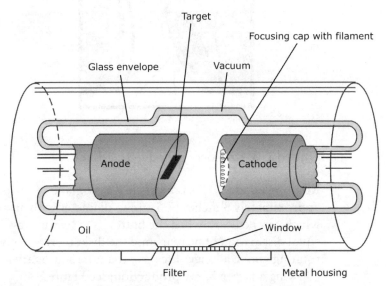

Figure 7.2 Tube head.

Stationary and rotating anodes

A method of removing heat from the target is essential. This is done by means of an anode. The anode can be of two forms:

• **Stationary anode** – The tungsten target is set in a block of copper. Copper is used as it is a good conductor of heat and removes heat to the surrounding oil where it is absorbed. Wider focal spots are also needed to disperse the heat as much as possible. Low X-ray production is the disadvantage with these types of anodes and they are mainly found in portable machines and dental radiography machines; see Figure 7.3.

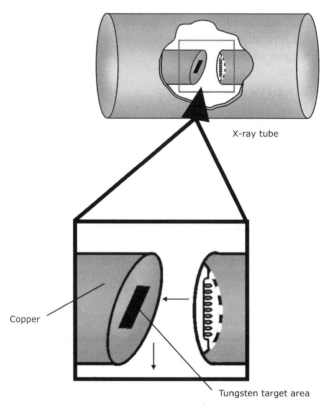

X-ray tube

Copper

Tungsten target area

Figure 7.3 Stationary anode.

Rotating anode – This is a bevelled disk made of tungsten approximately 3 inches (7.5 cm) in diameter with an audible spin, which can be heard when the button is in 'warm stage'. This allows equal dissipation of heat around the disk, therefore giving the rotating anode a longer life span than the stationary anode and allowing a larger X-ray production; see Figure 7.4.

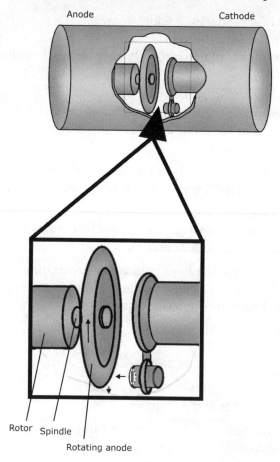

Anode

Cathode

Rotor Spindle

Rotating anode

Figure 7.4 Rotating anode.

Both anode types are made of tungsten because of its high melting point and its high atomic number.

Absorption of X-rays

It is the degree of absorption of X-rays that produces the varying shades from white to black on a developed film. Degree of absorption depends on:

- **The atomic number of the tissue**
  - The higher the atomic number of the tissue the more X-rays are absorbed, producing a white image, eg bone.
  - The lower the atomic number of the tissue the fewer X-rays are absorbed, producing a black image, eg air.
- **The specific gravity of the tissue**
  - The higher the specific gravity the more X-rays are absorbed, air has a low specific gravity so fewer X-rays are absorbed, producing a black image. Bone has a high specific gravity so more X-rays are

absorbed, producing a white image.
- **The thickness of the tissue**
  - Thicker areas of tissue absorb more X-rays than thinner areas.

Kilovoltage

The kilovoltage refers to how fast the electrons are accelerated from the cathode to the anode and therefore it determines the penetrating power of the beam.

The kV affects the number of shades (black/grey/white) on the film (contrast) and the degree of blackening (density).

Increasing the kilovoltage increases the penetrating power of the beam, thereby increasing the degree of blackening (density) with very little contrast (too low contrast).

Decreasing the kilovoltage reduces the penetrating power of the beam, thereby producing black and white images as opposed to varying shades (too high contrast).

Factors affecting the kV include:

- species
- weight
- density (specific gravity) of the tissue
- atomic number of the tissue.

Generally, the higher the density and atomic number of the tissue the more kilovoltage is required.

Milliamperage

The milliamperage refers to the number of electrons produced at the cathode, which determines the number of X-rays in the beam (ie the intensity of the beam).

Altering the milliamperage will either decrease or increase the intensity of the beam so the degree of blackening overall is decreased or increased but contrast between tissues remains the same.

Factors affecting the milliamperage are:

- thickness of the tissue
- density (specific gravity) of the tissue
- atomic number of the tissue

Time

Time refers to the length of exposure and is measured in seconds. The number of electrons and the length of time they will be exposed work in conjunction with one another and are expressed in milliamp seconds (mAs).

• milliamperage (mA) × time (s) = mAs

Film speed

See 3.7.05.

Film focal distance (FFD)

This refers to the distance between the focal spot and the radiographic film. As the FFD is increased the intensity of the beam reduces.

• If a long FFD is used the mAs will need to be increased.
• If a short FFD is used the mAs can be deceased.

new mAs = old mAs × [(new distance)^2 / (old distance)^2]

This is known as the **inverse square law** – the intensity of the beam varies inversely as the square of the distance from the source.

3.7.04   Exposures

What you need to learn

🐾 You need to be able to describe the procedure for setting up an X-ray machine for use with consideration to exposure factors:
  🐾 Types of X-ray machines – portable, mobile and static
  🐾 Line voltage – mA/kV/time
  🐾 Species – thickness, density, screen, film
  🐾 Details – species, date, part X-rayed, result
  🐾 Exposure factors – mA, kV, FFD.
🐾 Describe how to make a suitable exposure chart for an X-ray machine for the following species:
  🐾 dogs/puppies
  🐾 cats/kittens
  🐾 other small species.

There are three types of X-ray machines:

• **Portable** – These are very common. They have low output (usually an output of 10–30 mA, 40–70 kV) and need longer exposure times but they can be used for field radiography.
• **Mobile** – These are more powerful than portable machines and can have a range up 60–120 mA and 40–120 kV. They can be moved between rooms.
• **Fixed (static)** – These are the most powerful, up to 500 mA (300 mA–1250 mA) and 200 kV, but are very expensive to

purchase. They are fixed to the floors and mounted on rails on the walls or ceilings.

Procedure for setting up the X-ray machine

- Turn the power on.
- Check the line voltage and adjust if necessary. Bigger machines will have an autotransformer which will do this for you.
- Select the correct mA, s and kV – this can be done by looking at previous recordings for the same procedure or by judging the thickness and density of the tissue (use callipers to measure the tissue).
- Select the correct screen and film type.
- Label the cassette or radiograph – see 3.7.05.
- Use a grid if required.
- Record the following details in a day book (the day book should contain all details of any radiographic procedure):
  - species
  - date
  - area/part radiographed
  - result/comments
  - mA
  - s
  - kV
  - FFD
  - weight
  - owner's surname
  - patient's name.

Exposure charts

A separate exposure chart should be produced for dogs, cats, puppies, kittens and other small species. The chart can be complied as follows:

- Carry out a series of test exposures on a single patient (freshly dead animals can be used).
- Note the best exposures for various parts as they are encountered.
- Apart from the kV, s and mA keep all other parameters the same, eg FFD, screen/film combination.
- Measure the thickness of the tissue using callipers.
- Record findings, the exposure chart can then be built up over a period of time.
  Exposure charts are machine-specific; if there is more than one X-ray machine a separate exposure chart will need to be compiled

3.7.05 Recording apparatus

What you need to learn

* You need to be able to describe the structure of X-ray film, and film type differences to include reasons for film type selection:
  * patient
  * area to be X-rayed
  * exposure factors
  * screen and non-screen types of film
  * varying speeds of film.
* Describe the structure of varying speeds of screen film and adjust exposure factors accordingly.
* Describe the effects of varying factors on photographic emulsions, before, during and after developing:
  * temperature
  * light
  * pressure
  * humidity
  * chemicals
  * radiation.
* Describe the correct methods of safe storage and care of X-ray film.
* Describe the structure of X-ray cassettes and intensifying screens and their care.
* Describe the structure of varying speeds of intensifying screens, including fluorescent colour, and understand suitable speed selection. Structure types:
  * rare earth
  * calcium tungstate.
* Describe the structure of different grid types and outline their difference. Stationary types:
  * parallel
  * focused
  * pseudo-focused
  * crossed.
* Grid types: moveable and stationary.
* Describe grid factor and grid ratio and calculate exposure changes.
* Describe labelling methods for X-ray films and outline their advantage/disadvantages:
  * lead markers
  * lead impregnated tape
  * light markers
  * post exposure labelling.
* Identify the labelling requirements of the British Veterinary Association (BVA)/Kennel Club (KC) Hip Dysplasia Scheme.

Structure of radiographic film

The structure of radiographic film is shown in Figure 7.5.

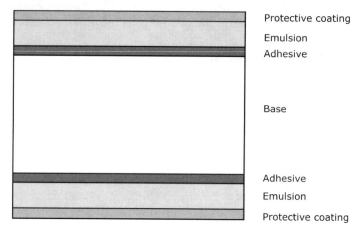

Protective coating
Emulsion
Adhesive

Base

Adhesive
Emulsion
Protective coating

Figure 7.5 Structure of double-sided radiographic film.

Types of radiographic film

- **Screen film** is the most commonly used. It is used with cassettes with screens, details are less than on non-screen film but exposure factors can be reduced.
- **Non-screen film** is used when finer detail is needed, eg intraoral work. Higher exposure factors are needed.
- **Orthochromatic film** has dye added to the emulsion to include green and yellow parts of the visible spectrum. It is used with green-emitting, rare-earth-intensifying screens.
- **Monochromatic film** is sensitive to blue light and is used with calcium tungstate screens.
- **Single-sided emulsion film** is used in cassettes with single screens. It was originally used for mammography but can be used if highly detailed images are required.

Film speeds

- **Fast (ultra speed) film** requires low exposure factors because of the large silver halide crystals but detail is compromised. It is susceptible to scatter radiation but is useful with low output machines.
- **Medium (standard) film** is the most commonly used. It requires higher exposure factors than fast film but gives better detail.
- **Slow (fine detail) film** produces good detail but requires up to twice the exposure of standard film because of the smaller silver halide crystals.

Fault on radiographic film

- Black crescent marks from fingernails
- Lighting effect from static electricity, eg pulling the film out of the box too quickly
- White marks – dirt, hair and dust on the screens. These marks will be on the same area consistently (can also be spilt contrast medium)
- Black marks – splash marks from spilt developer
- Blurred areas – loss of film/screen contact.

Methods of storage and care of the radiographic film

Radiographic film should be stored in the original packaging, in a light-proof container inside a light-proof hopper.

It should be stored away from:

- the X-ray area
- processing chemicals and water
- high temperatures and humidity; if necessary it should be refrigerated.

All radiographic film must be stored vertical and handled with care (usually by one corner) to avoid scratches, finger-nail marks and bending. It must be used before the expiry date.

Radiographic cassettes

Care of cassettes

- Cassettes should be cleaned with disinfectant after each use – special vigilance should be applied if contrast agents have been used because these will appear on future films if they are not cleaned off correctly.
- Check the hinges are working correctly and that the locks click in to place when re-loading.
- Check for any damage.
- It is good practice to keep the cassette loaded with film.

Intensifying screens

Care of intensifying screens

As a rule, screens should be cleaned every six weeks or more often if required.

- Open the cassette (having removed the film in the darkroom previously).
- Lint-free swabs should be used with the cleaner recommended by the manufacturer.

- Start in the centre and work outwards removing any hair, dust, or marks.
- Stubborn dirt or hairs can be blown out using air.
- Leave to dry for at least 10 minutes.
- Check for any damage or loss of contact.
- Re-load with film.

Types of intensifying screens

Intensifying screens are of two types: **calcium tungstate screens** are blue-emitting while the **rare-earth screens** are green-emitting, eg gadolinium oxysulphide and lanthanum oxysulphide.

The phosphors used in rare-earth screens are much more efficient at converting light to X-rays than the originally used phosphor calcium tungstate.

Speed of intensifying screens

- **Fast (high speed) screens** require low exposures because of the large phosphor crystals emitting more light, however detail is compromised.
- **Medium (regular speed) screens** are the most commonly used because they provide a good compromise, requiring fairly low exposures but giving better detail than fast screens.
- **Slow (ultra detail) screens** require high exposures because of the small phosphor crystals emitting less light, however they give greatly increased detail.

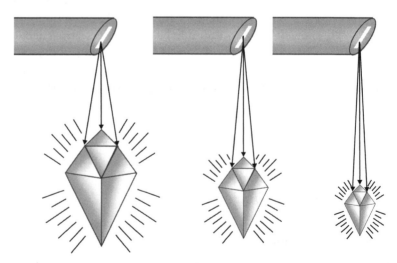

Figure 7.6 The amount of light emitted by crystals.

Grids

Types of grid

Grids are either stationary or moving

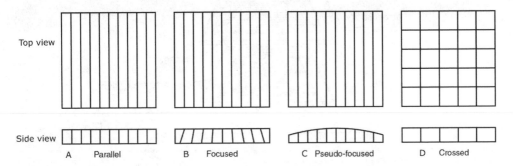

Top view

Side view

A   Parallel   B   Focused   C   Pseudo-focused   D   Crossed

Figure 7.7   Stationary grids.

Stationary grids can be:

- parallel (lead strips are parallel)
- focused (lead strips are angled towards the centre)
- pseudo-focused (lead strips are vertical but become shorter towards the edge)
- crossed (two grids either parallel or focused superimposed on one another).

Moving grids use a Potter-Bucky diaphragm which creates an electronic connection between the moving grid and the X-ray machine. They eliminate the parallel lines that are visible on the radiograph when stationary grids are used; see Figure 7.8.

Calculating exposure factors

- **Grid factor** is the amount by which the exposure needs to be increased (to compensate for loss of the primary beam).

The mAs needs to multiplied by the grid factor which is usually between 2 and 3.

- **Grid ratio** is the ratio of the height of the lead strips to the distance of the radiolucent interspace. The larger the ratios the more efficient it is at absorbing scatter.
- **Lines per cm** denotes the number of lines per cm the grid possess. The greater the number of lines, the fewer the grid lines that appear on the radiograph.

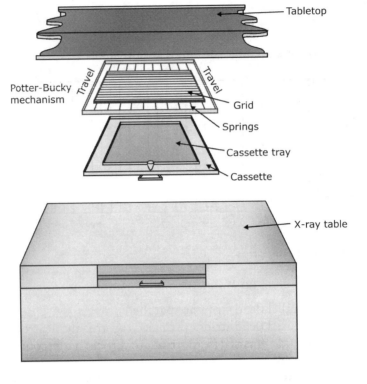

Figure 7.8 Potter-Bucky Grid radiography.

Labelling X-rays

The following identification should appear on each radiograph:

- patient's name including surname
- date
- left/right marker
- time if performing contrast studies.

Methods of applying identification

Identification labelling can use the following techniques:

- Lead letters and numbers can be placed on before exposure. This is a simple method but needs a holder to prevent movement of the characters.
- Lead-impregnated tape (X-rite® tape) can be placed on before exposure. It is easy to use but may become 'unstuck' from the cassette.
- Light marker can be placed on after exposure. The imprint must be on the correct corner of the radiograph.

• The radiograph can be written on with a pencil or other pointed device after development. This is not ideal but can be used if identification was forgotten earlier.

Labelling requirements of the hip dysplasia scheme

The following must be identified on the radiograph before processing for X-rays taken for the British Veterinary Association/Kennel Club Hip Dysplasia Scheme:

• The kennel club registration number or appropriate form of identification if not registered with the kennel club
• Date
• Left/right marker.

The radiographs will be returned if this information is not visible.

3.7.06 Darkroom

What you need to learn

❧ You need to be able to describe the principles of basic darkroom design and identify common faults.
❧ Outline darkroom protocol to include equipment handling and storage:
   ❧ film hangers (channel/suspension)
   ❧ processing chemicals
   ❧ film
   ❧ cassettes.
❧ Describe suitable conditions for the storage and handling of films and cassettes:
   ❧ film – hanger channel and suspension
❧ Describe the use of safelights, different coloured filters and light traps.

Darkroom design

The following are characteristics required of a darkroom.

• It must be lightproof.
• There should be a water supply, drainage and an electricity supply.
• It should be of a reasonable size.
• Ventilation should be provided.
• The decor of the room should be white or cream.
• There should be a wet area and a dry area.
• There must be a safelight.

Common faults in darkroom design include:

- leakage of light
- chemical spills or splashes
- incorrect colour of safe light or wattage of bulb
- incorrect decor of the darkroom
- wet areas left from radiographs drying (when using wet development)
- working area too small.

Darkroom protocol

Film hangers can be channel or clip (suspension) type.

- Ensure the hangers are kept clean and dry.
- Check for damage daily.
- Store vertically.
- Store dry hangers in the dry area of the darkroom.

Processing chemicals should be handled as follows:

- Store in the labelled containers supplied by the manufacturer.
- Store in the wet area of the darkroom.
- Wear gloves when using the chemicals.
- Avoid accidental mixing of developer and fixer when refilling tanks
- Avoid splashes and spills onto work areas, or onto exposed and unexposed film; wipe any spills up immediately.
- Check tank levels daily and re-fill as required.
- Check the temperature of developer daily if using wet development.
- Check waste chemicals daily and empty into correct waste containers as required.

Film should be cared for as follows:

- Store in a light-proof container in the dry area of the darkroom.
- Store vertically in the dry area of the darkroom.
- Store away from chemicals and heat.
- Handle by one corner only with minimal pressure, avoid using finger nails.
- Check when re-loading cassettes that only one film has been removed from the packaging.

Cassettes should be cared for as follows:

- Store vertically.
- Store in the dry area of the darkroom.
- Ensure they are clean and dry.
- Remove the film by handling only one corner, it may help to gently shake the cassette.
- Close the cassette if not re-loaded immediately.

- Re-load the cassettes with film each time they are used, handle using one corner only with little or no pressure.
- Lay the film in the cassette ensuring it is correctly positioned.
- Check the locking clips are working and that there is no damage.

The darkroom should be kept clean tidy and organised; it is helpful to have a waste paper bin, tissue paper (for wiping spills and splashes) and a timer (if using wet development).

When using the film hangers the following procedure should be used:

- Channel hangers
  - Handle one corner of the film only.
  - Slide the film down the sides of the hanger.
  - Ensure the film is inserted correctly.
  - The area of the film inside the channels will not develop.
  - After washing the film remove it from the hanger and clip onto the drying line in the wet area of the darkroom.
  - Wash and dry the hanger.
- Clip (suspension) hangers
  - Handle one corner of the film only.
  - Turn the hanger and film upside down and clip the bottom of the film.
  - Turn the hanger and film the correct way and clip the top of the film.
  - After washing the film, the hanger with the film still attached can be hung up to dry in the wet area of the darkroom.
  - Wash and dry the hanger after use.

Safe lights can be indirect or direct. The light bulb should be no more than 15 watts.

The correct colour filter needs to correspond with the colour of the film being used, ie a brown filter for blue-sensitive film, a dark red filter for green-sensitive film (this colour may also be used for blue-sensitive film). The wrong colour filter will result in film fog.

The safe light needs to positioned at least 4 feet (1.2 m) away from the working area to avoid film fog.

3.7.07   Processing

What you need to learn

- You need to be able to describe ways of heating chemical solutions for processing in practice:
  - water baths
  - thermostatic heaters.

☙ Describe the structure and working of an automatic processor.
☙ Describe how to make up developer and fixing solutions for automatic processors:
  ☙ developer
  ☙ fixer
  ☙ replenishers
  ☙ hardeners – dilutions
  ☙ acid stop baths.
☙ Describe correct measures for disposal of processing chemicals, taking into account COSHH Regulations.
☙ Identify the chemical constituents of processing solutions, their functions, and reasons why they become exhausted:
  ☙ manual and automatic developing solutions.
☙ Describe the processing of a radiograph.
☙ Describe the chemical reactions of developer on photographic emulsion at a given temperature.
☙ Describe the preparation of developer before processing to include correct times and temperatures.
☙ Describe correct storage for chemicals.
☙ Outline the need for careful washing and drying of films after wet processing.

Heating chemical solutions

Methods of heating chemicals include **water baths** – with a heating element placed inside the tank with a thermometer (manual processing), or **thermostatic heaters** – a thermostatically controlled heating system used in automatic processors. The temperature is constantly monitored and controlled.

Automatic processors

Automatic processors operate at approximately 35°C. The film is fed into the processor tray which leads the film into the rollers. The rollers are driven by a motor which transports the film through the developer tank, fixer tank and wash tank allowing the correct amount of time for each. Any excess chemicals are 'squeezed' out by the rollers. There is no wash procedure in between developing and fixing.

Making up solutions for an automatic processor

• **Developer and fixer** are available in ready-to-use formulae or as liquids or powders that require mixing with water. The developer receives fresh solutions at a set rate from the store of the chemicals. This is activated when the film has been fed into the processor.

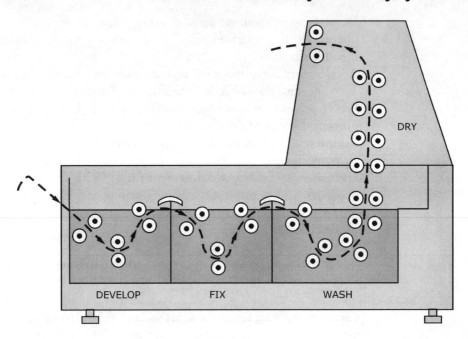

Figure 7.9 Automatic processor.

Chemicals should be replaced every 12 weeks regardless of whether they have been used or not.

- **Replenisher** is used to replenish the developer and acts as top-up fluid. It is not the same as developer but can be used to replace developer as levels fall within the tank.
- **Hardeners** are added into developer during manufacture for use with automatic processors. They prevent excessive swelling of the film emulsion (if the film emulsion has swollen the rollers could cause damage) and harden the film.
- **Acid stop bath (stop bath)** chemicals such as acetic acid can be added to the rinse tank, as an alternative method for stopping development.

Disposal of chemicals

The regulations stated in COSHH must be adhered to.

- Wear gloves when handling chemicals.
- Developer and fixing waste should be collected and retained in appropriate containers that are disposed of by authorised companies. Silver can be recovered from waste fixer. **Developer and fixer cannot be disposed of down sinks or drains.**

Processing solutions

Developer contains the following chemicals.

- **Developing or reducing agent** contains hydroquinone or phenidone. It converts exposed grains of silver halide to black metallic silver.
- **Accelerators** contain potassium carbonate or sodium carbonate. They increase the efficiency of the developer by increasing the pH.
- **Preservatives** contain sodium sulphite. They reduce oxidation and prevent staining of the film emulsion.
- **Restrainers** contain potassium bromide and limit the action of the reducing agents.
- **Hardeners** are added into developer for use with automatic processors. They prevent excessive swelling of the film emulsion (if the film emulsion has swollen the rollers could cause damage) and harden the film.
- **Solvent** (ie water) is used to dissolve the chemicals.
- **Fungicides** may be added to prevent growth of fungi.

Fixer contains the following chemicals:

- **Clearing or fixing agent** contains sodium thiosulphate or ammonium thiosulphate and is used to dissolve and remove unexposed silver halide crystals from the film.
- **Preservatives** contain sodium sulphite and prevent deterioration of the fixing agent.
- **Hardeners** contain aluminium salt. They prevent excess swelling and softening of the film emulsion and also shorten the drying time.
- **Acidifiers** are acetic acid. They neutralise any alkaline developer carried over to the fixer tank and accelerate the action of other chemicals.
- **Buffers** maintain the pH.
- **Solvent**, ie water, is used to dissolve the chemicals.

Processing a radiograph by wet development (by hand)

The following is the process followed for wet development of a radiograph.

- Check chemical levels.
- Ensure developer is at 20°C.
- Stir each chemical tank with separate 'paddles'.
- Remove the film from the cassette.
- Place film into a hanger.
- Insert the film into the developer and agitate.
- Replace the lid and begin timing (usually 3–5 minutes), agitating periodically.
- Re-load cassette with new film.
- When completed in the developer, place the film into the rinse tank and agitate for approximately 20 seconds.

- Place the film into the fixing tank and agitate.
- Leave the film in the fixer for 10 minutes (use a timer). The door may be opened or lights turned on after 1 minute.
- When time is completed in the fixer, remove the film and place in the wash tank (with running water) for 15–30 minutes.
- Finally, hang the films up to dry (remember if channel hangers have been used you will need to remove the film).

Chemical reactions of developer

The developer converts the exposed silver bromide crystals into black metallic silver and releases the bromide ions into the solution. This is known as reduction. The time required to develop the film is between 3 and 5 minutes.

If the film is developed over the recommended time then unexposed silver bromide crystals will also be converted into black metallic silver causing an overall darkening of the film (development fog).

It is important that the temperature is kept constant as development is dependent on both time and temperature – usually 20°C.

Preparation of developer

When preparing the developer ensure that the temperature is 20°C and that it is maintained at this. Stir the developer before use with a 'paddle' specifically kept for developer. Replenish or re-fill the developer if required.

Development time is between 3 and 5 minutes; the actual correct time will be stated by the manufacturer.

Storage of chemicals

Storage of chemicals in the darkroom should follow these guidelines:

- Store in the wet area of the darkroom.
- Store in the original labelled containers supplied by the manufacturer.
- Store away from film and cassettes.

Washing and drying of films

Rinsing film

This is performed between development and fixing, for 20 seconds. It is required to stop development and to remove developer from the film as the alkaline developer would neutralise the acidic fixer. A chemical solution, eg acetic acid, may be added as an alternative method of stopping development. This is known as a stop bath.

Washing

After fixing for 15–30 minutes it is necessary to wash the film to remove any processing chemicals. If this procedure is not carried out correctly and for the correct amount of time, the image on the radiograph will develop yellow-brown stains, discolour and fade.

Drying

After the wash process films developed in channel hangers need to be removed for drying, otherwise the areas under the channels will not dry correctly. They should be clipped onto a drying line (like a washing line) over a sink in a dust-free area. Ensure the radiographs are not touching one another. Drying cabinets and drying frames are available.

3.7.08 Quality of radiographs

What you need to learn

- You need to be able to define terms associated with radiographic quality:
  - density
  - contrast
  - sharpness/definition
  - under/over exposure
  - under/over development.
- Outline the relationship between exposure factors which create contrast and density of an X-ray image on a photographic emulsion:
  - kV
  - mAs.
- Describe the effects of improper processing on contrast, definition and density:
  - dirty intensifying screens
  - double exposure
  - static electricity
  - over/under development
  - developer and fixer splashes
  - crimp marks
  - developer temperature.
- Describe the effects of white light on photographic emulsion before and during processing.
- Describe and recognise the effects of movement during exposure and measures taken:
  - patient
  - apparatus

❧ film
❧ anaesthesia
❧ sedation
❧ breathing
❧ positioning aids.
❧ Describe the effect of poor screen contact or dirty intensifying screens on photographic image.
❧ Explain the value of the use of grids to improve detail and quality of image and describe the implications of incorrect use of grids.
❧ Outline film faults due to the imbalance of the chemical constituents of the developer.
❧ Outline film faults caused by incorrect handling of films during processing.
❧ Outline film faults as a result of incorrect washing and drying.
❧ Describe the effects of distance on the quality of radiographs:
  ❧ FFD
  ❧ patient-film distance.

Radiographic quality

- **Density** – the degree of blackness on the radiograph
- **Contrast** – the difference between shades on the radiograph
- **Sharpness** (or **definition**) – the clarity of the visible structures on the radiograph
- **Underexposure** – the image is too white but the background of the radiograph is black
- **Overexposure** – the image is too dark and the background on the radiograph is black. Items such as metal markers will remain white.
- **Underdevelopment** – the image and the background are too light and have a grey appearance. If a radiograph is underdeveloped then your fingers will be visible if placed behind the radiograph
- **Overdevelopment** – the image and background are too dark.

Contrast and density

Density, the degree of blackness, is primarily affected by the mAs. The higher the mAs the more X-rays are present, so a blacker film is created, contrast however remains unchanged. Kilovoltage will also affect the density but the contrast is affected along with the density.

Contrast, the difference between shades, is primarily affected by the kilovoltage. If the difference in shades is great, eg black and white, the contrast is high, if the difference in shades is smaller, eg lots of greys, the contrast is low. The higher the kilovoltage the lower the contrast.

Effects of improper processing on contrast and density

The following problems in the processing will affect the contrast and density.

- Dirty intensifying screens – dust, dirt and hairs can affect the amount of light reaching the film thereby reducing both contrast and density. They will also appear as white marks on the film which will be visible in the same place on each radiograph.
- Double exposure – when two exposures have been made on the same film. This will increase density and contrast and the exposure would have to be repeated on a new film.
- Static electricity – this looks like lightning across the radiograph; it can be caused by pulling the film out of the box too quickly, or if the film has been near nylon material/clothes.
- Overdevelopment – this will cause increased density, including items such as metal markers.
- Underdevelopment – this will cause decreased density and contrast, producing a grey film and background (fingers will be visible if placed behind the background of the film).
- Developer and fixer splashes – these can be viewed as white, grey or black patches.
- Crimp marks – these appear as black or white crescent-shaped marks and are caused by bending the film or using finger nails.
- Developer temperature – if the temperature is too high the film will be overdeveloped, resulting in increased density. If the temperature is too low the film will be undeveloped, resulting in reduced density and contrast.

Effects of white light

If the whole film is exposed to white light before processing then the whole film will be black following processing.

If part of the film is exposed to white light, eg the lid is left off the film box or the cassette is faulty, then only that part will be black following processing. The remaining film will show the rest of the image.

If the film is exposed to white light before completing the clearing time in the fixer then the whole film will be black. After the clearing time has completed, white light does not affect the film.

When using an automatic processor, if the whole film has not been allowed to be fed into the rollers and is exposed to white light then that specific part will be black.

Effects of movement

Movement blur can be caused by:

- movement of the patient, eg physical movement, excessive breathing
- movement of the X-ray table
- movement of the tube head
- movement of the cassette containing the film – more common in equine radiography.

Movement caused by any of the above factors causes blurring of the film.

Measures to rectify movement blur include:

- anaesthesia
- sedation
- controlled breathing – inflate the lungs before exposure or expose on the peak of inspiration for thoracic radiography; expose on expiration for abdominal radiography
- positioning aids, eg sandbags, cradles.

Faults with intensifying screens

Poor screen–film contact will appear as areas that lack sharpness. This will show on the same area each time the cassette and screens are used.

To test for screen–film contact:

- Prepare the X-ray machine to take an exposure.
- Place the cassette on the table and align the beam.
- Place either a piece of mesh wiring or a single layer of paper clips on top of the cassette.
- Make an exposure and develop the film; any areas with poor contact will appear unsharp (almost blurring).

Dirty screens can cause marks on the radiograph as follows:

- Dust and dirt will appear as white marks.
- Hairs will appear as white lines (that can be mistaken for fractures).
- Exposure to fluid will produced unexposed areas on the film.

Screens that have been damaged by pressure, fluids, or abrasion cannot be repaired and should be replaced. Screens with poor film contact should also be replaced.

Grids

Grids improve the detail and quality of the image as they absorb scatter radiation. Scatter radiation produces fogging on the film, resulting in general darkening and lack of contrast and definition. Grids are used when the thickness of the tissue is 10 cm or more.

Incorrect use of stationary grids

- Be sure to use the grid the right way up – it will produce coarse grid lines if used upside down.
- Be sure to align the primary beam correctly when using focused or pseudo-focused grids.
- Do not drop the grid as this can damage the edges.
- If the lead strips become bent then an artefact will present on all radiographs.
- Be sure to increase the mAs by multiplying the mAs by the grid factor.

Film faults due to developer imbalances

If the developer has not been changed or replenished then it becomes exhausted, ie there is no longer sufficient reducing agent present to develop the silver bromide crystals in the film. The film following processing will be undeveloped – see contrast and density 3.7.08. If the film density is patchy it indicates that the developer was not stirred or that the film was not agitated.

Film faults due to incorrect handling

Incorrect handling of the film can cause faults. Examples of such handling include:

- static electricity
- crescent-shaped marks as a result of finger-nail pressure or bending
- greasy finger marks
- processing chemical marks caused by splashes and spills.

Film faults due to incorrect washing and drying

If the washing and drying are inadequate or incorrect the following problems can occur:

- Dichroic fog – yellow-brown stains are caused by inadequate washing.
- Wet edges occur if the film was not removed from the channel hanger before drying.
- Ingrained dust can occur if the film was not left to dry in a dust-free area.

Effects of distance

FFD

This refers to the distance between the focal spot and the radiographic film. If the FFD is increased, the intensity of the beam reduces and the film will appear underexposed. If the FFD is decreased the intensity of the beam is greater and the film will appear overexposed. The mAs should be adjusted accordingly if the FFD is altered. The standard FFD is 75 cm (see page 283).

Patient–film distance

This refers to the distance between the film and the part of the patient being radiographed. It is important to keep the parts being radiographed as close to and as parallel to the film as possible to prevent:

- magnification
- distortion
- foreshortening.

3.7.09   Positioning

What you need to learn

- You need to be able to outline the standard positioning for all common radiographic examinations of:
  - thorax
  - abdomen
  - spine (cervical, thoracic, lumbar)
  - pelvis
  - forelimbs
  - hind limbs
  - joints
  - skull.
- Recognise and use positioning aids appropriately:
  - cradles
  - sandbags
  - foam pads
  - ties
- Outline the different views needed and the reasons for their requirement.
- Explain the clinical considerations which should be taken into account when positioning an animal for radiography.
- Describe how poor positioning can affect the final radiograph

- movement
- incorrect positioning
- incorrect collimation.

- Explain the need to restrain, sedate or anaesthetise the patient to achieve accurate positioning without movement.

Standard positioning

- **Thorax** – lateral (right lateral recumbency is the standard but both right and left lateral views may be required); dorso-ventral (DV); ventro-dorsal (VD); but do not use if the patient is dyspnoeic.
- **Abdomen** – lateral (left or right); VD
- **Spine** (cervical, thoracic and lumbar) – lateral (left or right); VD
- **Pelvis** – lateral (left or right); VD; use a VD relaxed frog-leg position if a pelvic fracture is suspected.
- **Forelimbs** – lateral; craniocaudal (CrCd)
- **Hind limbs** – lateral; CrCd
- **Shoulder** – lateral; caudocranial (CdCr)
- **Elbow** – lateral (flexed and extended); CrCd or CdCr
- **Carpus and metacarpus** – mediolateral; CrCd; oblique views
- **Phalanges** – lateral; CrCd
- **Stifle** – lateral; CrCd or CdCr
- **Hock (tarsus)** – lateral; CrCd or CdCr
- **Metatarsals** – mediolateral; CrCd; oblique views
- **Phalanges** – lateral; CrCd
- **Skull** –
  - lateral; DV; VD;
  - lateral oblique; rostrocaudal
  - open mouth; rostrocaudal; DV intra-oral; VD intra-oral; 20° VD open mouth

Aids to help with positioning

There are various aids to help with positioning:

- cradles
- sandbags
- foam pads/wedges
- rope ties
- physical positioning (moving of the patient)

Clinical considerations

The following should be taken into account when positioning patients:

• cardiac disease
• respiratory disease
• fractures
• dislocations/luxations
• wounds
• dressings/splints.

Poor positioning

Movement caused by the patient will result in movement blur.

Incorrect positioning will result in subsequent radiographs having to be taken.

Incorrect collimation – if over tight the area of interest may not be included and the radiograph would have to be repeated.

Scatter radiation will result in fogging of the radiograph resulting in loss of contrast and density.

To maintain correct positioning the patient should be either restrained using positioning aids, eg rope ties, sandbags, sedated, or anaesthetised.

Maintenance of correct positioning:

• reduces the need for repeated radiographs
• reduces the amount of personnel exposure
• produces a good image of the part being radiographed.

3.7.10   Contrast radiography

What you need to learn

☙ You need to be able to describe the different contrast media, and their radiographic densities:
  ☙ positive
  ☙ negative
  ☙ double.
☙ Outline the use for each type of contrast medium and their appropriate use.

❦ Describe equipment preparation and procedures for common contrast techniques:
  ❦ pneumo-cystogram
  ❦ intravenous urography (IVU)
  ❦ myelography and arthrography.
❦ Describe patient preparation and management for common contrast techniques to include health and safety.

Contrast media

There are three types of contrast media.

- **Positive contrast media** are more radiopaque than the surrounding tissue, eg barium sulphate, iodine compounds.
- **Negative contrast media** are more radiolucent than the surrounding tissue, eg oxygen, room air, nitrous oxide, carbon dioxide.
- **Double contrast** involves using a small volume of positive contrast followed by negative contrast.

Types of contrast media

- **Barium sulphate:**
  - used in alimentary studies, eg megaesophagus, obstructions [It cannot be used if perforation of the intestines is suspected.]
  - insoluble
  - good contrast
  - cheap
  - can cause granulomatous reaction or aspiration pneumonia
  - messy.
- **Ionic media**, eg Conray®, Urografin®:
  - used for angiographic studies and to outline the kidneys, ureters and the bladder [Cannot be used for myelography]
  - more uses than barium
  - water soluble so can be used intravenously
  - rapidly excreted
  - is irritant if injected perivascularly
  - can cause vomiting and anaphylactic reactions because of high osmotic pressure
  - needs to be stored in the dark
  - expensive
  - versions of ionic media are available to use for gastrointestinal studies if perforation of the intestines is suspected, eg gastro Conray, gastro graffin, however they provide poor contrast and are very bitter to taste.
- **Non ionic media**, eg Niopam, Omnipaque:
  - used in myelography

- low osmotic pressure which reduces side-effects such as vomiting
- needs to be stored in the dark
- **Air, oxygen, nitrous oxide, carbon dioxide:**
  - less contrast and mucosal detail is obtained than when positive agents are used
  - easy to administer
  - cheap
  - readily available.

Common contrast techniques

Pneumocystogram

The patient is starved for 12 hours before the procedure is required.

Equipment required comprises:

- negative contrast agent
- urinary catheter
- three-way tap
- syringe
- kidney dish
- universal container with or without boric acid.

The technique is performed as described:

- Sedation or general anaesthetic will be required.
- Place the animal in a lateral recumbency position.
- Take a plain radiograph first.
- Insert catheter into the bladder and collect urine.
- Dispense urine into containers if required.
- Attach three-way tap and syringe.
- Inflate with air (or other negative contrast) until the bladder is moderately distended.
- Take a lateral view of the caudal abdomen.
- A ventrodorsal view may be required in some circumstances.
- Remove the air and catheter once the procedure is completed.

Intravenous urography (IVU) – low volume, rapid injection

The patient will require starving for 24 hours and an enema should be administered 2–3 hours before the procedure

Equipment required comprises:

- ionic contrast agent
- syringe and needle
- intravenous catheter.

The technique involves the following,

- General anaesthesia will be required.
- Insert and secure the intravenous catheter.
- Place the animal in the dorsal recumbency position.
- Take a plain radiograph first.
- Align the primary beam and set the exposure factors so that the radiograph can be taken immediately.
- Inject the dose of the agent rapidly via the catheter.
- Take a radiograph immediately after administration.
- Subsequent radiographs are then taken at 1-, 5-, 10-, 15- and 20-minute intervals.
- Usually the ventrodorsal view is used but the lateral view may be used in some circumstances.

A contrast agent is infused over 10–15 minutes through an intravenous catheter. The contrast agent is more dilute than that used in the low volume rapid injection technique. Lateral and ventrodorsal views should be taken at 5, 10 and 15 minutes.

Myelography (cisternal puncture)

The animal is starved for 12 hours before the procedure is required.

The equipment required includes:

- non-ionic contrast agent
- hypodermic needle with a short bevel or spinal needle
- clippers
- surgical preparation solution
- sterile container.

The technique involves the following:

- General anaesthesia is essential.
- Take plain radiographs first of the whole spine.
- Place the animal in lateral reumbency.
- Clip a 10 cm × 10 cm area over the base of the skull and the wings of the atlas.
- Prepare as you would for a surgical procedure.
- Tilt the table to elevate the head (if available).
- By flexing the neck, direct the nose downwards towards the shoulder blades and hold, so it is at right angles with the spine (beware of kinking endotracheal tubes).
- The needle is then placed into the subarachnoid space.
- Cerebrospinal fluid (CSF) will flow back and should be collected into a sterile container if analysis is required.
- Inject the contrast agent slowly and remove the needle once completed.
- Tilt the head and/or the table to assist caudal flowing of the agent.

• Take lateral and ventrodorsal views of the whole spine, oblique views may be required in some circumstances.

Arthrography

The animal is starved for 12 hours before the procedure is required. The equipment required includes:

• positive, negative, or double-contrast agent (positive most commonly used)
• syringe and needle.

The technique involves the following:

• General anaesthesia is required.
• Position for recumbency will depend on the joint being investigated.
• Take plain radiographs first.
• Prepare as you would for a surgical procedure.
• Inject contrast agent into the joint.
• Remove the needle and manipulate the joint.
• Take two views of the joint, again this will depend on the joint been investigated.

Patient preparation and management

• The ionising regulations should be adhered to.
• All patients should have an intravenous catheter (and a three way tap if required).
• Ensure the bladder and bowels have been emptied if not contraindicated.
• Check if the patient has eaten/drunk that morning.

3.7.11   Ultrasound

What you need to learn

❧ You need to be able to define the basic principles and understand how to use the ultrasound machine:
  ❧ time adjustment
  ❧ display modes A, B and M.
❧ Describe the selection and preparation of ultrasound equipment with respect to investigation procedures:
  ❧ transducer
  ❧ linear and curved array scanners
  ❧ image displays.
❧ Outline the advantages and disadvantages of ultrasound.
❧ Outline patient preparation for ultrasound procedure.

Basic principles of ultrasonography

Sound waves are produced and received by piezo-electric crystals (in the transducer).

A voltage is applied to the crystal which deforms its shape and produces a sound wave; this happens on an intermittent basis (short pulses of sound). In between the pulses, the crystal receives returning echoes which deform its shape. These are recognised and converted onto the screen (or other visual display) and seen as the image. Frequencies used are in the 2–10 MHz range.

There are three image display modes:

- **A-mode** (amplitude mode)
  - This is the simplest form and is rarely used.
  - It only shows position of tissue interfaces.
  - The horizontal axis represents the depth of the echo.
  - The vertical axis represents the strength of the echo.
- **B-mode** (brightness mode)
  - This is the most commonly used mode.
  - Returning echoes are represented as dots.
  - The position of the dot represents the point of origin of the echo.
  - The brightness of the dot represents the strength of the echo.
  - This produces a two-dimensional, cross-sectional image.
  - Movement of structures can be seen.
- **M-mode** (time–motion)
  - Most B-mode machines can also be used to produce M-mode.
  - This mode uses a single ultrasound beam.
  - Echoes are represented as dots in a vertical line on the left hand side of the screen.
  - The brightness of the dot indicates the strength of the echo.
  - The distance along the line indicates the origin of the echo.
  - Details are continuously updated.
  - This mode is used commonly in cardiology.

How to use ultrasound

When using ultrasound on a patient, the following procedure should be used:

- Prepare the patient.
- Position the patient as required.
- Dim the lighting.
- Set the ultrasound machine at the highest frequency.
- The power should be set as low as possible.
- Use the time gain compensator to adjust the brightness.
- Place the transducer on the patient with enough pressure to

maintain contact.
- Scan slowly and in a methodical order.

Selection and preparation of ultrasound equipment

Transducers can be of three types:

- **Linear and curved array transducers** contain crystals that are arranged in a line and activated in small groups in sequence. They produce a rectangular view and are used mainly in large animal work.
- **Mechanical sector transducers** have either one crystal that oscillates backwards and forwards or three to five crystals mounted on a rotating wheel. They produce a pie-shaped view.
- **Phased array sector transducers** contain approximately 60 piezo-electric elements that do not move. They produce a pie-shaped view but are very expensive.

Image displays can be A, B or M mode as already described.

Advantages of ultrasound

- No sedation or anaesthesia is required.
- There is no risk to personnel.
- Ultrasound can differentiate between fluid and soft tissue.
- Ultrasound can provide information on structure and movement of organs.

Disadvantages of ultrasound

- Skill is needed to operate the machine.
- Skill is needed in diagnosing from and interpreting the results.
- Ultrasound cannot be used for imaging bones or gas-filled areas.
- Artefacts can be produced.
- The patient has to be clipped.

Patient preparation

- Sedation or anaesthesia are rarely required.
- Withhold food for a few hours before the procedure if scanning the gastrointestinal tract.
- If scanning the bladder, uterus or prostate, prevent urination for 1–2 hours before the procedure.
- Clip and clean the area to be scanned.
- Apply coupling gel to the patient and/or the transducer, avoiding air bubbles.
- Keep the patient comfortable as they are then more likely to stay still.

3.7.12   Endoscopy

What you need to learn

* You need to be able to outline the principles of endoscopy techniques and their appropriate use.
* Describe the correct procedure for the cleaning and maintenance of different endoscopes:
  * rigid
  * flexible.

Principles of endoscopy

Endoscopes are used to examine the internal structures of a cavity or organ and facilitate obtaining biopsies from these cavities or organs. They use combinations of glass fibre optics, mirrors and lenses coupled with a light source.

Light is transmitted from the light source through the endoscope to the tissue and then the image is carried back so it can be visualised by the operator. The image can be viewed on a television screen.

Care of rigid and flexible endoscopes

* Prepare the endoscope-friendly disinfectant.
* Wash the outside of the tubing in detergent.
* Clean the biopsy channels using special brushes; flush through with disinfectant and repeat with water.
* Clean the lenses with cotton buds or lens tissues.
* Lay the tubing in the disinfectant but not the eyepiece (the eyepiece is immersible if a blue ring is present). Special endoscope-cleaning tables are available.
* Following disinfection, rinse the endoscope in water.
* Store vertically; if transporting use the original packing case.
* Endoscopes can be sterilised using ethylene oxide if available.

3.7.13   Imaging techniques

What you need to learn

* You need to be able to state the other methods available:
  * computer aided tomography (CAT)
  * magnetic resonance imaging (MRI)
  * nuclear imaging (scintigraphy).

Other imaging techniques available include:

* computer-aided tomography (CAT) for use of scanning X-rays.

- magnetic resonance imaging (MRI) – (high frequency radiowaves pass through the body and are analysed by the computer to create images of organs and tissues of the brain).
- nuclear imaging (scintigraphy – image map produced by scanning and distribution of a high energy radiation tracer).

Multiple choice questions

1. Which of the following measures will not reduce scatter?
   - ☐ A using a high kV
   - ☐ B beam collimation
   - ☐ C use of a grid
   - ☐ D using a horizontal beam

2. The Radiation Protection Advisor (RPA):
   - ☐ A defines the controlled area
   - ☐ B ensures that local rules are complied with
   - ☐ C reports faults directly to the HSE
   - ☐ D is a person appointed within the practice

3. Protective clothing in the form of X-ray gloves:
   - ☐ A protect against the primary beam
   - ☐ B should be folded for ease of storage
   - ☐ C should be more than 0.35mm (LE)
   - ☐ D can be less than 0.25mm (LE)

4. Energy which forms the primary beam is known as:
   - ☐ A atomic energy
   - ☐ B electrons
   - ☐ C quanta
   - ☐ D the atomic number

5. The filament is heated by:
   - ☐ A thermionic emission
   - ☐ B mA supplied to the cathode
   - ☐ C a step down transformer
   - ☐ D kV applied to the anode by a high tension transformer

6. Which of the following is NOT true:
   - ☐ A the focal spot is the target on the cathode
   - ☐ B a smaller focal spot produces a sharper image
   - ☐ C the focusing cup is composed of molybdenum
   - ☐ D the kV provides the penetrating power of the beam

7. The filament usually made of tungsten because it:
   - ☐ A is a light metal
   - ☐ B has a high melting point
   - ☐ C is a good conductor of heat
   - ☐ D efficiently disperses the heat

8. A relatively white X-ray image would be due to the tissue in question possessing:
   - ☐ A a high atomic number
   - ☐ B a low specific gravity
   - ☐ C little fat
   - ☐ D a low density

9. A high contrast radiograph with black and white images could be improved by:
   - ☐ A decreasing the kV
   - ☐ B increasing the kV
   - ☐ C decreasing the mA
   - ☐ D increasing the mA

10. If a short Film Focal Distance is to be used for a radiograph, then a suitable image could be produced by:
    - ☐ A increasing the time
    - ☐ B reducing the mAs
    - ☐ C squaring the old mAs
    - ☐ D dividing the distance squared by the new distance squared

11. Which type of X-ray film will require the highest exposure?
    - ☐ A orthochromatic
    - ☐ B ultra fast
    - ☐ C single sided emulsion screen film
    - ☐ D fine detail

12. X-ray film should be stored:
    - ☐ A in a light proof container in the freezer
    - ☐ B in a hopper in the controlled area
    - ☐ C in an airtight container at 5°C
    - ☐ D horizontally in the dark room

13. If a grid with a grid factor of 3 was used, then:
    - ☐ A 3 would represent the number of lines per cm.
    - ☐ B The difference between the height and width of the lead strips would be 3cm
    - ☐ C The mAs should be multiplied by 3
    - ☐ D The kV should be divided by 3

14. Fixer:
    - ☐ A contains hydroquinone
    - ☐ B is acidic
    - ☐ C converts exposed silver halide grains
    - ☐ D contains a preservative to prevent oxidation

15. An increase in film density may be caused by:
    - ☐ A under development
    - ☐ B movement blur
    - ☐ C static electricity
    - ☐ D exposure to white light during processing

16. In contrast radiography, ionic iodine compounds:
    - ☐ A are less radiopaque than the surrounding tissues
    - ☐ B are used for myelography
    - ☐ C appear black on the radiograph
    - ☐ D can be used for intestinal studies in cases of suspect gastric and intestinal perforation

17. Cisternal mylography consists of injection of a suitable contrast media into the:
    - ☐ A space between the atlas and axis
    - ☐ B foramen magnum
    - ☐ C subarachnoid space
    - ☐ D epidural space

18. Which type of ultra sound display mode produces a two dimensional cross sectional image:
    - ☐ A time-motion mode
    - ☐ B brightness mode
    - ☐ C amplitude mode
    - ☐ D continuous mode

19. Regarding ultra sound investigation which of the following is NOT true?
    - ☐ A sound waves are produced in the transducer
    - ☐ B the patient must be catheterised before scanning the bladder
    - ☐ C coupling gel insures close contact
    - ☐ D the lungs will not image well

20. The production of cross sectional radiographs is known as:
    - ☐ A magnetic resonance imaging
    - ☐ B scintigraphy
    - ☐ C obliquie positioning
    - ☐ D tomography

Level 3: Unit 8

General surgical nursing

3.8.01   Local inflammation and healing

What you need to learn

* You need to be able to define inflammation and describe the changes which occur in an inflamed region and the results of these changes in:
  * dogs
  * cats
  * other species eg birds, rodents, lagomorphs, reptiles.
* Describe wound classification:
  * puncture
  * avulsed
  * incised
  * lacerated
  * abrasion
  * shear.
* Understand wound classification by degree of contamination
  * clean
  * clean contaminated
  * contaminated
  * dirty.
* Describe types of wound closure and methods of skin apposition.
* Describe the treatment methods of inflammation:
  * antiseptics
  * cleansing solutions
  * dressings.
* Describe healing by first and second intention, the formation and function of granulation tissue.
* Describe the outcomes of wound healing:
  * resolution
  * regeneration
  * organisation.
* Describe the role of inflammation in healing.
* Describe the aftercare of a surgical wound and state the reasons for wound breakdown and delayed healing.
* Outline how wound breakdown and delayed healing may be prevented and treated in

- mammals
- birds
- exotics.
- Describe the general cause of a contaminated wound and state the treatment, including the type of dressing used:
  - dressings types: (see Level 2, 2.4.12)
  - lavage
  - antiseptics.
- Describe types of surgical drain and explain the function and use of a drainage tube:
  - passive
  - active
  - intra-thoracic
  - intra-abdominal.
- Describe the care of drainage tubes while in position:
  - antiseptics
  - cleansing solutions
  - dressings
  - mutilation prevention.
- Describe the difference between fistula and sinus:
  - subcutaneous
  - congenital
  - acquired.

Inflammation is the reaction of tissues to injury. It can be acute or chronic.

Changes seen in an inflamed region include:

- Fluid (high in protein and white blood cells) enters the tissue spaces.
- There is an increase in blood flow to the inflamed tissues.
- There is guarding of the area.
- There is increased pressure on nerve endings.

These changes result in:

- swelling
- redness
- heat
- loss of normal function
- pain.

Wound classification

There are various criteria with which to classify wounds. They can be classified by type of wound:

- **Puncture wounds** are produced by a sharp object, eg a tooth. They tend to be perpendicular to the skin, creating an entry wound only (no exit wound).

- **Avulsed wounds** are where tissue has become separated from its attachments.
- **Incised wounds** are produced by sharp objects, eg glass. They are parallel to the skin.
- **Lacerated (degloving) wounds** involve the tearing (peeling) away of skin (like removing a glove from your hand).
- **Abrasions** are wounds in which the epidermal and dermal layers are damaged.
- **Shearing wounds** are similar to a laceration but may involve bones and joints.

Wounds can also be classified by degree of contamination:

- **Clean wounds** are wounds made under aseptic conditions, eg surgical incisions not involving the respiratory, gastrointestinal, or urogential tracts.
- **Clean-contaminated wounds** are wounds made under aseptic conditions, eg surgical incisions involving the respiratory, gastrointestinal, or urogential tracts.
- **Contaminated wounds** are traumatic wounds under six hours old or surgical wounds in which aseptic technique has been compromised.
- **Dirty wounds** are traumatic wounds over six hours old or surgical wounds with infection already present.

Types of wound closure

Wounds can be closed in various ways:

- suturing
- staples
- tissue glue
- dressings to support second intention healing (see text that follows).

Treating inflammation

The following can be used to aid treatment of inflammation.

- **Antiseptics**, eg Savlon, can be used for cleaning the surface area of the inflammation.
- **Cleansing solutions**, eg sterile saline, can be used for flushing wounds with inflammation.
- **Dressings** are used to provide protection and allow second intention healing.
- **Non-steroidal anti-inflammatory drugs (NSAID)** help to reduce inflammation.

- **Antibiotics** are used to reduce bacteria that are present causing the inflammation.

First intention healing

First intention healing occurs in clean surgical wounds that are sutured and it occurs over a period of 14 days.

- Blood clots seal the wound.
- The epithelium heals by regeneration.
- Macrophages remove dead tissue.
- Granulation tissue and collagen fibrils fill the space below the epithelium.
- Regression of blood vessels commences and the collagen begins to contract.

Second intention healing

Second intention healing happens when the wound edges cannot be sutured together because of tissue loss.

- The base and margins of the wound are filled with granulation tissue.
- The debris is gradually removed.
- Granulation tissue moves from the wound edges towards the centre.
- Re-epithelialisation begins on the granulation tissue already present.
- Wound contraction begins by fibroblasts in the granulation tissue contracting.
- The last two processes continue until the wound has healed.

Outcomes of wound healing

- **Resolution** – the tissue returns to its original state where it was damaged by inflammation.
- **Regeneration** – the tissue is replaced with like tissue where it was damaged by inflammation.
- **Organisation** – tissue is replaced with scar tissue (connective tissue) where it was damaged by inflammation.

The role of inflammation in healing

Inflammation has two main roles in healing. It provides a blood supply to the area, which encourages and aids healing and it provides white blood cells to help fight infection.

After-care for wounds

- Observe for any bleeding, swelling, discharges, smells, redness, pain, or heat.
- Check sutures are not too tight or too loose.
- Change dressings if required, note down any exudates.
- Prevent self-interference.
- Monitor demeanour, temperature, pulse and respiratory rate.

Causes of wound breakdown (wound dehiscence)

Dehiscence of wounds can occur for a variety of reasons:

- poor suturing technique
- poor aseptic technique leading to infection
- infection already present
- poor surgical technique
- poor post-operative care
- decreased blood supply to the wound.

Causes of delayed healing

Delayed healing can occur because:

- the patient is in poor health
- the patient is elderly
- the patient has diabetes mellitus
- poor suturing technique or incorrect material was used
- the patient has had medication such as steroids
- the patient has had radiation therapy
- the location of the wound, eg over a joint, makes healing difficult.

Prevention of wound breakdown and delayed healing

Mammals

In mammals wound breakdown and delayed healing can be minimised by the following procedures:

- Theatre protocols should be followed, especially aseptic technique.
- Infectious patients should be housed away from healthy patients.
- Good surgical and suturing techniques should be used.
- In poorly patients further preparation may be needed before the operation, eg medication, fluids.
- Medication may have to be adjusted, eg steroids may be graduated down and then stopped.

Treatment for wound breakdown involves covering with a dressing (sterile dressing if evisceration has occurred) until the wound can be flushed with sterile fluid and re-sutured.

Exotics

Wound healing is generally similar in exotic species as in dogs and cats. Similar principles in care of the wounds apply. It is often difficult to prevent self-inflicted trauma during wound healing but suitable Elizabethan collars are available for birds and small mammals.

Wound healing is slower in poikilothermic animals due to their reduced metabolic rates.

Birds, reptiles and rabbits have heterophils rather than neutrophils. These don't contain lysoenzyme and so these species are unable to break down cat gut and this should therefore be avoided in these animals.

Reptiles are more susceptible to gram negative bacterial infections during wound healing. These should be treated with antibiotics as necessary.

Wound contamination

Contamination of a wound can occur from debris entering the wound at a road traffic accident, from poor aseptic technique and prolonged exposure to the environment.

Dressings for contaminated wounds vary (see also 2.4.12):

• hydrogels
• hydrocolloids
• alginates
• dry/dry
• wet/dry
• foam dressings.

Management of the contaminated wound involves the following procedure:

• Flush the wound (lavage) using high volumes of fluids at 8 pounds per square inch (PSI) (achieved by using a 20-ml syringe and 21-gauge needle).
• Dry the wound as much as possible.
• Antiseptics may be applied if necessary.
• Debride the wound if required (particularly if the wound is over six hours old).
• Contaminated wounds are often left to heal by second intention

rather than suturing them, dressing of the wound is therefore required.
- Administer antibiotics and pain relief.

Surgical drains

Drains can be either passive or active.

Passive drains rely on gravity, capillary action and overflow from the wound and are placed in a dependent area through a separate stab incision. They drain down the outside and inside, (placing fenestrations in the drain decreases the surface area and therefore decreases drainage). Examples of passive drains include Penrose, Corrugated and Yeates.

Active drains provide drainage by using pressure either continuously using a suction device or intermittently by a syringe. The tube has to be rigid so it does not collapse under the pressure. Active drains are used when there is extensive fluid or air. Examples include: Heimlich valve (intra-thoracic) and sump drain (intra-abdominal).

Care of drainage tubes

- Clean the area with an antiseptic solution.
- Solutions of povidine-iodine and water or chlorohexidine and water may be used.
- Dress the drain and wound to prevent ascending infection.
- Prevent patient interference.
- Empty the reservoirs as needed.
- Drains are usually kept in place for 3–5 days.

Fistula vs sinus

A **fistula** is an abnormal tract connecting the skin and a mucosal surface. It can be acquired, eg anal furunculosis, or congenital, eg rectovaginal fistula.

A **sinus** is a tract with one entrance lined with granulating tissue. It can be subcutaneous, eg abscess, or deep within the tissues, eg caused by orthopaedic implants. They are acquired not congenital.

3.8.02   General cutaneous

What you need to learn

- You need to be able to define an abscess and state the factors which may lead to abscess formation:
  - dogs

- cats
- exotics
- small mammals.
- Describe the clinical signs of an animal suffering from a cutaneous abscess and state methods of treatment:
  - lancing
  - compresses
  - surgical removal.
- Describe a cold abscess and understand the reasons for its development and its treatment:
  - treatment
  - drainage
  - removal of cause.
- Describe an ulcer, the different types, causes and their treatment:
  - infection
  - trauma
  - pressure
  - neoplasm.
- Describe a haematoma and the factors which will cause a haematoma.
- Outline the treatment of a haematoma:
  - aural haematoma
  - surgical and non-surgical treatments
  - aftercare bandaging.
- Outline conditions of the skin amenable to surgery and understand the principles of skin grafting.
- Describe methods of skin grafting and post operative care:
  - pedicle grafts
  - free skin grafts.
- Outline the reasons for graft non-adherence.
- Describe common conditions of the external ear amenable to surgery:
  - haematoma
  - aural resection
  - ablation.

Abscess formation (dogs and cats)

An abscess is an area of pus associated with localised inflammation. Cutaneous abscesses occur as a result of bacterial infection, eg from cat bites, from bacteria entering a wound, or from chemical or mechanical irritants in the tissue.

Signs and treatment of cutaneous abscess

The signs of cutaneous abscess are as follows:

- heat and erythema
- swelling
- pain
- pus may be seen if the abscess has 'burst'
- loss of function depending on location, eg the patient may not be able to walk on the limb if the abscess is on the foot.

Cutaneous abscesses can be treated by lancing, compresses, or surgical debridement.

- **Lancing** involves the following techniques:
  - Sedation or anaesthesia is usually required.
  - Clip and prepare the site as you would for a surgical wound.
  - Lance the abscess with a blade – an incision is made in a ventral direction so pus is allowed to drain with gravity and not against it.
  - Remove all pus.
  - The abscess is then flushed through the incision with sterile saline or antiseptic solution.
  - A drain such as a Penrose may be placed to aid drainage further.
  - The hole is then left open so drainage can continue and the wound heals by second intention.
  - Commence antibiotic treatment if needed.
- **Hot compresses** can be use to aid 'bursting' of the abscess and after lancing to aid drainage.
- Occasionally abscesses will be **surgically removed** by dissection; this would certainly be the case if the abscess was within the abdominal or thoracic cavity.

Cold abscess

A cold abscess has pus present but no inflammation. Its treatment involves surgically excising the abscess as a whole.

Abscesses in rabbits are treated in the same way as in other mammals. Rabbit pus is very thick and caseous. Abscesses can therefore be difficult to lance and drain. Abscesses in the facial area in rabbits are likely to be related to dental disease. These abscesses are very difficult to treat. There is often associated osteomyelitis in the mandible. Aggressive antibiotic treatment or euthanasia are often necessary.

Abscesses are very common in reptiles. Again the pus is usually thick and caseous. Skin abscesses can be lanced or removed surgically. Radiographs should be taken if the abscess involves a limb as there may be bony involvement. If there is osteomyelitis in the bone amputation may be necessary as treatment is extremely difficult.

Ulcers

An ulcer is a loss of tissue on the skin's surface or on any mucous membrane. The types include:

• decubital ulcers (pressure sores) – ulcers over the elbows, etc
• ulcers of the gingiva or mouth – trauma, infection
• gastric ulcers – certain drugs, neoplasia (mast cell tumours)
• corneal ulcers – infections, trauma
• rodent ulcers (eosinophilic granulomas) – allergy – immune mediated.

Ulcers can be treated in the following ways:

• Remove the cause of the ulcer, eg stop NSAID.
• Protect skin ulcers with dressings, flush mouth ulcers with antiseptic solutions. The third eyelid may be sutured over in corneal ulcers.
• Treat bacterial and viral infections.

Haematomas

A haematoma is a collection of blood under the skin. It can be caused by trauma eg after a road traffic accident, severe bruising, or head shaking.

Treatment of an aural haematoma can be either surgical or non-surgical. Also see 3.8.12.

Surgical treatment of haematoma will require the following:

• General anaesthesia is required.
• The hair on both sides of the ear should be clipped and the skin should be surgically prepared.
• An incision is made on the inner surface of the ear and all the blood is expressed.
• Sutures or buttons are then placed vertically on either side of the incision; drains may also be used.
• The ear may bandaged or an Elizabethan collar supplied.
• Drains are removed three to five days later; sutures and buttons are removed 7-14 days later.

Non-surgical treatments include draining the haematoma with a syringe and needle and treatment with long-acting steroids.

The cause of the haematoma should also be investigated and treated, eg if the patient is head shaking because of ear mites, the ear mites must be treated or the haematoma will return.

After-care of the treated haematoma involves the following.

- Prevent patient interference with the wound.
- If the ear is bandaged, change the dressings as required.
- If the ear is not bandaged keep the ear and Elizabethan collar clean by bathing in warm water.
- Administer any medication, eg pain relief, antibiotics.

Bandaging

Non-adherent dressings, such as impregnated gauze, should be used for the primary layer. A head bandage can be adapted to include the ear. This can be done with the ear in its natural position or with the ear over the top of the head. It is important to make a note on the bandage itself and on the patient records if this is case, to avoid the ear being cut on removal. Elastoplast should be used for the territory layer as self-conforming bandage can tighten and may obstruct the neck causing breathing difficulties.

Conditions of the skin amenable to surgery

- wounds, eg lacerations
- lumps/masses – benign and malignant
- warts
- skin disease/infection requiring biopsy.

Principles of skin grafting

Some wounds may not heal because there has been a significant loss of skin and tissue or there may be too little mobile skin to provide apposition of the wound edges. Skin grafts are used to provide skin for the wound to heal and can be obtained in one of three ways.

- **Autogenous graft** – skin is taken from a separate area on the same patient (most commonly used)
- **Allograft** – skin is taken from another patient but of the same species
- **Xenograft** – skin is taken from a patient but of another species.

Methods of skin grafts

Pedicle grafts (skin flaps) involve an area of skin being rotated from part of the body to another part including its blood supply. Donor areas include the skin over the shoulder blade and ventral abdomen.

Free skin grafts involve an area of skin being transferred from part of the body to another part but without a blood supply. They can be classified as either:

- full thickness – contain all dermal structures; or
- split thickness – contain the epidermis and part of the dermis.

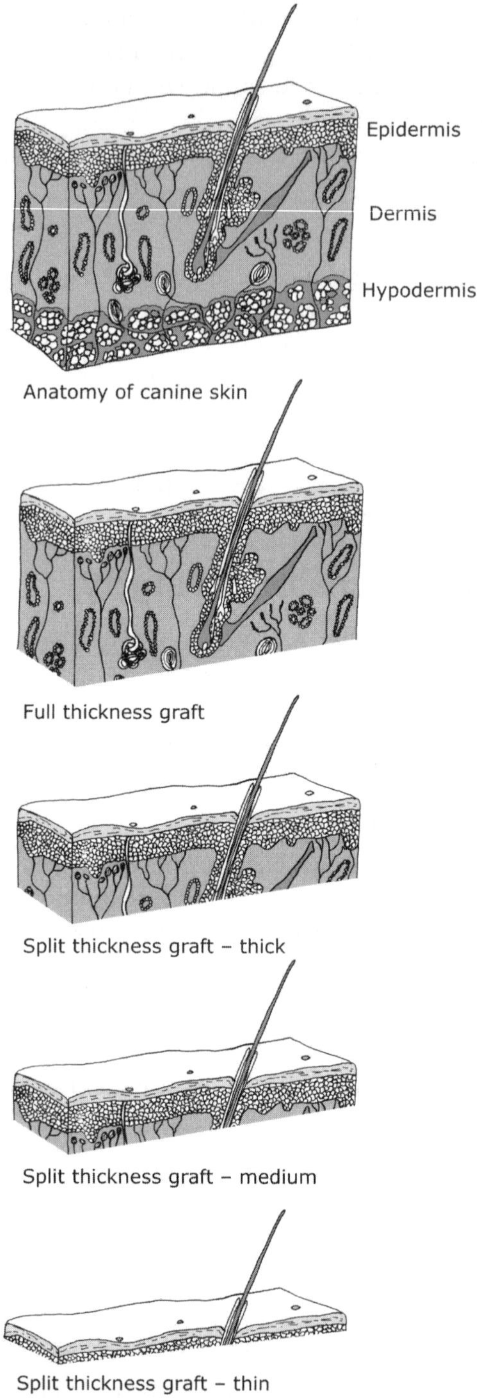

Epidermis

Dermis

Hypodermis

Anatomy of canine skin

Full thickness graft

Split thickness graft – thick

Split thickness graft – medium

Split thickness graft – thin

Figure 8.1 Skin grafts.

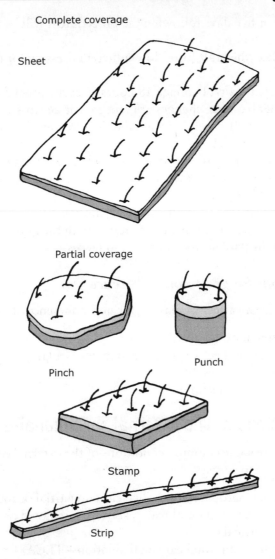

Complete coverage

Sheet

Partial coverage

Pinch

Punch

Stamp

Strip

Figure 8.2 Sheet and pinch skin drafts.

Free skin grafts can be further classified by their preparation into:

• sheet (meshed or unmeshed) grafts – which cover the whole wound and
• pinch, punch, stamp and strip grafts – which cover part of the wound.

Post-operative care for skin grafts

• The graft on the limb or body part needs to be immobilised for several weeks for it to take correctly.

- Four or five days following the procedure it will be visible if the graft is 'taking'.
- Bandage the graft (use a low-adherent dressing for the primary layer).
- Change the first bandage 48 hours after the procedure.
- Further bandage changes are repeated at 24- to 48-hour intervals.
- Be extremely careful when removing dressings as the graft has not fully developed.
- Examine the graft at each dressing change for exudates (exudates interfere with the graft and provide a medium for bacteria) and colour changes.
- Administer medications, such as pain relief, as required.
- Prevent the patient from interfering with the graft.
- Keep the patient free of urine and faeces.

Reasons for graft non-adherence

There are a variety of reasons for non-adherence of the graft.

- movement of the graft
- the recipient bed was not adequately vascularised
- infection
- poor surgical technique.

Common conditions of the external ear amenable to surgery

There are some common conditions of the external ear that are amenable to surgery.

- aural haematoma (blood-filled ear flap partial or total)
- aural resection (lateral wall resection) – removal of the lateral part of the vertical canal
- aural ablation (total ear canal ablation – TECA) – the horizontal and vertical canals are both removed
- vertical canal ablation (VCA) – removal of the vertical canal.

3.8.03   Alimentary tract

What you need to learn

❧ You need to be able to outline the common conditions of the alimentary tract amenable to surgical correction:
  ❧ gastric torsion (GDV)
  ❧ foreign body removal
  ❧ intussusception
  ❧ enterectomy
  ❧ enterotomy.

☙ Outline common conditions/diseases of the rectum and anus amenable to surgical correction:
  ☙ neoplasia
  ☙ polyps
  ☙ anal furunculosis
  ☙ anal sac disease
  ☙ perineal rupture/hernia.

Surgical diseases of the stomach and intestines

Gastric dilatation/volvulus (GDV)

(Also called **gastric torsion**):

- Dilatation of the stomach with or without a **volvulus** (torsion or twist)
- GDV is a life-threatening condition which requires emergency treatment.
- The stomach becomes distended with food and gas. This affects blood flow by pressing on the vena cava.
- The dilated stomach can twist so that the outflow is occluded. More gas is produced.
- The animal very quickly becomes shocked and will die if the condition is not corrected surgically.
- Symptoms include:
  - Unproductive retching (animal tries to vomit but is unable due to the volvulus).
  - Bloated abdomen. Often feels like a balloon on palpation.
  - Restlessness and discomfort
  - Respiratory distress
  - Shock
  - Death.
- Breeds which have a deep chest are most commonly affected because the stomach has more room to move (and therefore becomes twisted). Examples of commonly affected breeds are Great Danes, Wolfhounds, Greyhounds, Dobermans, Weimaraners.
- However, GDV can occur in any breed and sometimes in cats.
- GDV usually occurs when overfeeding is followed by exercise.
- First-aid treatment is aimed at reducing the pressure in the gas-filled stomach, and treating shock.
- Attempts should be made to pass a tube through the mouth into the stomach. If the stomach is not fully twisted the stomach tube will pass into the stomach and release some of the gas.
- If passage of a stomach tube is not possible the gas can be released by passing a wide-bore needle through the body wall into the distended stomach (**gastrocentesis**).

- Fluid therapy should begin as soon as possible. The animal will usually be in shock.
- Surgery to correct the disorder should then be performed as appropriate.
- Surgery involves untwisting the stomach and anchoring it to the abdominal wall (**gastropexy**) so that it is unable to twist again.
- In uncomplicated cases the stomach contents are removed using a stomach tube only.
- In more complicated cases the stomach may need to be opened (**gastrotomy**) in order to remove the contents. There is a risk of contamination and peritonitis so the prognosis is less favourable for these animals.
- If the torsion has been present for a few hours the blood supply to the stomach wall may have been compromised. Any devitalised parts of the stomach should be removed surgically. The prognosis is less favourable for these animals.
- Occasionally the spleen is involved in the torsion. If its blood supply has been compromised for any length of time the spleen may need to be removed (**splenectomy**).

Foreign body removal

Gastric foreign bodies:
- These are very common in both cats and dogs.
- Most gastric foreign bodies cause intermittent occlusion of gastric outflow.
- Symptoms may include:
  - Intermittent vomiting
  - Drooling
  - Haematemesis
  - Weight loss
- Some animals may have gastric foreign bodies for years without showing any clinical signs.
- Diagnosis is usually by radiography. Contrast studies such as barium swallows may be necessary to detect radiolucent foreign bodies.
- Treatment involves correcting any dehydration and removal of the foreign body by:
  - Inducing vomiting – only for recently ingested, smooth foreign bodies.
  - Endoscopic removal – using grasping attachment on endoscope
  - Surgery.
- Surgical treatment involves a ventral midline incision and opening the stomach (**gastrotomy**) to remove the foreign body.
- Care is taken to avoid spillage of gastric contents into the abdomen (risk of peritonitis).

Small intestinal foreign bodies

- These are also very common in dogs and cats.
- Symptoms are usually more dramatic because the small intestine is often completely occluded.
- Symptoms may include:
  - Acute, persistent vomiting of both food and liquids
  - Diarrhoea – seen in more distal obstructions.
  - Abdominal pain – adopting the 'praying' position
  - Anorexia, depression
  - Dehydration, shock
- Diagnosis can sometimes be made by palpation of the foreign body accompanied by loops of gas-filled gut. Radiography is often necessary to confirm the diagnosis. Contrast studies such as barium swallows may be necessary to detect radiolucent foreign bodies.
- Treatment involves:
  - Stabilising the animal's condition using fluid therapy and antibiosis.
  - Surgical removal of the foreign body.
- Surgery involves a ventral midline incision and opening the small intestine (**enterotomy**) to remove the foreign body.
- If there has been severe damage to the area of intestine where the object has been lodged it may be necessary to remove a section of intestine (**enterectomy**) and then reattachment of the healthy ends (**anastamosis**).
- A different form of foreign body obstruction is sometime seen in cats. This is obstruction with a **linear foreign body** (such as string or thread). In these cases the obstruction is initially only partial so there are symptoms of intermittent vomiting and abdominal pain. The linear foreign body causes the intestine to gather into pleats, and eventually may cut through the gut rather like a cheese wire. These foreign bodies are difficult to detect. Surgery to remove them often requires multiple enterotomies as pulling on the foreign body can cause the cheese wire effect.

Intussusception

- This condition is seen most frequently in younger animals, often following diarrhoea.
- The contracting piece of gut is forced into the lumen of the next section of gut rather like a telescope.
- The blood vessels are usually occluded so that the affected gut becomes devitalised.
- Symptoms are often similar to that a gut obstruction and may include:
  - Vomiting
  - Diarrhoea – often bloody

- Abdominal pain
- Diagnosis can be through palpation of the thickened gut or by radiography.
- Treatment involves:
  - Stabilising the animal's condition using fluid therapy and antibiosis.
  - Surgery to correct the disorder. This involves a ventral midline incision. Gentle traction is used to reduce the intussusception. If the damage is severe or the intussusception can't be reduced an enterectomy and anastamosis may be necessary.
  - The condition is prone to recurring. Some surgeons anchor the gut in folds so that the condition can't recur. This is called **enteroplication**.
  - The underling condition (often diarrhoea) must be treated to prevent recurrence.

Surgical diseases of the rectum and anus

Neoplasia:

- Tumours which may affect the rectum and anus include:
  - Lymphosarcoma
  - Adenocarcinoma
  - Leiomyosarcoma
  - Polyps, which are benign proliferations of tissue, can also cause problems in the rectum.
- Symptoms may include:
  - Dyschezia and tenesmus – caused by mechanical obstruction.
  - Haematochezia
  - Vomiting – particularly if the animal has become constipated
- Diagnosis may involve:
  - Palpation of a more distal mass
  - Radiography, possibly using contrast (barium enema) to highlight more proximal lesions.
  - Proctoscopy (using the endoscope per rectum)
  - Biopsy
- Treatment depends on what kind of mass has been detected and where it is situated.
- More proximal masses can be removed by laparotomy (ventral midline abdominal incision)
- More distal masses may be removed per rectum. This can involve a **rectal pull through** technique to carefully prolapse a small portion of rectum out through the anus so that surgery can be performed.
- Some tumours may respond to chemotherapy.
- Surgery to the rectum and anus is often contaminated with faecal material.

• Patients should be starved for 24 hours before surgery and should be given enemas before surgery to reduce faecal contamination of the surgical site.

Anal furunculosis:

• This disease is characterised by multiple chronic ulcerated sinuses and fistulous tracts in the peri-anal area.
• It occurs mainly in German Shepherds.
• The cause is unknown but factors which contribute may include dietary intolerance, immune mediated disease, anal gland disease and low tail carriage.
• Symptoms may include:
  • Dyschezia
  • Haematochezia
  • Excessive licking of the perineum
• Diagnosis is through physical examination, usually under general anaesthesia. Biopsy can be used to confirm the diagnosis.
• Treatment can be:
  • Medical – antibiotics and suppression of immune-mediated component using corticosteroids or cyclosporine.
  • Surgery – To remove all of the diseased tissue and often the anal glands. Surgery is difficult and associated with post-operative conditions such as recurrence, incontinence and stricture formation.

Anal sac disease:

• This is a very common condition in the dog, and is occasionally seen in the cat.
• May involve impaction, inflammation, infection, abscessation and occasionally neoplasia of the anal sacs.
• Impaction often leads to inflammation (**sacculitis**) and infection. Animals on low fibre diets or with narrow ducts tend to be predisposed to disease.
• Symptoms may include:
  • Foul smell
  • Licking at perineum
  • Scooting perineum along floor
  • Dyschezia
  • Abscessation appears as an infected ulcerated sinus next to the anus.
• Treatment can be:
  • Medical – gentle expression of both glands, appropriate antibiotic therapy, improved fibre content in diet. Some animals benefit from having the glands flushed and packed under general anaesthesia.
  • Surgical – Removal of the anal sacs (**anal sacculectomy**). Surgery is

reserved for animals with recurrent or unresponsive cases of anal sacculitis and in cases of anal sac neoplasia. The anal sac is pre-filled with viscous material so that it can be easily palpated by the surgeon. The animal is placed in sternal recumbency and the tail elevated. The entire anal sac is removed through the skin adjacent to the anus by careful dissection leaving the transected duct only

- Post-operative complications are uncommon but can include faecal incontinence (if sphincter muscles damaged), dyschezia and infected sinus tracts from remaining duct tissue.

Perineal hernia:

- This is a condition which usually affects middle-aged to elderly entire male dogs.
- It is an acquired hernia where the muscular support of the rectal wall fails so that the caudal rectum becomes stretched and weak.
- It is usually unilateral but the opposite wall will probably be weakened and may herniate in the future.
- It is thought that an enlarged prostate contributes to faecal tenesmus and predisposes animals to this condition.
- Symptoms may include:
  - Swelling to one side of anus, often quite large.
  - Dyschezia, tenesmus and constipation.
  - Occasional dropping of faeces without the animal being aware
  - Occasionally the bladder can become involved in the hernia resulting in urinary obstruction.
- Diagnosis is usually by physical examination and rectal palpation. Radiography may be necessary in cases where there is suspected bladder involvement and to assess the size of the prostate gland.
- Treatment may be:
  - Medical – increased dietary fibre, castration, occasional manual removal of impacted faeces from the hernia sac.
  - Surgical – The animal is placed in sternal recumbency and the tail elevated. An incision is made over the hernia. The hernia is reduced and support for the rectal wall is provided by suturing two or three of the adjacent muscles together over the rectal wall.
  - Possible post-operative complications include wound breakdown, incontinence, tenesmus, rectal prolapse and recurrence of the original condition.

NB The patient should be castrated to minimise the risk of recurrence.

3.8.04 **Urogenital**

What you need to learn

☙ You need to be able to outline common conditions of the urinary tract amenable to surgical correction and explain associated terms:
  ☙ cystotomy
  ☙ urethrotomy
  ☙ urethrostomy
  ☙ nephrotomy
  ☙ nephrectomy
  ☙ ovariohysterectomy
  ☙ castration
  ☙ Caesarian section.

Surgery of the kidneys

There are a number of reasons for performing surgery on the kidneys. These include kidney biopsy, tumour, removal of a kidney and removal of a kidney stone.

Nephrectomy:

• This is the removal of a kidney
• It may be necessary to treat:
  • Neoplasia
  • End stage kidney disease such as following obstruction, severe infection, trauma.
  • Renal haemorrhage which can't be controlled in any other way.
• Before attempting surgery the animal's renal function should be fully assessed to ensure that the animal is capable of recovering with a reasonable quality of life.
• An incision is made in the ventral midline and the kidney to be removed should be identified. The renal artery and vein are ligated. The ureter is transected at the level of the bladder neck.

Nephrotomy:

• This is surgically opening the kidney.
• It may be necessary to remove a kidney stone if the stone cannot be dissolved medically.
• An incision is made in the ventral midline and the kidney to be operated on should be identified. The renal artery and vein are temporarily occluded. The capsule is carefully opened and the surgeon dissects through the parenchyma to the renal pelvis and the stone is removed. The ureter should be flushed to check it is still patent and the kidney is sutured closed. The blood flow is restored through the artery and vein.

• Post-operatively the animal may have haematuria for a few days.

Surgery of the lower urinary tract

• Surgery of the ureters may be necessary to treat ureteral obstruction or rupture and to treat ectopic ureters.
• Surgery of the urethra may be necessary to treat urethral obstruction or rupture.
• Surgery of the bladder may be necessary for removal of bladder stones (cystic calculi), removal of bladder tumours or biopsy of the bladder wall among other things.

Urethrotomy:

• This is opening into the urethra temporarily.
• It is necessary for removal of calculi which block the urethra.
• It is more likely to be necessary in male animals because the urethra is longer and narrower than in females, and therefore more likely to become obstructed.
• In male dogs the usual incision site is just caudal to the os penis. The animal is placed in dorsal recumbency and the urethra is catheterised so that it is easily palpable. An incision is made through to the urethra and the calculus is removed. The urethra is flushed repeatedly to ensure all calculi have been removed. The urethra may be sutured or can be left to heal by second intention.
• Post-operative complications include marked haematuria and occasional stricture formation.

Urethrostomy:

• This is creating a permanent opening from the urethra to the outside of the body.
• It is performed in animals with recurrent urethral obstruction with calculi, severe penile trauma and following penile amputation in cases of urethral neoplasia.
• There are a number of sites where the urethrostomy can be performed. The most common sites are the pre-scrotal urethrostomy in dogs and the perineal urethrostomy in cats.
• The urethra is catheterised so that it is easily palpable. An incision is then made over the site of the urethrostomy. Distal tissues are removed and the urethra is opened out and surgically attached to the skin.

Cystotomy:

• This is surgical opening of the bladder.
• It is necessary for removal of bladder stones (**cystic calculi**), removal

of bladder tumours or biopsy of the bladder wall, etc.
- The animal is placed in dorsal recumbency. A ventral midline incision is made and the bladder exteriorised. An incision is made into the bladder and the procedure performed (biopsy, stone removal or lump removal). The bladder is the sutured closed.

Surgery of the reproductive tract

Ovariohysterectomy (neutering of the female animal, spaying):

- This is the surgical removal of the uterus and both ovaries in the female animal.
- This is performed for a number of reasons including:
  - Prevention of reproduction
  - Pyometra, mucometra, metritis (types of infection of the uterus)
  - Uterine prolapse, torsion or rupture.
  - To facilitate treatment of diseases such as diabetes mellitus which are affected by female hormones.
- In the bitch it is usually performed with the patient in dorsal recumbency through a ventral midline incision.
- In the queen it is usually performed through a left flank incision with the animal in right lateral recumbency.
- Once the incision has been made each ovary is located and elevated. The blood vessels and ligaments attached to each ovary are clamped and ligated, then transected. The cervix is then located, ligated and then transected. The abdomen is examined to check that there is no bleeding from the ligated stumps and the abdomen is closed.
- Possible complications include bleeding, recurrent oestrus due to retained ovarian tissue, urinary incontinence, weight gain and occasionally accidental ligation of a ureter.

Castration (neutering of the male animal):

- This is the surgical removal of both testicles.
- It is performed for a number of reasons including:
  - Prevention of reproduction and modification of behaviour
  - Neoplasia
  - Retained testicle (**cryptorchidism**)
  - Testicular trauma or torsion
  - Treatment of testosterone-related diseases such as peri-anal adenomas, perineal hernias and prostatic disease.
- In the dog the incision is made just cranial to the scrotum in the ventral midline, with the dog in dorsal recumbency. The testicle is pushed forwards into the wound. It can be removed within its tunic (closed castration) or the tunic can be opened (open castration). The

testicle is elevated and the spermatic cord is clamped, ligated and transected. This is repeated for the other testicle and the wound is sutured.
- In the cat an open castration is performed through an incision in each scrotum, usually with the cat in lateral recumbency.
- Complications include haemorrhage and weight gain.

Caesarian Section:

- This is the surgical removal of neonatal animals through a surgical incision into the uterus while the dam is anaesthetised.
- It is necessary during **dystocia** (difficulty in parturition) for a number of reasons:
  - Uterine inertia (failure of the uterus to contract)
  - Foetal oversize
  - Anatomical abnormality of the birth canal
  - Malformed foetus
- A ventral midline incision is made with the patient in dorsal recumbency, and the uterus is exteriorised. An incision is made into the body of the uterus. The foetuses are milked into the wound and removed. If possible the placenta is gently removed with each foetus. The offspring are handed to an assistant for resuscitation. Once the uterus is empty and the birth canal has been checked for foetuses the uterus is repaired. In some cases the uterus is removed as described for ovariohysterectomy. The abdominal wound is closed and the animal allowed to awaken.

3.8.05   Obstetric

What you need to learn

- You need to be able to outline the indications for Caesarian section:
  - general surgical principles
  - anaesthetic choice.
- Describe the care of neonates immediately following Caesarean section:
  - neonate care (see Level 2, 2.3.77/78).

Dystocia is the term used to describe difficulty in parturition.

- Dystocia can be obstructive or non-obstructive.
- **Obstructive dystocia:**
  - A puppy or kitten has become stuck in the birth canal (usually due to oversized foetus or narrow birth canal)
  - The dam will strain unproductively
  - If the pup/kitten can't be removed by careful traction a caesarian

section operation will be necessary.

- **Non-obstructive dystocia:**
  - The uterus is failing to contract strongly enough to expel the foetuses (known as primary uterine inertia).
  - The symptoms can vary. Usually the owner will be concerned because the dam has entered the first stage of labour but not progressed. There is sometimes a green discharge at the vulva indicating placental separation.
  - Various treatments are used to encourage the uterus to contract.
  - Caesarian section may be necessary if the foetuses become distressed.
- First-aid treatment involves keeping the dam comfortable and quiet while the situation is assessed by a veterinary surgeon. Placing the animal in a dark kennel will reduce stress.
- Older animals or those for which labour has been prolonged may require supportive treatment such as fluid therapy.
- If the foetuses have died there is a risk of infection and endotoxic shock, so the dam must be monitored carefully.
- A caesarian section should be recommended if the animal is failing to pass the foetuses or if there is health risk to the dam and the offspring without performing surgery.
- The anaesthetic must be selected carefully, taking care that:
  - The anaesthetic is short-acting so that the dam can be reunited with her offspring as soon as possible after the operation.
  - There is minimal effect of the anaesthetic on the offspring (such as respiratory and cardiovascular depression)
- For further information see anaesthesia 3.10.01-13
- The surgical procedure has been briefly described.

Care of the neonate following Caesarian section

Also see 2.3.77/8.

- Lack of oxygen (**hypoxia**) is the main cause of death of neonates at birth.
- Apnoea (not breathing) occurs fairly commonly in neonates.
- Neonates therefore often require resuscitation, particularly after delivery by caesarian section.
- The neonates should be removed from the foetal membranes.
- Fluid from the nose and mouth should be cleared. Suction or gentle swinging with the head down can help.
- Respiration can be encouraged by gentle chest compressions.
- A respiratory stimulant such as doxapram may be administered (usually under the tongue).
- Artificial respiration can be performed by blowing gently into the mouth and nose of the neonate.

- External cardiac massage may be used if the heart is not beating.
- Once the neonates are breathing well they should be kept warm in a lined box until they are returned to the dam.
- The neonates should be examined carefully for congenital defects such as cleft palate, umbilical/inguinal hernias or obvious deformities.
- **Fading puppy/kitten syndrome** can result in high mortality rates. Signs of general weakness can appear within hours of birth. The animals are usually dehydrated and fail to suck. Treatment is unrewarding and the puppy or kitten usually dies. Possible causes are parvovirus infection, low birth weight, trauma during parturition, and congenital abnormalities.

Management of the orphaned newborn

- Neonates can become orphaned for a number of reasons including illness or death of the mother; inability of the mother to cope with feeding the whole litter or simply being rejected by the mother.
- Hand rearing orphans can be extremely difficult.
- A selection of commercial kitten and puppy milk substitute are available. Examples are Welpi® and Cimicat®. Initially the orphans will need small amounts of concentrated milk substitute. As the animal grows a greater volume of more diluted milk can be provided.
- Special feeding bottles with small rubber teats are available for feeding orphans.
- The orphan will need feeding every two hours including through the night.
- The orphan will need to be encouraged to pass urine and faeces. The mother would do this by licking the perineum of the puppy/kitten. When hand-rearing this can be simulated by wiping the perineum gently with a moist cotton bud. This should be done after every feed. Failure to do this can result in failure to thrive and even death.
- It is sometimes possible to find a foster mother for the orphans.
- A foster mother can be a mother:
  - who has lost her own litter but is still lactating
  - who has plenty milk and only a small litter
  - whose own offspring have been weaned but who still has plenty milk.
- Care must be taken to ensure the orphans are not rejected by the foster mum as injury can result.
- Before introducing the orphans attempts should be made to rub the smell of the bitch onto the pups/kittens. This can be done by allowing the orphans to sleep on a blanket belonging to the bitch.

What you need to learn

☙ You need to be able to outline common conditions of the respiratory tract amenable to surgical correction and explain associated terms:
- ☙ tracheotomy
- ☙ pneumothorax
- ☙ thorocotomy
- ☙ collapsed trachea
- ☙ ruptured diaphragm.

Surgery of the upper respiratory tract

Collapsing trachea:

- This is a common condition in toy breeds of dog, particularly the Yorkshire Terrier.
- The tracheal cartilages are weakened and the muscular part of the trachea becomes stretched and flaccid.
- Symptoms typically include a dry chronic, dry, 'honking' cough. Overweight dogs are generally more seriously affected.
- Diagnosis is through the clinical signs and radiography.
- Medical treatment can involve:
  - Bronchodilators, antibiotics, expectorants, rest.
- Surgical treatment can involve:
  - Folding (plication) of the dorsal muscular part of the trachea
  - External prosthetic support of the tracheal cartilages.
- Surgery is often avoided because although 80–90% of cases are successful, the unsuccessful cases tend to die from post-operative complications.

Tracheotomy:

- This involves creating a temporary opening into the trachea.
- It may be performed for a number of reasons:
  - To relieve upper respiratory tract obstruction (emergency procedure)
  - To aid in the removal of respiratory secretions
  - To provide a route for inhaled anaesthetic gases during complicated oro-facial surgery.
- During the emergency procedure there is not time to surgically prepare the area.
- The animal is placed in dorsal recumbency and a longitudinal incision is made caudal to the larynx. The trachea is elevated and an incision made transversely between tracheal rings. A tracheotomy tube is placed into the trachea and secured in place.

- Care must be taken that the end of the tube is kept clean. Inspired air should be humidified.

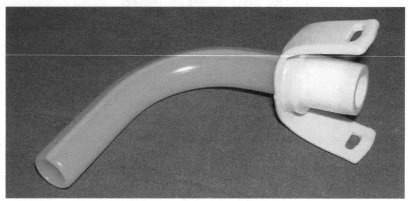

Figure 8.3 Tracheotomy tube.

Surgery of the lower respiratory tract and thorax

Thoracotomy:

- This is creating a surgical opening into the thoracic cavity.
- Great care must be taken with the anaesthetic for these patients as they require artificial respiration.
- Reasons for performing a thoracotomy may include:
  - Removal of pulmonary abscesses, cysts, tumours or bullae (air filled pockets)
  - Removal of a lung lobe (due to torsion, consolidation or neoplasia)
  - Cardiac surgery
- The thorax can be opened in a number of ways:
  - Sternotomy – splitting and retracting each side of the sternum.
  - Entry through the intercostal muscles between the ribs

Treatment of pneumothorax

- Occasionally a pneumothorax can be caused by the presence of blebs and bullae within the lungs. These are air-filled spaces which can leak air into the pleural cavity, causing a pneumothorax.
- This condition is initially treated by inserting an indwelling chest drain for 2–3 days and drawing off the air.
- If this is unsuccessful a thoracotomy is performed. The bleb or bulla is identified and the affected portion of lung is surgically removed.

Ruptured diaphragm:

- Tears in the diaphragm are usually seen as a result of a road traffic accident.

- Tears in the diaphragm should be repaired as soon as possible as complications can include the movement of abdominal contents through the tear into the thorax.
- The animal is very carefully anaesthetised. Patients are often dyspnoeic and may require artificial respiration. The patient is placed in dorsal recumbency and a ventral midline abdominal incision made. Any herniated abdominal contents should be replaced in the abdomen and the defect in the diaphragm is sutured closed.
- The surgery causes a pneumothorax to develop as air from the atmosphere can travel through the diaphragmatic tear into the thorax. For this reason a chest drain is often necessary to remove air from the pleural space post-operatively.

3.8.07   Fractures

What you need to learn

- You need to be able to describe the classification of fractures:
  - complete
  - incomplete
  - simple
  - compound
  - complicated
  - comminuted
  - multiple
  - pathological
  - acquired.
- Outline the causes and signs and common sites of fractures.
- Outline the principles of bone healing.
- Describe the principles of fracture fixation.
- Outline factors in selection of a method of fracture treatment.
- Describe types and limitations of splints.
  - flexible
  - rigid
  - moulded
  - extension.
- Describe the principles and application of a Robert Jones bandage.
- Describe the First Aid treatment of an animal with a suspected fracture (see Level 2, 2.4.33):
  - handling
  - restraint
  - medication
  - reduce further injury.

Classification of fractures

Fractures can be:

- **Complete** – the bone is fractured across both cortices.
- **Incomplete** (or **greenstick**) – the bone is fractured across one cortex only.
- **Simple** – the bone is fractured across one line without damage to the surrounding areas. This is further classified into the direction of the line – spiral, oblique, or transverse.
- **Compound (open)** – the broken bone penetrates through the skin.
- **Complicated** – there is other serious injury involved, eg rib causing a punctured lung.
- **Comminuted** – there are multiple fracture lines and multiple fragments.
- **Multiple** – there is more than one fractured bone.
- **Pathological** – a fracture arising from normal use, of a diseased bone.
- **Acquired** – a fracture resulting from trauma.
- **Avulsion** – a bone prominence is detached as a result of the force of a muscle or tendon, eg avulsion of tibial tuberosity.
- **Depressed** – a fragment of bone is driven below its normal; this usually occurs in the skull.

Causes of fractures

Fractures can be caused by **direct trauma**, eg a road traffic accident, by **indirect trauma**, when an excessive force is used on the bone, or by **pathological disease**, eg tumours, or calcium or vitamin D deficiency.

Signs of fractures

The signs of a fracture are:

- loss of function
- pain
- swelling
- heat
- bone may be visible or deformed
- crepitus
- bruising
- abnormal movement.

Common sites of fractures

- physeal (Salter Harris fractures, these are graded)
- diaphyseal

• epiphyseal
• condylar
• supracondylar.

Bone healing

When a bone fractures, blood vessels and the periosteum are torn (Stage 1), which leads to a haematoma developing at the ends of the fracture, in between it and for a short distance along the side of the bone ends – see Figure 8.4.

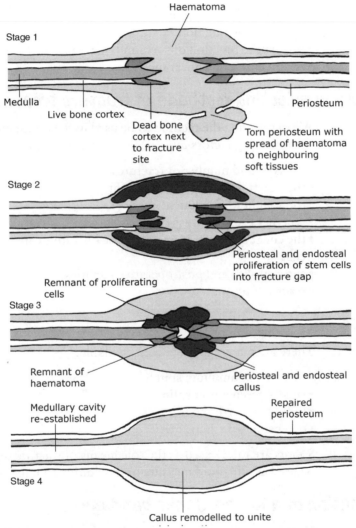

Figure 8.4 Bone fracture.

Granulation tissue, stem cells and new blood vessels replace the haematoma (stage 2).

A callus is formed around the ends of the bone. This callus eventually becomes harder as a result of the higher content of bone and cartilage. When the bone ends meet this is known as clinical union (stage 3).

Haversian remodelling begins to eliminate the callus and new bone is produced. It is during this process that if the bone is not aligned correctly then re-shaping of the bone will occur (stage 4).

Principles of fracture fixation

The principles of fracture fixation are to:

• encourage bone healing
• restore bone function
• restore the function of surrounding tissues
• regain cosmetic appearance.

Factors in selecting methods of fracture treatment

When selecting the method to be used in the treatment of a fracture the following factors must be taken into account:

• the type and number of fractures
• the age and activity of the patient
• the weight of the patient
• whether the fracture is open or closed
• the client's co-operation with post-operative care
• cost
• surgical skill and post-operative facilities
• return of normal function.

Splints

There are many types of splint available.

• flexible – aluminium splints
• rigid – green gutter splints
• moulded – orthoboard
• extension – metal frames.

Splints are rarely used as the sole means of fracture repair. They can be used as a first-aid measure or in addition to internal fixation.

Application of a Robert Jones bandage

The principle of a Robert Jones bandage is to provide support and protection (pre- and post-operatively) or as a means of treatment.
• The affected limb should be uppermost.
• The affected limb may be clipped.
• Apply stirrup strips to the cranial and caudal areas of the limb.

- Pad the toes with cotton wool.
- Apply cotton wool or Soffban® from the mid-femur to the toes (do not include the toes) and ensure the third and fourth digits are visible.
- Apply a layer of conforming bandage over the padding and place the stirrup strips over the dressing.
- Steps 4 and 5 should be repeated twice more.
- A territory layer is then applied, either Elastoplast or self-conforming material, eg Vetrap®.
- The bandage should be three times the diameter of the limb and when flicked should sound like flicking a water melon.

For first aid treatments, see Level 2, 2.4.33.

3.8.08 External fixation

What you need to learn

- You need to be able to describe external methods of fracture fixation:
  - splints
  - extension splints.
- Casting materials are:
  - plaster of Paris
  - polyurethane
  - resins
  - fibreglass
  - thermoplastic polymers.
- Outline the indications for use and the general advantages and disadvantages of external immobilisation.
- Outline the preparation and application of casting materials.
- Describe the advantages/disadvantages of alternative casting materials:
  - species variations
  - size
  - weight of animal.
- Describe the maintenance and removal of the various casting materials.

External methods of fracture fixation

The following materials can be used to provide external fixation:
- plaster of Paris
- polyurethane
- resins
- fibreglass

- thermoplastic polymers
- flexible splints – aluminium splints
- rigid splints – green gutter splints
- moulded splints – orthoboard
- extension splints – metal frames.

Indications for external immobilisation

External immobilisation is indicated:

- to provide first-aid support and immobilisation of distal limbs
- to provide extra support and immobilisation following internal fixation of distal limbs
- to provide patient comfort
- to decease soft tissue damage
- if internal fixation is too costly
- if there is a lack of orthopaedic surgery experience.

Advantages and disadvantages of external immobilisation

Advantages of external immobilisation are:

- It is quick and simple to apply.
- It is cheaper than internal fixation.
- It is suitable for greenstick fractures.
- Less orthopaedic skill is needed.
- It can be used for primary stabilisation.
- It can aid internal fixation.

Disadvantages of external immobilisation are:

- It is not suitable for open fractures.
- Plaster of Paris is heavy.
- It cannot be used for fractures of the humerus or femur as the cast or splint acts as a pendulum.
- Bone alignment may be poor if it is used as the sole means of fracture fixation.

Preparation and application of casting materials

Prepare all equipment and have it close to hand before starting to apply the cast.

- The patient will require general anaesthesia to allow closed fracture reduction.
- Wear gloves when applying the material.
- Clip the limb using electric clippers if the patient has long hair.
- Apply stirrups to the cranial and caudal sides if using fibreglass material.

- Apply a layer of cast stockinette.
- Apply two layers of cast soft padding.
- Remember to provide extra padding to areas of thin tissues or bony prominences.
- Apply a layer of conforming bandage.
- If using plaster of Paris unroll a short amount, place in water (the warmer the water the shorter the setting time) and expel excess water.
- The overlap of plaster of Paris is approximately 50%.
- Apply to the patient, beginning at the toes and working proximally (the third and fourth toes should be visible).
- Once sufficient layers are applied, smooth and mould the cast.
- If using fibreglass, soak the roll in warm water and apply as for plaster of Paris.
- Apply two or three layers of fibre glass depending on the size of the dog, apply the cast material quickly, as it sets in approximately 5 minutes.
- Apply a layer of Elastoplast® or self-conforming bandage and invert the stirrups and stick onto this outer layer.

Casting materials available are:

- plaster of Paris
- polyurethane
- resins
- fibreglass
- thermoplastic polymers.

The manufacturer's instructions should always be read carefully before preparing any casting material.

Advantages and disadvantages of casting materials

Advantages of casting materials include the facts that they can be used on most cats and dogs and they are suitable for thin and average weight patients.

Disadvantages of casting materials include the facts that they are unsuitable for small furry animals and birds and large dogs may find the cast heavy and cumbersome particularly if plaster of Paris is used. They are unsuitable for overweight or heavy patients as the three remaining limbs may suffer carrying the extra weight.

Maintenance and removal of the cast

The following need to be monitored regularly until removal:

- Check there are no smells; these would indicate infection.
- Check the cast is not over-tight.

- Check the cast is not too loose or it may slip down or come off.
- Check there is no swelling above or below the cast; this would indicate that it was too tight.
- Check there are no pressure sores – red, sore and ulcerated areas. Some are seen at the top or bottom of the cast, others will only be visible on removal. Check for these at each re-dress. Use extra padding in bony/thin-skinned areas.
- Check the toes are not cold; this indicates poor circulation and an over-tight cast.
- Check there is no weeping of the tissues or exudate around and under the cast; this would indicate infection.
- Check there is no redness or heat around the surrounding areas; this indicates inflammation or infection.
- Check for signs of pain or anxiety.
- Ensure that the cast is dry at all times; a wet cast will be cold, will induce sore skin and will not provide adequate support. Change the cast immediately if it becomes wet. A plastic bag or an old drip bag can be placed over the cast with an elastic band.
- Ensure that the patient can walk and rest correctly.
- Check with the veterinary surgeon if there are limits on the amount of exercise or movement and adhere to this.

Care of the cast

To ensure that the cast is cared for correctly:

- Protection – keep it dry, place a plastic bag over the cast.
- Exercise – limit to lead exercise only.
- Observation – monitor the cast as described.

Removal of the cast

When removing the cast use an oscillating saw or plasters shears. A mask should be worn. The lateral and medial sides should be cut and then the cast should be removed.

3.8.09   Internal fixation

What you need to learn

- You need to be able to state the general advantages and disadvantages of internal fixation.
- Describe the principles, use and nursing of internal/external fixation:
  - ASIF/AO
  - bone plates
  - screws
  - pins

☘ wires
☘ Kirshner Ehmer apparatus/Ilazirov fixator
☘ Ilazirov fixator.

☘ Describe the commonly used orthopaedic implants, internal and external fixators:
  ☘ ASIF/AO
  ☘ bone plates
  ☘ screws
  ☘ pins
  ☘ wires
  ☘ Kurshner–Ehmer apparatus\Ilazirov fixator.

☘ Describe the care and storage of orthopaedic implants (see Surgical nursing – instrument care).

☘ Outline the aftercare required by both nurse and owner of patients following fracture repair using internal/external fixation:
  ☘ exercise
  ☘ wound care
  ☘ self-mutilation prevention
  ☘ fixator movement.

☘ Describe the commonly used orthopaedic instruments, their care and storage (see Surgical nursing – instrument care):
  ☘ packing
  ☘ sterilisation
  ☘ storage.

☘ Describe the factors that influence the rate of fracture healing and the complications of internal fixation:
  ☘ fixator movement
  ☘ inappropriate use of fixator
  ☘ animal variation due to lifestyle.

☘ Describe callus formation and how the rate of fracture healing can be assessed.

☘ Describe the terms malunion, delayed union, non-union and osteomyelitis.

Advantages of internal fixation

Internal fixation has many advantages over external techniques.

- It allows accurate reduction.
- The fixation is stable.
- It promotes early use of the limb.
- It is suitable for most fracture sites.
- A greater range and type of fractures can be repaired.
- The patient cannot interfere with it.
- After-care is reduced.

Disadvantages of internal fixation

There are, however, disadvantages to internal fixation.

• Open reduction is usually required.
• Strict asepsis is needed to prevent infection.
• Orthopaedic skill is needed.
• It is expensive.
• It incurs soft tissue damage.

Association of the Study of Internal Fixation (ASIF)/AO

Bone plates (dynamic compression plates) are specially made to produce compression across a fracture line.

• They have an oval hole as opposed to a round hole.
• They can be used as compression plates, buttress plates, or neutrilisation plates.

Nonself tapping or tapped screws are used with these plates and can be identified by the hexagonal screw head. They are suitable for use in cats and dogs.

Procedure for applying tapping screws into ASIF bone plates:

• drill
• countersink
• measure
• tap
• insert.

Traditional bone plates

Bone plates, along with self-tapping screws, are used to hold the bone ends or fragments together. They are available in various lengths (indicated by the number of holes) and in various hole diameters. The diameter of the holes determines the screw size that will be accepted, for example a 2.7 mm bone plate will accept 2.7 mm screws.

These bone plates are suitable for use in both cats and dogs.

Screws

Screws are used with bone plates to hold the plate in place. They can also be used by themselves as a lag screw. Screws are available in various lengths and diameters and as cancellous or cortical screws.

Screws are suitable for use in cats and dogs.

Pins (intramedullary pins)

These are placed down the medulla cavity of a bone and across the fracture line to hold the bone ends or fragments together. They are suitable for use in cats and dogs.

Two pins of the same diameter should be available in a sterile pack; one is used for internal fixation and the second is used for measurement against a radiograph.

Wire

Wire can be used alongside internal fixation to improve stability (cerclage/hemicerclage wiring). It can be used on its own, eg to wire a fractured jaw (inter-fragmentary wiring). It can also be used in a a a figure of eight to counteract the pull of muscles, tendons and ligaments, (tension band wiring).

Wire is available in various diameters and is suitable for use in both cats and dogs.

Kirschner wires

These wires are used to repair fractures of the epiphysis (growth plate) and other small fractures. One end has a trocar point and the other is flattened in a diamond shape. Kirschner wires are available in various diameters and are suitable for use in cats and dogs.

Arthrodesis wires

Arthrodesis wires can be used as intramedullary pins in small bones. Both ends have a trocar point and the wires are available in a few diameters but all small sizes. They are suitable for use in both cats and dogs.

Kirschner–Ehmer apparatus/Ilazirov fixator

Pins are placed through the skin and through either one or both cortices of the bone. The pins are attached to an external frame, giving the appearance of a scaffold. This technique is used in complicated or open fractures. It is suitable for use in cats and dogs.

Commonly used implants

External fixators

External fixators comprise connecting bars, clamps (single or double), pins either threaded at one end, threaded in the middle or with a trocar point at one end.

They can be applied as unilateral (uniplanar or unilateral biplanar) or bilateral (uniplanar and bilateral biplanar).

A dynamic compression plate (DCP) is shown in Figure 8.5 with oval holes.

Tapped screws, either cancellous or cortical, have a hexagonal screw head. A hexagonal screwdriver is required to apply these screws.

The tap is used to pre-tap the hole before the screw is applied. This

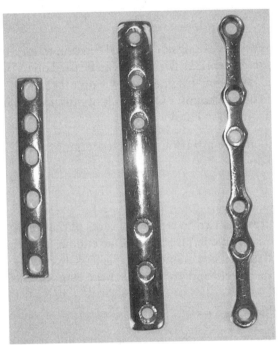

Figure 8.5 Bone plates: Dynamic compression plate, Venables plate and Sherman plate.

prevents micro-fractures as the screw is not cutting it is own thread as self-tapping screws do.

Bone plates such as the Venables plate (Figure 8.4) are traditional (not ASIF). They use self-tapping screws, either cancellous or cortical, and round holes.

A Sherman plate is shown in Figure 8.4. This type of plate uses self-tapping screws, either cancellous or cortical. It is a traditional technique (not ASIF) with round holes.

The Sherman plate is an indented plate, making it particularly weak.

Finger plates can be used on the metacarpels/metatarsals. Acetabular plates can be used in surgery on the acetabulum.

Screws

Screws can be of various types.

- **Self-tapping screws** do not require tapping as they cut their own thread when inserted using a screwdriver. This can cause micro-fractures and the fit may not be as snug as it is with tapping screws. These are identified by the flat or Phillips screw head.
- **Tapped screws** require to be tapped using a special piece of equipment called a tap. These screws provide a snug fit and prevent micro-fractures. They can be identified by their hexagonal head.
- **Cancellous screws** are used in the soft spongy bone found in the ends of long bones. The pitch is much wider than that of a cortical screw, which aids their grip in the spongy bone. They can be either partially or fully threaded.
- **Cortical screws** are used in hard bone, eg the midshaft of bones. The pitch is much narrower to provide a good secure fit with the hard bone. They can be partially or fully threaded.

Pins

The **Steinmann pin** is used as an intramedullary pin in long-bone fractures. Both ends have a trocar point; one end may also be threaded.

Kirshner wires are used to repair fractures of the epiphysis (growth plate) and other small fractures. One end is a trocar and the other is flattened in a diamond shape.

Arthrodesis wires can be used as intramedullary pins in small bones. Both ends have a trocar point.

Wire is made from stainless steel and is used for tension band wiring, intrafragmentary wiring and cerclage wiring. It is usually available on a reel.

Care and storage of orthopaedic implants

See 3.9.03.

After-care needed from nurses

- The patient is normally restricted to cage rest but instructions given by the veterinary surgeon on weight bearing, exercise limitations and rest should be followed.
- Examine the wound daily for redness, swelling, discharges and suture placement.
- Prevent self-mutilation.
- Post-operative radiographs are usually required to check adequate fixation has been achieved.
- Provide adequate analgesia (under the instructions of the veterinary surgeon).

- Administer any medication such as antibiotics.
- Monitor for signs of pain and restlessness.
- Monitor temperature, pulse and respiration rate and pattern.
- Keep the patient dry and comfortable.
- Take dogs out for short frequent walks if indicated.
- Cat litter can be supplied in the corner of the kennel on newspaper so that the cat does not have to climb into a litter tray.

After-care needed from the client

- The animal is normally restricted to house rest with short lead walks to urinate and defaecate. Any instructions from the veterinary surgeon on weight bearing, exercise limitations and rest must be fully explained to the owner.
- The client should examine the wound daily for redness, swelling and discharges.
- The owner must prevent self-mutilation. Elizabethan collars could be supplied; paws may be bandaged. Other pets in the household should be discouraged from licking or attacking the wound.
- Regular post-operative checks are required to examine stability, eg in external fixators the pins can be prone to movement or plates can bend. Radiographs will be performed periodically to inspect callus formation and healing.
- Instruct the owner on any medication.

Commonly used orthopaedic instruments

See 3.9.03.

Rate of fracture healing

The following will delay healing:

- movement of external fixator pins, bending of plates or snapping or pins
- the use of the wrong type of internal or external fixation, eg a bone plate used in the presence of infection (from a open fracture), external fixation would have been more appropriate
- inappropriate exercise
- owner non-compliance, eg patient is not receiving medication or exercise is not restricted
- poor diet
- infection.

Complications of internal fixation

Internal fixation can have complications associated with it.

- Inadequate orthopaedic skill may create poor alignment of the bone

ends.
- The wrong type of fixation may be used or necessary equipment may not be available.
- Osteomyelitis may develop.
- The implant may fail to work.

Callus formation

See 3.8.07.

Assessing fracture healing

There should be regular post-operative checks to examine weight bearing, limb function and pain. Also, regular post-operative radiographs should be taken to examine callus formation and the implant.

Problems with healing of a fracture fall into several categories.

- **Malunion** describes a fracture that heals in poor alignment caused by inadequate reduction and/or fixation.
- **Delayed union** occurs when clinical union is not achieved within the expected time (12–16 weeks) ie healing progress is slow.
- **Non union** describes the complete failure of the fractured ends of a bone to unite.
- **Osteomyelitis** can occur; this is an infection of the bone.
- **Clinical union** describes the state when the fractured ends of the bone have united correctly.

3.8.10   Dislocations

What you need to learn

- You need to be able to describe the terms luxation and subluxation.
- Outline the common luxations and describe their first aid treatment:
  - carpus/tarsus
  - hip
  - elbow
  - stifle (patella)
  - restraint
  - handling
  - reduction of further injury.
- Describe open and closed reduction of luxations and outline their postoperative management (see Surgical nursing – Theatre practice):
  - preparation for operation
  - instruments

❀ medication
❀ manipulation.

❀ Describe the care of a patient following reduction of a luxation and outline the possible complications which may follow treatment of luxations.

Luxation (dislocation) is the complete displacement of a bone from its normal position involving a joint. It can be either acquired or congenital.

Sub-luxation (sub-dislocation) is the incomplete displacement of a bone from its normal position involving a joint. It can also be acquired or congenital.

Common luxations

Common positions where luxations occur are:

• carpus joint
• tarsus joint
• hip joint
• elbow joint
• stifle joint (patella).

First-aid treatment

• Restrain the patient with care, avoid handling the affected joint.
• Prevent further injury of the dislocated joint by providing stabilisation (splints or slings).
• Provide the patient with cage rest until reduction can be performed.

Open and closed reduction

See 3.6.06 and 3.9.07.

Following reduction of a luxation

After reduction of a luxation these procedures should be followed.

• Perform post-operative radiography to confirm reduction of the luxation.
• Restrict exercise.
• Apply slings or supporting bandages.
• Administer medication, eg analgesia, antibiotics.
• Monitor for signs of pain and restlessness.
• Monitor temperature, pulse and respiration rate and pattern.
• Keep the patient dry and comfortable.
• Take dogs out for short frequent walks if indicated.

• Cat litter can be supplied in the corner of the kennel on newspaper so the cat does not have to climb into a litter tray.
• Prevent self-mutilation by the patient.

Complications after luxation

After a luxation there can be complications:

• re-luxation
• damage to surrounding nerves and soft tissue
• infection.

3.8.11 Ophthalmic

What you need to learn

☙ You need to be able to outline the common conditions of the eye amenable to surgery:
  ☙ eyeball prolapse
  ☙ comeal damage
  ☙ enucleation
  ☙ perforation
  ☙ cataracts
  ☙ tumours
  ☙ entropion/ectropion
  ☙ distichiasis
  ☙ prolapsed meibomian/harderian gland.
☙ Describe principles of patient and instrument preparation for ophthalmic surgery.

Eyeball Prolapse

• This is anterior displacement of the globe so that the eyelids are not able to close over it.
• It is usually associated with blunt trauma such as an RTA.
• In some brachycephalic breeds with prominent eye (such as the Pekinese) very minor trauma can cause prolapse of the globe.
• This condition requires very prompt treatment if the eye is to be saved.
• Cold compresses should be applied to the eye by the owner while the animal is transported to the practice. This reduces swelling.
• The globe can rarely be replaced with manual pressure alone so surgery must be performed if the animal is well enough for a general anaesthetic.
• A lateral canthotomy is performed. This involves making a transverse cut at the lateral canthus. This enables the globe to be

replaced to its normal position. The cut is then sutured. Usually the eyelids are then sutured closed over the eye for 10–14 days.
- Possible complications are infection and wound breakdown. It is not uncommon for the patient's vision to be permanently damaged due to stretching of the optic nerve.

Corneal Injury

- Corneal injury is very common in small animal practice.
- It can range in severity from superficial scratches through to perforations of the cornea.
- Corneal ulceration can occur following trauma (often scratch from cat claw), foreign body and eyelash abnormality (entropion, distichiasis).
- Injury to the cornea can be detected using the dye Fluorescein.
- Superficial injuries are treated with topical treatment (antibiotic) only.
- Deep lacerations should be examined under general anaesthesia. Topical medication should not be used if a perforating injury is suspected.
- Tears can be repaired using very fine suture material.
- Foreign bodies should be removed with great care under general anaesthetic and any tears repaired.
- A **third eyelid flap** can be performed to provide protection for the healing cornea. This involves suturing the third eyelid to the dorso-lateral conjunctiva.
- **Conjunctival pedicle flaps** can also be used to provide protection for the healing cornea where there is a large defect. This involves sliding a strip of conjunctiva with an intact blood supply over the defect and suturing it in place.

Cataracts

- A cataract is an opacity of the lens.
- In more complete cataracts the vision may be severely affected or lost altogether.
- Surgical treatment may be necessary in these more severely affected animals.
- This may involve:
  - Lens extraction (lendectomy) – the attachments of the lens are broken down and either the whole lens or the anterior capsule is removed.
  - Phaecoemulsification – ultrasonic breakdown of the affected part of the lens followed by the removal of the cataract material through a small corneal incision.
- Care must be taken that only animals which have still got normal

retinal function and which are not suffering from uveitis are selected for this surgery.
- Medical treatment is ineffective.

Entropion

- Inversion of the eyelid with in-rolling of the eyelashes so that they cause corneal irritation.
- Symptoms include:
  - Blepharospasm
  - Epiphora
  - Keratitis, corneal oedema and corneal ulceration
- Commonly affects breeds with lots of facial skin folds such as Shar-peis, Chows, Clumber spaniels, Rottweilers, Golden retrievers and numerous other breeds.
- Entropion is sometimes secondary to painful ocular conditions which cause blepharospasm. Correcting the primary condition results in resolution of the entropion.
- Treatment of primary entropion is usually a surgical procedure during which a small strip of skin is excised to return the eyelid to its normal position.

Ectropion

- Eversion of the eyelid, often related to the conformation of the breed.
- Breeds which are commonly affected include St Bernards, Bloodhounds, Bassett Hounds, Mastiffs and other similar breeds.
- Causes fewer problems than entropion as the eyelashes are not in contact with the cornea.
- Can result in keratitis and chronic conjunctivitis in severe cases as the animal is unable to closes its eyelids properly.
- In severe cases surgery may be necessary to correct the condition.
- Surgery involves removing skin from around the eye to reduce the length of the eyelids.

Distichiasis

- Common congenital abnormality in dogs
- Extra cilia (eyelashes) emerge from the meibomian glands on the eyelid margin.
- Symptoms include:
  - Epiphora
  - Keratitis, corneal oedema and corneal ulceration
  - Blepharospasm
- Treatment may involve

- Plucking the cilia – temporary measure as these will regrow
- Electrolysis
- Surgical excision of the affected strip of meibomian glands
- A similar but less common condition occurs where **ectopic cilia** grow from the palpebral conjunctiva. This condition is treated with surgery to remove the haired area of conjunctiva.

Prolapse of the nictitans gland

- Prolapse of the nititans gland so that it appears as a smooth red swelling at the medial canthus.
- Also known as '**Cherry Eye**'.
- Commonly affects breeds including Bulldogs, Mastiffs, Rottweilers, American Cocker Spaniels.
- Treatment involves suturing the gland back into place. **NB** the gland should not be removed as it contributes to the tear film.

Enucleation

- This is the surgical removal of the globe.
- It is performed for a number of reasons including:
  - Neoplasia (melanoma, malignant melanoma, squamous cell carcinoma).
  - Severe trauma or infection
  - Pain relief where the vision has already been lost (eg non-responsive glaucoma)
- Enucleation is usually performed by removing the globe and all the other contents of the orbit. This ensures that there is no spillage of infection or tumour material into the surrounding tissues.
- The eyelids are sutured closed. An incision is made all the way round the eyelids. The tissues are carefully dissected away within the conjunctival sac. Eventually the only remaining attachment is the optic nerve and blood vessel. This is clamped, ligated and transected. The wound is then closed. **NB** packing material should not be used to pack the hole as this acts as a source of infection.

Preparation for ophthalmic surgery

- Ophthalmic surgery occasionally requires the eye to be completely still. An example is cataract surgery. Neuromuscular blocking agents may be necessary for this type of surgery.
- Some patients may require treatment with atropine to reduce tear production during ophthalmic surgery.
- See 3.9.03 for instrument preparation for ophthalmic surgery.

3.8.12   Aural

What you need to learn

☙ You need to be able to outline common conditions of the ear amenable to surgery:
  ☙ aural haematoma
  ☙ lateral wall and vertical canal resection
  ☙ ablation.

Aural haematoma

Also see 3.8.02.

- This is the development of a blood-filled pocket within the pinna.
- It is usually caused by head shaking which indicates damage to a small blood vessel. This vessel then bleeds into the space between the cartilage and the skin.
- The haematoma can be left to resolve naturally but this takes some time and often results in a distorted 'cauliflower' ear. There is also a risk of infection if left untreated.
- Surgical treatment involves making an incision on the internal surface of the pinna which is from end to end of the haematoma. The blood is therefore released. Sutures are the used to close the dead space which was created by the haematoma. There are many methods in use to reduce this dead space such as stitching buttons, X-ray plate or lengths of plastic piping onto the ear. Some surgeons prefer to use thick suture material only. The animal should be maintained on antibiotics until the sutures are removed after 10–14 days.
- Any underlying condition (usually otitis externa) should be treated to prevent further head shaking.

Lateral wall resection (LWR)

- This is used to treat animals with chronic persistent otitis externa.
- It is indicated particularly in animals which have chronically stenosed (narrowed) canals.
- The purpose of the LWR is to widen the canal and improve air flow. It should only be performed if all efforts at medical treatment of the condition have failed.
- Surgery involves removing the lateral wall of the external ear canal so that the vertical canal opens directly to the skin.
- Post-operative complications include infection and wound breakdown.

Vertical canal ablation (VCA)

- This is used for treatment of chronic persistent otitis externa.

- It is indicated particularly in animals which have chronically stenosed (narrowed) canals.
- It involves complete removal of the vertical canal. The aim is to remove all the diseased tissue so this procedure should be avoided if there is infection in the middle or inner ear.
- Post-operative complications include infection and wound breakdown.

Total ear canal ablation (TECA)

- This is used for treatment of chronic otitis externa and media.
- It is indicated particularly in animals which have chronically stenosed (narrowed) canals.
- It involves complete removal of both the vertical and horizontal canal.
- The aim is to remove all the diseased tissue.
- A bulla osteotomy (removal of the lining of the tympanic bulla) is often also performed.
- Hearing is severely impaired in the ear following this procedure.
- Post-operative complications include infection and wound breakdown.

3.8.13 Dental

What you need to learn

- You need to be able to describe common dental diseases.
- Describe the meaning of dental calculus and explain its formation.
- Outline the removal and prevention of dental calculus in dogs and cats:
  - hand scaling
  - mechanical scaling and polishing
  - ultrasonic scaling.
- Outline the care of patients during a scaling operation and describe their aftercare:
  - anaesthetic considerations
  - feeding and medication.
- Identify common dental instruments and describe their care and maintenance.

Common dental diseases

- Gingivitis
- Stomatitis
- Periodontitis

• Abscesses
• Feline neck lesions (resorptive lesions)
• Caries

Dental calculus

Calculus begins with the formation of plaque. Plaque is formed from bacteria within the mouth and lines the tooth surface. As the bacteria multiplies and grows, so does the plaque which will begin to cause gingivitis. Salvia contains inorganic substances which are deposited onto the layer of plaque. This will then form dental calculus (tartar). Dental calculus (if not removed or treated) will cause periodontitis.

Removal and prevention of dental calculus

Hand scaling – this involves removing the calculus from the supragingival area (above the gingival margin) with an instrument called a supragingival scaler. The instrument is always used in the direction of the gingiva to the tip of the crown. A curette is used to remove calculus from the subginginval area (below the gingival margin) and is moved in a circular fashion around the gingival margin

Mechanical scaling and polishing – mechanical scaling involves the use of a scaler using either ultrasonic (piezoelectric or magnetostrictive) or sonic, units. By using electrical currents the scaler tip vibrates (oscillates) and breaks up the calculus. It is advisable that large areas of calculus are removed with calculus forceps first to protect the scaler tip. A constant supply of water is needed when using this equipment as a great amount of heat is generated. This heat is controlled by the supply of water otherwise the heat will cause damage to the tooth's enamel. The scaler tip should not be used for more than 15 seconds per tooth to prevent heat damage (you may return to the same tooth if needed). The point on the scaler tip must be never be used to scale teeth as this creates grooves in the enamel allowing bacteria to take residence and therefore creating more plaque.

Polishing must always following scaling; polishing is performed at a much lower speed than scaling and smoothes the enamel which has been roughed by scaling. It also removes the last layer of plaque. Various types of polishing cups are available.

Prevention of calculus

• Brushing
• Chewing (eg raw hides, dental chews, toys)
• Feeding dried food

Care during the dental procedure

- Ensure the patient is intubated with a cuffed endotracheal tube
- Ensure the body is raised above the head by using blankets or tilting table. This should also continue in recovery until the patient is in sternal recumbency.
- Pack the throat. It is essential that a pack with a visible tie is used so it is not forgotten at the end of the procedure (tampax tampons are a cheap alternative!)
- Always turn the patient under rather the over to avoid water and debris entering the airways

Aftercare

- It is advisable to feed the patient soft/mushy food for 3-5 days especially following extractions
- Often antibiotics and analgesia will be required (palatable versions of each are available if tablets prove difficult to administer)
- Continue or begin brushing to help prevent the build-up of calculus and plaque

Dental instruments

See Figure 9.11.

Explorer/measuring probe

Used for examining the enamel and measuring the sub gingival pocket depth.

Subgingival curette

Used for removing tartar from the subgingival area (below the gum line). The points on the end of the curette and rounded and blunt.

Supragingival scaler

Used for removing tartar from above the gum line (the crown). The points on the end of the scaler are shaped and pointed.

Luxators

Used for detaching the tooth from the periodontal ligament.

Elevators

Used for elevating the tooth from the socket.

Extraction forceps (calculus forceps)

Used for removing the tooth and calculus.

Care of dental instruments

- Wash and dry after each procedure using a suitable detergent
- Sharpen using a sharpening stone. Sharpening dirty instruments will contaminate the sharpening stone.
- Protect sharp edges.
- Sterilise the instruments.

Instruments such as luxators and elevators are prone to chipping and breaking. Care should be used not to drop them or let them bang against other instruments. Repair and sharpening of instruments can be carried out by dental equipment suppliers.

3.8.14   Circulatory

What you need to learn

- You need to be able to state common conditions of the cardiovascular system amenable to surgery:
  - portosystemic shunts
  - congenital heart defects.

Portosystemic shunts (PSS)

- A portosystemic shunt is a blood vessel which shunts blood from the hepatic portal vein to the major systemic veins such as the vena cava. This causes the blood to bypass the liver.
- Can be congenital or acquired (secondary to liver disease).
- Clinical signs reflect impairment of liver function:
  - Stunted growth in young animals
  - Anorexia, depression, weight loss.
  - Intermittent vomiting and diarrhoea.
  - Neurological signs caused by hepatic encephalopathy (caused by high blood ammonia levels). Neurological signs are usually worse following a meal.
  - Uric acid urinary calculi.
- Diagnosis is through blood samples: mild hypochromic anaemia, hypoproteinaemia, elevated ammonia and bile acids. Contrast study of the hepatic blood vessels confirms diagnosis.
- Treatment involves medical treatment of hepatic encephalopathy (lactulose reduces blood ammonia levels) followed by surgery to ligate the shunting blood vessel. Blood pressure in the portal circulation must be monitored during the surgery and if this becomes too high the shunting vessel may only be partly ligated.
- Acquired shunts often involve multiple small vessels. These cannot easily be ligated and the prognosis is very guarded.

• The prognosis is reasonable for young dogs following successful surgery.

Congenital heart defects

Patent ductus arteriosus (PDA)

• The ductus arteriosus is a foetal blood vessel which shunts blood from the pulmonary artery to the aorta in the foetus. This avoids unnecessary circulation in the as yet non-functional lungs.
• A PDA results from the failure of the ductus arteriosus to close after birth.
• Increased pressure in the aorta at birth causes the direction of blood flow to reverse in the PDA (changes to a left to right shunt). This results in left sided congestive heart failure if it is left untreated.
• Diagnosis is through auscultation (continuous machinery murmur) and visualisation of the shunting vessel using colour flow Doppler echocardiography.
• Treatment involves improvement of the dog's condition using medication to support cardiac function followed by surgery to ligate the PDA.
• The animal should be anaesthetised with care, and will need ventilating during the thoracotomy. Surgery involves a thoracotomy at the 4th left intercostal space. The shunting vessel is identified and very carefully ligated. Occasionally the ductus can tear, causing damage to the pulmonary artery or aorta. This complication is often fatal. A chest drain is placed to allow removal of air and the chest is closed.
• The success of this surgical procedure approaches 95% and animals treated early will lead a completely normal life.

Vascular ring anomalies

• This is a group of congenital conditions which result from malformation of the great vessels during development. It often results in ligamentous bands (remnants of blood vessels) which form strictures around the oesophagus. This causes regurgitation in young animals.
• Diagnosis is through radiography with contrast study (barium meal).
• Treatment is usually surgical transection of the ligamentous band.
• Surgery involves a thoracotomy at the 4th intercostal space, identification and ligation of the structure.
• The oesophagus may be able to recover some of its function in the weeks after surgery but the animal often requires dietary control (feeding liquid/soft food from head height) for the rest of its life.

3.8.15   Other surgical procedures and terms

What you need to learn

☙ You need to be able to define hernia and rupture:
  - ☙ reducible
  - ☙ irreducible
  - ☙ strangulated.
☙ Describe specific types of hernia and rupture:
  - ☙ umbilical
  - ☙ inguinal
  - ☙ perineal
  - ☙ diaphragmatic
  - ☙ ventral rupture.
☙ Understand the significance of diaphragmatic rupture and its anaesthetic requirements.

- A **hernia** is the protrusion of all or part of an organ through a defect in the wall of the cavity within which it lies.
- The term **hernia** is usually used for congenital defects.
- The term **rupture** is usually used for an acquired hernia.
- Hernias and ruptures are classified according to:
- **Anatomical site:**
  - **Umbilical** – defect where the umbilical vessels left the foetus through the ventral midline.
  - **Inguinal** – defect through inguinal ring.
  - **Perineal** – failure of rectal wall resulting in flaccid pouch in caudal rectum.
  - **Diaphragmatic** – Defect in diaphragm, usually acquired through trauma.
  - **Ventral body wall** – usually involved detachment of the body wall from its attachment at the prepubic tendon.
- **What is happening to the contents of the hernia:**
  - **Reducible** – The contents of the hernia can be easily replaced to their original position through the defect. This is commonly the case in small umbilical hernias.
  - **Irreducible (incarcerated)** – The contents can't be easily replaced. The contents may have developed fibrous adhesions which are holding them in place. This often occurs in long-standing hernias. NB in these hernias the blood supply to the hernia contents has not been compromised.
  - **Strangulated** – The blood supply to the contents of the hernia has become compromised, often because they have twisted. Strangulated hernias are painful and can be life-threatening if they involve an organ. They should be treated as an emergency.
- Hernias should be repaired surgically with the exception of small

umbilical hernias which are too small to allow a loop of gut to pass though.

Diaphragmatic hernias/rupture

- Tears in the diaphragm are usually seen as a result of a road traffic accident.
- Tears in the diaphragm should be repaired as soon as possible as complications can include the movement of abdominal contents through the tear into the thorax.
- The animal is very carefully anaesthetised. Patients are often dyspnoeic and may require artificial respiration. The patient is placed in dorsal recumbency and a ventral midline abdominal incision made. Any herniated abdominal contents should be replaced in the abdomen and the defect in the diaphragm is sutured closed.
- The surgery causes a pneumothorax to develop as air from the atmosphere can travel through the diaphragmatic tear into the thorax. For this reason a chest drain is often necessary to remove air from the pleural space post-operatively.

3.8.16   Tumours

What you need to learn

- You need to be able to define the terms tumour and neoplasia:
  - lipoma
  - papilloma
  - melanoma
  - sebaceous adenoma
  - mast cell tumour
  - basal cell tumour.
- Define benign and malignant tumours and explain their differences:
  - carcinomas and sarcomas
  - squamous cells carcinomas
  - lymphosarcomas.
- Describe the term metastasis.
- Outline the predilection sites of tumours:
  - dogs
  - cats
  - rodents
  - birds.
- Describe the complications associated with tumours:
  - hypercalcaemia
  - histamine release

* anaemia
* obstruction
* haemorrhage.

☙ Describe the term carcinogen and outline types of carcinogens.

☙ Outline the various types of treatments for neoplasia and tumours with an understanding of their common applications:

* surgical excision
* chemotherapy
* radiation therapy
* cryotherapy.

☙ Describe biopsy techniques and how different biopsies are taken:

* punch
* trephine
* incisional
* excisional.

☙ Describe the process of preparing a sample for cytology in the practice.

Tumour – describes any swelling of tissue, but usually reserved for neoplasia.

Neoplasia – uncontrolled growth and proliferation of new cells.

Cancer – term usually reserved for malignant neoplasia; use this emotive term with care.

Oncology – the study of neoplasms.

Metastasis – spread of neoplasm to another tissue or organ. Can happen through lymphatic system, blood system or by the seeding of neoplastic cells across a body cavity.

• Neoplasms are often classified as:
  • **Benign** – usually slow growing, encapsulated (do not invade adjacent tissues) and do not metastasise.
  • **Malignant** – usually faster growing, never encapsulated (but can appear to form a pseudocapsule which is merely compressed layers of adjacent tissue), invade local tissue and metastasise.
• Note that the situation is not always as clear cut as this. Some tumours (such as haemangiopericytomas) are locally invasive but do not metastasise; other tumours (such as mast cell tumours) can show a variation in behaviour from benign to malignant.
• Examples of usually benign tumours include:
  • Lipoma – benign tumour of adipose cell. Can grow quite large. Tends to occur in older animals and those which are overweight.
  • Papilloma – wart-like tumour of epithelial cells.
  • Melanoma – occasionally benign tumour of melanocytes in the skin and mucous membranes. Note, however, that many melanomas are malignant.
  • Sebaceous adenoma – benign tumour of the sebaceous gland cells.

- Perianal adenoma – benign tumour of the glands surrounding the anus. Occurs in older entire male dogs.
- Basal Cell tumour – benign tumour of the basal cell.
- Note that the suffix '**-oma**' often denotes a benign neoplasm.
- Malignant neoplasms of the epithelial tissues are often followed by the suffix '**-carcinoma**'
- Malignant neoplasms of the mesenchymal (connective) tissues are often followed by the suffix '**-sarcoma**'.
- Examples of usually malignant tumours include:
  - Squamous Cell Carcinomas – malignant tumour of the squamous epithelium. Commonly seen on the tips of the pinnae in cats.
  - Lymphosarcoma – malignant neoplasia of the lymph nodes commonly seen in dogs. Gut or thymic lymphosarcoma is often seen in cats which have been exposed to the feline leukaemia virus (FeLV).
  - Transitional cell carcinoma – malignant tumour of transitional epithelium of the bladder.
  - Adenocarcinoma – malignant tumour of glandular epithelium.
  - Osteosarcoma – highly malignant bone tumour. Metastasises readily to multiple organs.
  - Fibrosarcoma – malignant tumour of fibrous tissue.
- Mast cell tumours are tumours of the mast cells. They vary greatly in their behaviour and are graded as 1–3 with Grade 1 being benign and Grade 3 being aggressive and metastatic. This grading is performed by a pathologist from a biopsy sample.
- Mammary tumours are common, particularly in older entire bitches. They vary from benign mixed tumours to malignant adenocarcinomas and sarcomas. Metastasis often occurs through the lymphatic system.
- Mammary tumours in cats are less common but tend to be highly malignant.
- Neoplasia can occur in any tissue. It is a disorder in the control of the growth and division of a cell population.
- For this reason tissues which are rapidly dividing are more likely to suffer a neoplastic change. Rapidly dividing tissues include those in the gut, immune system and skin.
- More slowly dividing tissues such as muscle cells are much less frequently associated with neoplastic change.
- Some tumours occur more commonly at certain sites known as predilection sites. Common predilection sites in animals include:
  - Dogs – melanomas tend to occur in the mouth and on the toes; osteosarcomas tend to occur in the proximal humerus, distal radius, distal femur and proximal or distal tibia.
  - Cats – squamous cell carcinomas tend to occur on unpigmented areas on the face and pinnae of cats.

- Birds – tumours of the preen gland are occasionally seen, as are papillomas in the upper airways.
- Rodents – mammary tumours are extremely common in both male and female rats; entire female rabbits are very prone to uterine carcinomas.

Paraneoplastic disease

- Tumours can be associated with various medical complications which are caused either by the presence of the neoplasm in a tissue, or by the production of a substance by the neoplasm itself. This is called paraneoplastic disease.
- Paraneoplastic effects should be identified and treated as well as treating the primary neoplasm.
- Paraneoplastic effects can include:
  - **Hormonal effects**: adrenal and pituitary tumours can cause Cushing's disease; thyroid adenomas cause hyperthyroidism in cats, beta cell tumours of the pancreas (insulinomas) cause hypoglycaemia in dogs.
  - **Blood cell production effects** – neoplasia of the bone marrow can cause anaemia, thrombocytopaenia and various leukopaenias.
  - **Haemorrhage** – rupture of a vascular tumour (such as a splenic haemangiosarcoma), invasion of a tumour into a blood vessel, or indirect effects such as bleeding from a gastric ulcer caused by histamine release from a mast cell tumour.
  - **Hypercalcaemia** – various tumours produce a parathyroid hormone-like substance which causes hypercalcaemia. Examples include lymphoid and myeloid tumours and anal gland adenocarcinomas.
  - **Histamine release** – Cells from mast cell tumours degranulate releasing histamine. In severe cases this can result in anaphylactic shock. The histamine can also cause gastric ulceration.
  - **Physical effects** – such as obstruction of the gastrointestinal tract.
- A carcinogen is a substance which can affect the cell cycle in a way that causes neoplasia to develop.
- Examples of carcinogens include:
  - Viruses – papillomas virus, FeLV
  - Radiation
  - Ultraviolet light – causes some melanomas and squamous cell carcinomas
  - Chemical carcinogens – substances in cigarette smoke is thought to be carcinogenic in animals as well as humans.

Treatment of neoplasia

- Treatment of tumours depends on a number of factors

- Location
- Size
- Type of tumour
- Presence of metastases
- Health of patient
- Prognosis
- Possible treatments include:
  - **Surgery:** The most common treatment is surgical removal of all or part of the neoplasm.
  - **Wide excision:** If possible the tumour should be surgically removed, also excising a margin of healthy tissue on all sides and beneath the mass. The ensures that no neoplastic cells are left behind as tumour regrowth occurs from a single cell. When the mass is sent for histology this is called an **excisional biopsy**.
  - **Debulking:** Removal of the bulk of a neoplasm without taking clear margins is called debulking. It is often performed for large benign tumours which are causing a mechanical problem (eg large lipomas can impeded limb movement if they are situated in the axilla or inguinal area).
  - **Chemotherapy:** This is the use of medication to selectively destroy neoplastic cells. Chemotherapy drugs include cytotoxic drugs as well as corticosteroids and other anti-inflammatory medications. Choice of chemotherapy agent depends on the type of tumour and its susceptibility to treatment with those drugs.
  - **Radiotherapy:** This is the use of radiation energy to selectively destroy neoplastic cells. It is very effective for the treatment of certain tumours but is only available in a small number of specialist facilities.
  - **Cryosurgery:** This is the destruction of neoplastic cells using the application of extreme cold directly to the neoplasm. It is mainly used for small skin neoplasms such as papillomas.
- Treatment often involves a combination of two or more of the described methods. For example, the primary neoplasm is surgically removed and chemotherapy or radiotherapy is used to destroy any remaining cells or metastases. Occasionally the neoplasm is reduced in size using chemotherapy or radiotherapy before being excised surgically.

Biopsy techniques

- In order to successfully treat a neoplasm it must be identified and if necessary graded (as with mast cell tumours).
- This involves obtaining a sample of the mass for histological examination. Methods include:
  - **Excisional biopsy** – the whole mass is removed with margins and submitted for histopathology.

- **Punch biopsy** – A small circular plug of tissue is removed from the surface of the mass using a sharpened tool. This method is used for small superficial masses.
- **Trephine biopsy** – A hollow trephine biopsy needle is used to penetrate bone and obtain a core sample.
- **Incisional biopsy** – A small wedge of tissue is removed surgically, often using scissors or a scalpel blade. This method is used during exploratory laparotomy if a suspicious lesion is detected.

Preparing a cytology sample

- The biopsy sample is normally placed in a preservative solution before transport to the laboratory. The preservative solution prevents necrosis and degradation of the sample.
- The sample must be no more than 2–3 cm thick so that the preservative is able to penetrate the whole sample.
- When deciding which part of a tissue sample to send it is important to include the border between diseased and normal tissue. The centre of a large lesion is often necrotic and of little diagnostic value.
- When an excisional biopsy has been taken it is important to send the normal margins for histopathology. This is necessary for determining whether the whole lesion has been removed. If the lesion is a malignant tumour this information is vital for providing prognosis.
- If a whole organ has been removed (usually the spleen, kidney or a gland or lymph node) small (< 2 cm) representative samples only must be preserved and sent for histopathology.
- Body fluids can be preserved by making a fixed smear as described earlier; or by adding a drop of formal saline to 1ml of fluid. This preserves the morphology of any cells.
- When collecting samples for histopathology care must be taken when selecting a container for transport.
- A suitable container must be large enough to contain the sample and the preservative fluid.
- Wide neck containers allow easy removal of the sample.
- It must be sealable so that liquid will not escape when the container is inverted.
- It must be strong enough to withstand reasonable handling. Fragile or easily breakable containers must be avoided (such as glass or brittle plastic).
- Preservatives which are commonly used in veterinary practice include:
  - **Formalin** – this is a 40% solution of dissolved formaldehyde gas. It fixes, or hardens, tissue samples. Formalin is irritant and COSHH rules must be followed when handling it.

• **Formal saline** – this is more commonly used than formalin. It consists of a 10% solution of formalin in a saline solution.
• **Neutral buffered formalin** – this is also a 10% solution of formalin in saline but is buffered to protect against changes in pH. This protects the sample from damage caused by changing acidity.

Multiple choice questions

1. The cardinal signs of inflammation do not include
   - ☐ A swelling
   - ☐ B heat
   - ☐ C ischaemia
   - ☐ D pain

2. A wound where tissue has become separated from its attachments is classified as a/an
   - ☐ A incised
   - ☐ B avulsed
   - ☐ C lacerated
   - ☐ D puncture

3. The outcome of healing where the tissue destroyed by the inflammatory process is replaced with similar functional tissue is known as
   - ☐ A organisation
   - ☐ B re-epithelialisation
   - ☐ C resolution
   - ☐ D regeneration

4. Dehiscence is
   - ☐ A erosion of the epithelial layer
   - ☐ B pus diffusely distributed throughout the tissues
   - ☐ C wound breakdown
   - ☐ D abnormal protrusion of an organ through a natural opening in a body cavity

5. Delayed healing is not usually associated with
   - ☐ A corticosteroid therapy
   - ☐ B diabetes mellitus
   - ☐ C pregnancy
   - ☐ D radiation therapy

6. An example of an active surgical drain is
   - ☐ A Heimlich
   - ☐ B Corrugated
   - ☐ C Yeates
   - ☐ D Penrose

7. An abnormal tract which connects two epithelial surfaces or an epithelial surface to the skin is known as a/an
   - ☐ A rupture
   - ☐ B abscess
   - ☐ C sinus
   - ☐ D fistula

8. The wound dressings most appropriate to dress a wound with heavy exudation and significant tissue loss are
   - ☐ A occlusive (hydrocolloid)
   - ☐ B hydrogel
   - ☐ C alginate
   - ☐ D wet packs

9. A skin graft which is taken from another patient of the same species to promote healing of a site of significant skin loss is a/an
   - ☐ A allograft
   - ☐ B autogenous graft
   - ☐ C pedicle graft
   - ☐ D xenograft

10. A split thickness skin graft comprises the
   - ☐ A epidermis and parts of the dermis
   - ☐ B epidermis and all the dermis
   - ☐ C epidermis
   - ☐ D epidermis and hypodermis

11. A large blood filled painless swelling is termed a
   - ☐ A lipoma
   - ☐ B seroma
   - ☐ C haematoma
   - ☐ D fibroma

12. In cases of GDV if a stomach tube cannot be passed to release the accumulated gas a needle can be passed through the body wall into the distended stomach. This procedure is known as a
   - ☐ A gastropexy
   - ☐ B gastrocentesis
   - ☐ C gastrotomy
   - ☐ D gastrectomy

13. The 'praying' position when adopted in dogs is indicative of
   - ☐ A dehydration
   - ☐ B tenesmus
   - ☐ C abdominal pain
   - ☐ D depression

14. Intussusception is seen most frequently in young animals commonly following
    - ☐ A diarrhoea
    - ☐ B vomiting
    - ☐ C cystitis
    - ☐ D constipation

15. Anal furunculosis is characterised by multiple chronic ulcerated sinuses and fistulous tracts in the peri-anal area and occurs commonly in
    - ☐ A Poodles
    - ☐ B Irish Setters
    - ☐ C Boxers
    - ☐ D German Shepherds

16. The term used to describe difficulty in parturition is
    - ☐ A dyspnoea
    - ☐ B dyschezia
    - ☐ C dystocia
    - ☐ D dysuria

17. A fracture which comprises of multiple fracture lines and fragments is
    - ☐ A complicated
    - ☐ B comminuted
    - ☐ C depressed
    - ☐ D greenstick

18. Inversion of the eyelid with in rolling of the eyelashes causing corneal ulceration is termed
    - ☐ A entropion
    - ☐ B ectropion
    - ☐ C epiphora
    - ☐ D enucleation

19. A chondroma is a
    - ☐ A benign tumour of glandular tissue
    - ☐ B malignant tumour of fibrous tissue
    - ☐ C benign tumour of cartilage
    - ☐ D malignant tumour of bone

20. The destruction of neoplastic cells using the application of extreme cold directly to a neoplasm is
    - ☐ A radiography
    - ☐ B cryosurgery
    - ☐ C chemotherapy
    - ☐ D debulking

Theatre practice

3.9.01   Asepsis and sterilisation

What you need to learn

- You need to be able to describe the common terms associated with asepsis and sterilisation:
  - asepsis
  - antisepsis
  - sterilisation
  - disinfection.
- Describe the principles of sterilisation.
- Outline the factors which affect the spread of infection.
- Describe why it is necessary to clean materials before sterilising:
  - surgical equipment
  - instruments
  - manual cleaning
  - electronic cleaning.
- Describe the methods of dry heat sterilisation and the use of a hot air oven:
  - basic oven
  - fan assisted.
- Outline the methods of moist heat sterilising:
  - autoclave.
- Describe the principles of an autoclave and its operation.
- Outline the different types of autoclave and identify the hazards in the use of an autoclave:
  - downward/upward
  - air displacement
  - vacuum assisted.
- Identify materials that can be autoclaved and state the temperature and pressure for different materials.
- Describe the materials used for packaging and explain the principles of preparing equipment/supplies for autoclaving.
- Describe the monitoring methods for assessing the effectiveness of sterilisation, their use and colour changes:
  - Bowie-Dick tape
  - Browne's tubes

- TST indicator strips
- indicator spots
- spore tests.
- Describe the method of gas sterilisation and state how to operate an ethylene oxide steriliser and the appropriate ventilating system.
- Describe what equipment can be sterilised by ethylene oxide and their preparation for ethylene oxide sterilisation.
- Identify the hazards associated with ethylene oxide sterilisation and describe the health and safety legislation related to its use.
- Outline what equipment is commonly sterilised by gamma radiation.
- Describe the use of cold chemical sterilisation.
- Describe the hazards and limitations associated with cold chemical sterilisation.
- Outline the most appropriate methods of sterilising different types of instruments.
- Describe the care, sterilisation and storage of surgical equipment/supplies/materials:
  - instruments
  - theatre clothing
  - swabs
  - rubber articles
  - dressings
  - ligatures
  - endoscopes
  - cryosurgical
  - orthopaedic equipment.
- Describe the correct storage and labelling of packs after sterilisation.
- Outline current health and safety legislation relevant to sterilisation procedures.

Common terms associated with asepsis and sterilisation are:

- **Asepsis** – freedom from all micro-organisms including spores
- **Antisepsis** – prevention of sepsis by inhibiting or destroying micro-organisms
- **Sterilisation** – the destruction of all micro-organisms including bacterial spores
- **Disinfection** – the removal of micro-organisms but not always bacterial spores
- **Antiseptics** – an agent that provides antisepsis and is safe to use on animal skin and tissue
- **Disinfectant** – an agent that provides disinfection. Disinfectants are available as skin disinfectants or environmental disinfectants. The latter are for use on inanimate objects only.

The principles of sterilisation are to:

• destroy all micro-organisms, including spores
• enable equipment to be used in a sterile manner
• prevent the spread of infection.

Factors affecting the spread of infection include:

• poor aseptic technique
• poor environmental cleaning
• overuse of antibiotics
• not isolating infectious patients from healthy patients
• length of surgery
• contamination of the surgical wound
• surgical technique.

Cleaning materials prior to sterilising

All surgical equipment, instruments and materials must be cleaned before sterilising. Micro-organisms can be concealed in blood and sterilisation is made more difficult as debris hinders the action of the steam, heat, gas, or liquid.

Methods of cleaning can be **manual,** involving the mechanical removal of debris with a brush and water containing a cleaning solution, eg Rapidex®, or **electronic,** in which debris is removed by cavitation (implosion of air bubbles) created by an ultrasonic cleaner (instruments must be lubricated after cleaning with this method).

Dry heat sterilisation

Dry heat sterilisation can be performed in hot air ovens. These can be of various types: the basic oven, convection ovens or high vacuum-assisted ovens.

The **basic hot air oven** kills micro-organisms by oxidative destruction of bacterial protoplasm. It is heated by an electrical element and is economical. High temperatures are needed for sterilisation – 150–180 °C as standard, 160 °C for 60 minutes. These ovens are used for glass, cutting instruments, drill bits, powders and oils but plastics, rubber and fabrics are damaged by this method. A long cooling period is required before the items can be used.

Fan-assisted hot air ovens (convection ovens) are the same as the basic oven just described but a fan is incorporated to provide a uniform temperature.

High vacuum assisted hot air ovens are the same as hot air ovens but are fully automatic and incorporate a vacuum, reducing sterilising time by 15 minutes.

Moist heat sterilising

Moist heat, provided by autoclaves, penetrates materials much more rapidly that dry heat because water conducts heat better than air. The temperature of the steam increases as the pressure is increased. As the steam meets the material being sterilised (which is cooler) the heat from the steam is transferred to the material. This process continues until the steam and material are the same temperature. All the air should be removed from the materials and packaging as air inhibits the steam from penetrating the material and reaching the correct temperature. Standard conditions for sterilisation are 15 pounds per square inch (PSI) at 121 °C for 15 minutes.

The principles of an autoclave is to achieve sterility by using steam under pressure.

Types of autoclave

An upward displacement autoclave can be horizontal or vertical.

- The steam is provided by heating water at the bottom of the chamber.
- A thermostat is present to maintain the correct temperature.
- A discharging valve is fitted at the top or on the side. This is left open at the beginning of the process until all the air is expelled, when it is then closed.
- Air is expelled by the steam by upward displacement.
- Only loose instruments can be sterilised in these autoclaves.

A downward displacement autoclave is usually horizontal.

- Steam enters the chamber at the top and displaces the air downwards out of a drain line.
- Condensation is removed by the drain line.
- The temperature of the drain line indicates when all the air is removed.
- Only loose instruments can be sterilised in these autoclaves; they are not suitable for fabrics and paper as they remain wet.

Vacuum-assisted autoclaves have the following characteristics.

- They work on the same principle as the downward displacement autoclave.
- A high vacuum pump is incorporated to remove the air rapidly at the start of sterilisation.
- High temperatures can be reached within shorter times.

- A second vacuum is incorporated at the end of the process to remove moisture and dry the load.
- These autoclaves are suitable for wrapped instruments, fabrics and hollow instruments.
- They are more expensive to purchase than the other two autoclaves.

Autoclaves are subjected to a test to withstand 50% greater pressure than their maximum. Many autoclaves are now presented with safety features but they should be inspected regularly.

Materials that may be autoclaved include:

- surgical instruments
- drapes, gowns, swabs and fabrics (vacuum-assisted autoclave)
- needles.

Table 9.1 lists the temperatures, pressures and times required for sterilisation in autoclaves.

Table 9.1 Temperatures, pressures and times required for sterilisation in autoclaves

Temperature (°C)	Pressure (PSI)	Sterilising time (minutes)
121	15	15
126	20	10
130	25	2.5
134	30	3

Materials used for packing

The following materials are suitable for use as packing in autoclaves:

- non-woven material, eg paper
- woven material, eg cotton muslin
- nylon film (on a roll and cut to size or as ready-made bags)
- plastic/paper seal-and-peel pouches
- boxes and cartons
- metal drums
- perforated metal trays for loose instruments.

Preparing equipment for autoclaving

The following procedure should be followed:

- Wash equipment with detergent in warm water or soak in instrument cleaner – the temperature must not exceed 60 °C.
- If using an ultrasonic cleaner rinse equipment in warm water and place in the bath.

- Dry the instruments and lubricate.
- Check all instruments for corrosion; check that ratchets are locking correctly, that teeth/tips meet and that screws/pins are not loose. Scissors should be able to cut through four layers of swabs with their tips and needle holders should hold a needle without it rotating. Complex instruments, eg Balfour retractors, should be disassembled.
- Arrange instruments within the pack in the order the surgeon will use them.
- Curved instruments should be placed nose down.
- All instruments should be sterilised open.
- Containers should be placed open end up or horizontal.
- Any cloth items, eg drapes, should be concertinaed when folding to allow circulation of the steam.

Monitoring methods

There are various monitoring methods where sterilisation has been successful.

- **Bowie-Dick tape** changes from beige to black/dark brown, indicating that it has been exposed to a temperature of 121 °C. However, it gives no indication of exposure time. It can be used in the autoclave and with ethylene oxide, when it changes from beige to green.
- **Browne's tubes** change from red to green. Tubes are available which change at 121 °C, 126 °C, 134 °C, 160 °C, or 180 °C. The colour indicates that a particular temperature has been reached but again gives no indication of exposure time. These tubes can be used in both the autoclave and hot air ovens.
- **TST strips** (time, steam, temperature) have an indicator spot placed at the end of the strip that changes from yellow to purple once it has being exposed to the correct temperature for the correct amount of time. These strips can be used in the autoclave and with ethylene oxide.
- **Spore tests** are strips of paper impregnated with a controlled amount of bacterial spores, usually *Bacillus stearothermophilius*. The strip is placed in the centre of the load and then cultured for 72 hours after sterilisation. If the sterilisation has been successful there will be no growth. Spore tests are the most accurate method but there is a delay before obtaining the results. They can be used in the autoclave, with ethylene oxide and in hot air ovens.

Gas sterilisation

Ethylene oxide (EO) is currently the gas used for sterilisation; it destroys micro-organisms by inactivating their DNA, preventing further cell reproduction.

The steriliser consists of a chamber with a ventilation system. It should be kept away from the working area and the temperature needs to be at least 20 °C.

Use of an ethylene oxide steriliser follows this procedure:

- Ensure all items are clean and dry.
- Remove any bungs or caps from items.
- Place items in the appropriate packaging, eg peel-and-seal pouches (nylon film cannot be used as it is poorly penetrated by the gas).
- Place all items to be sterilised in the plastic liner within the chamber.
- Place an ampoule containing ethylene oxide, eg anprolene, into the plastic liner and seal the liner with a tie.
- Snap the ampoule within the liner; this releases the gas and the liner inflates.
- Close and lock the door and turn on the ventilation system.
- At room temperature the sterilising process takes 12 hours.
- Items then need 24 hours to allow the ethylene oxide to dissipate.

The following factors affect the efficiency of ethylene oxide sterilisation:

- temperature
- humidity
- pressure
- concentration
- time.

Equipment that can be sterilised by gas includes:

- endoscopes
- hollow tubing, eg suction tubes
- delicate instruments, eg ophthalmic instruments
- plastic equipment, eg catheters
- high-speed drills.

Equipment must be clean and dry before sterilisation; grease and protein will slow the sterilisation process and water can reduce the effectiveness of the gas. Any bungs and caps should be removed.

Hazards of ethylene oxide are that it is toxic, is irritant to tissues and is highly flammable.

COSHH regulations must be followed which may make it impractical for use in some practices.

Equipment sterilised by gamma radiation

Some equipment can be sterilised by gamma radiation, eg suture material, surgical gloves and scalpel blades.

Cold chemical sterilisation

Cold chemical sterilisation involves submerging the items in a liquid (using a container with a lid to avoid evaporation) for a specific period of time. This method should be thought of as disinfection as opposed to sterilisation. The liquids used are usually glutaraldehyde, chlorohexidine or alcohol.

The concentrations recommended by the manufacturer must be followed and care should be taken as these chemicals can be irritant to tissues.

Methods of sterilising different equipment

Table 9.2. lists different items and the preferred methods for their sterilisation.

Table 9.2 Methods of sterilisation used for veterinary equipment

Equipment	Method of sterilisation
Surgical instruments	Moist heat, vacuum or non-vacuum
Endoscopes	Ethylene oxide or cold sterilisation
High-speed drills	Ethylene oxide
Powders and oils	Hot air oven
Glass syringes	Hot air oven
Plastic tubing	Ethylene oxide
Cutting instruments	Hot air oven
Drapes and gowns	Moist heat, vacuum

Care, sterilisation and storage of equipment and materials

Theatre cloths and drapes

- Wash and dry – check for any fraying and holes.
- Remove any hair with a sticky-paper roller.
- Fold correctly – see description in 3.9.02.
- Pack in either material, peel-and-seal pouches, drums, nylon film, or cartons with an indicator.
- Sterilise using a vacuum autoclave or ethylene oxide.
- Store in closed cabinets if possible.
- Most gowns and cloth drapes can withstand 75 washes.

Swabs

- Swabs can be purchased sterile or non-sterile.
- Use a consistent set number of swabs per pack.
- Pack in either material, peel-and-seal pouches, drums, nylon film, or cartons with an indicator.

- Sterilise using a vacuum autoclave or ethylene oxide.
- Store in closed cabinets if possible.

Rubber articles

- Wash and dry.
- Pack in seal-and-pouches uncoiled with an indicator.
- Sterilise using ethylene oxide.
- Store in closed cabinets if possible.

Dressings

- Pack in material, peel-and-seal pouches, drums, nylon film, or cartons with an indicator.
- Sterilise by vacuum autoclave or ethylene oxide.
- Store in closed cabinets if possible.

Ligatures

- Pack in material, peel-and-seal pouches, nylon film, drums, or cartons with an indicator.
- Sterilise by vacuum autoclave or ethylene oxide.
- Store in closed cabinets if possible.

Endoscopes

- Clean according to the manufacturer's instructions.
- Sterilise by ethylene oxide (ensure all parts are clean and dry) or cold sterilisation (check the hand-piece can be submerged).
- Store in a vertical position.

Cryosurgical equipment

Some cryoprobes can be sterilised using an autoclave. Check with the manufacturer regarding sterilising procedures.

Orthopaedic equipment

- Wash and dry.
- Pack in material, peel-and-seal pouches, nylon film, cartons, drums, or on a tray with an indicator.
- It is always wise to check sterilising procedures with the manufacturer. Most equipment can be sterilised with a vacuum or non-vacuum autoclave.
- Cutting instruments can also be sterilised in a hot air oven, eg drill bits.
- All power-driven tools and plastic handles/cases can be sterilised by ethylene oxide.

• Store in closed cabinets if possible or use immediately if perforated trays are used.

Storage and labelling of packs

• Label all packs with the date, the contents and the person's initials.
• Ideally store in closed cabinets away from the floor.
• Store at an even room temperature.
• If stored on open shelves damp-dust daily with disinfectant.
• Avoid dropping the packs or placing them where they can easily fall.
• Although storage time does depend on the packaging material re-sterilise every 6–8 weeks if not regularly used.

All regulations stipulated by COSHH and the Health and Safety Act must be understood and followed.

3.9.02   Theatre practice

What you need to learn

❧ You need to be able to outline the meaning of an aseptic theatre and understand the correct method of preparing the environment correctly for surgical procedures:
  ❧ elective surgical procedures
  ❧ emergency surgical procedures.
❧ Describe correct cleaning protocol to maintain an aseptic theatre.
❧ Outline the importance of temperature regulation in the theatre.
❧ Describe the advantages and disadvantages of theatre fans/ventilation:
  ❧ ventilation systems
  ❧ types of gas scavenging.
❧ Describe types of anaesthetic gas scavenging systems and reasons for their use:
  ❧ passive
  ❧ active.
❧ Outline the correct procedures for equipment maintenance:
  ❧ heating
  ❧ lighting
  ❧ ventilation
  ❧ electrosurgical
  ❧ diathermy
  ❧ anaesthetic equipment/patient monitoring.
❧ Describe the correct routine for preparation of the operation site using suitable disinfectants/antiseptics:
  ❧ skin disinfectants/antiseptics

* electric clippers.
* Describe the correct procedure for scrubbing up using suitable disinfectants/antiseptics.
* Describe gowning and gloving procedures using both open and closed methods.
* Outline good personnel conduct in theatre to maintain sterility and asepsis of equipment materials and personnel during surgical procedures.
* Identify common materials used for drapes and gowns and describe suitable folding and packing techniques:
    * reusable
    * disposable.

The operating theatre

The operating theatre needs to be an end room and should not be used to gain access to another room. Traffic in and out of the theatre must be minimal with only designated staff actually in the theatre; ideally a one-way system should be set in place.

Correct attire must be worn at all times. The walls and floor must be easily cleaned; ideally the walls should be painted with a light colour waterproof paint. There should be minimal shelving and furniture and extra lighting should be provided in the way of operating lights. There should be a source of heat present. Two wall clocks are needed, one for timing surgery and one for use during monitoring anaesthesia.

Any windows and doors should remain closed. Piped gas outlets and an air supply for power tools should be available and a scavenging system is required.

A radiographic viewer should be present, ideally recessed into the wall. Any electrical sockets should ideally be recessed onto the wall.

The operating table should be adjustable and easily cleaned.

Preparing for elective surgical procedures

* Damp-dust all surfaces with disinfectant including any operating lights.
* Organise the operating list starting with clean surgery.
* Prepare the equipment needed for preparing the operative site.
* Prepare the instrument trolley for the first procedure, including surgical kit, gowns, patient drapes, gloves, swabs and any extra instruments.
* Check that the floor is clean.

When preparing for emergency procedures the above protocol cannot be followed because there is usually no time to do so. It is imperative therefore that the cleaning protocol is followed.

Cleaning protocol for theatre

- Damp-dust all surfaces with disinfectant, including any operating lights, each morning.
- Between operations all equipment and the floor should be checked for cleanliness and cleaned if necessary. Instruments should be removed and taken for cleaning.
- After operating has finished, all instruments should be cleaned and re-sterilised.
- All equipment, shelves, cupboards and the operating table, including the operating lights, should be cleaned with disinfectant.
- The scrub sink should be cleaned with disinfectant and any loose hair should be removed.
- All bins should be emptied and new liners put in place.
- Any mobile equipment should be moved out of the room and the floor should be vacuumed.
- The walls and floors should be cleaned with disinfectant; once they are dry the equipment may be returned.

Temperature regulation

It is important to maintain the theatre temperature between 21 and 23 °C to prevent heat loss and hypothermia in the patients. Heating can be provided by radiators (although these collect dust), electric heaters, or under-floor heating.

Theatre ventilation

Ventilation should be provided in the operating theatre with air filters to remove bacteria.

Air changes should be approximately 300 per hour; ideally the theatre should be at high pressure and the preparation area at low pressure.

Opening windows should be avoided as this both cools the theatre and breaks asepsis. To remove waste anaesthetic gases use either a passive or active scavenging system.

Scavenging systems

These systems remove waste gas from the expiratory limb of the anaesthetic circuit. There are two types:

- **Passive systems** comprise a piece of tubing attached to the expiratory valve on the circuit, the other end is then placed through a hole in the wall to the outside atmosphere or to an activated charcoal system (these do not absorb nitrous oxide).

• **Active systems** comprise a piece of tubing attached to the expiratory valve on the circuit, the other end of which is then attached to further tubing, to an extractor fan and then finally to the outside atmosphere. The extractor fan generates negative pressure which enables the gas to move along the tubing. An air brake receiver is incorporated to prevent excessive negative pressure being enforced on the patient and to prevent a build-up of excess pressure if the system fails.

Several anaesthetic systems can be scavenged using the same system.

Maintenance of equipment

Heating equipment – ensure that any heating equipment is kept clean and dust-free. If a fault occurs call an appropriate engineer.

Lighting should be kept clean and dust free; replace immediately any light bulbs that are not working. If a fault occurs call an electrician.

Ventilation – ensure that regular maintenance checks are carried out by professionals. If a fault occurs call an appropriate engineer.

Electrosurgical and diathermy equipment should be kept clean, dust free and dry. Change the fuses in plug sockets as required. If a fault occurs call the manufacturer.

Anaesthetic equipment should be kept clean and dust-free. Circuits should be checked daily for leaks. Flow meters should be checked daily; if the bobbin is not spinning or rising there could be a fault and the appropriate services should be called. Vaporisers should be serviced once a year.

Patient monitoring equipment – ensure that there is a daily check that it is working correctly. All leads and devices should be kept clean, dust free and dry. Change the fuses in plug sockets as required. If a fault occurs call the manufacturer.

Preparation of the operative site

Initial preparation should be carried out in the preparation room, not in the operating theatre.

• Clip the hair using electric clippers, leaving a 10-cm diameter around the incision site.
• Vacuum the hair from the patient and the table.
• Mix the chosen skin disinfectant with a small amount of warm water.

- Wear non-sterile gloves.
- Using lint-free swabs and the above solution begin at the centre of the incision and work outwards towards the hair in a circular motion. Once the hair is reached, discard the swab.
- Repeat approximately five times or until clean.
- Transfer the animal to theatre and repeat the described procedure using sterile gloves, swabs and water.
- A final preparation is then performed by the sterile scrub nurse using sterile swabs and sterile Rampley sponge-holding forceps.

Skin disinfectants that can be used are chlorohexidine gluconate, povidine-iodine, or isopropyl alcohol.

Surgical scrub method

- Put on the theatre cap and mask.
- Remove all jewellery, push cuticles back and clean nails. Nails should not be longer than the finger.
- Adjust the hot and cold taps to a comfortable temperature.
- Wet hands and arms and wash with hand soap, allowing the water to run from the hands to the elbows.
- Apply surgical scrub agent from a dispenser using only the elbows and wash hands and arms.
- Using a sterile scrubbing brush and the scrub agent, scrub hands and arms for 5–7 minutes for the first scrub. Pay particular attention to fingers and palms; use only the elbows to dispense the scrub agent.
- The block technique can be used where each side of the fingers, hands and arms is considered a block and each side is scrubbed ten times and repeated three times.
- Rinse hands and arms allowing the water to run from the hands to the elbows.
- Keep arms above waist height.
- Dry hands and arms with a sterile towel.

Surgical scrub agents are chlorohexidine gluconate, povidine-iodine and tricolsan.

Gowning procedure

- Ensure hands and lower arms are dry.
- Pick up the inside of the gown at the shoulders and let it unfold.
- Place a hand into each sleeve and push the hands forward by opening your arms. Never pull the sleeves up with your hands.
- The hands should remain within the sleeves.
- An unscrubbed assistant can adjust the gown from the inside so it fits correctly over the shoulders.

For back-tying gowns the ties are usually at the front or side. These may then be held out to the side and the unscrubbed assistant can secure them at the back.

For side-tying gowns, the unscrubbed assistant takes the paper tape (attached to the tie and passed to them by the scrubbed assistant) and takes the tie around the back of the gown to the other side. The scrubbed assistant then pulls the tie and the unscrubbed assistant is left with the paper tape. The scrubbed assistant then ties the two ties at the side.

Open gloving

The technique for open gloving is shown in the Figure 9.1. The hands are extended out of the gown:

- Step 1 – The sterile glove packet is opened by an unscrubbed assistant.
- Step 2 – Handling the inside of the glove only (the turned down cuff area) pick up the right glove with the left hand.

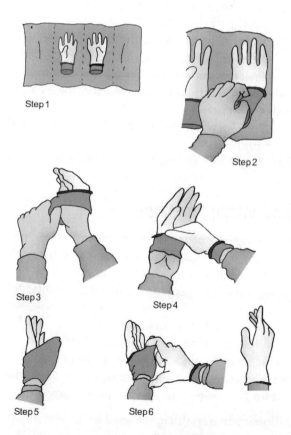

Figure 9.1 Open gloving.

- Step 3 – Pull onto the right hand using the inside of the glove. Do not unfold the cuff at this point.
- Step 4 – Place the gloved right fingers under the cuff of the left glove and pull onto the left hand touching the outside of the glove, not the inside.
- Step 5 – The cuff of the left glove is left hooked over the thumb, so the cuff of the gown can be adjusted.
- Step 6 – Pull the cuff of the left glove over the cuff of the gown using the right hand fingers.
- Repeat Steps 4 to 6 for the right hand.

Closed gloving

- The hands remain inside the gown:

- Step 1 – The sterile glove packet is opened by an unscrubbed assistant.
- Step 2 – Turn the packet round so that the fingers are pointing downwards – the right glove is now on the left and the left glove is now on the right.
- Step 3 – Pick the right glove up (on the left hand side) with the right hand at the rim of the cuff.
- Step 4 – Turn the hand over so the glove is lying on the palm and the fingers are facing towards your body.
- Step 5 – Pick the rim up with the left hand.
- Step 6 – The rim is then passed over the fingers and pulled down towards the wrist.
- Step 7 – Push forward with the hand at the same time and insert the fingers into the correct parts.
- Repeat Steps 3 to 7 for the left hand (using the opposite glove and hand).

Personal conduct within the theatre

- Wear appropriate attire at all times (scrub suits, hats, masks and white clogs, or sterile gown, hat, mask and white clogs).
- If unscrubbed do not touch anything sterile.
- Walk behind the surgeon or scrubbed assistants and not in front of them.
- Keep traffic to a minimum in theatre.
- Keep door opening to a minimum.
- Talk, sneeze and cough as little as possible.
- If the surgeon begins a procedure sitting down he/she should remain seated for the entire length of the procedure.

The following materials can be used for gowns and drapes:

- non-woven, eg paper, these are disposable

• woven, eg cotton, these are reusable
• polyester and cotton, these are reusable
• clear plastic, these are waterproof and disposable.

Table 9.3 lists the advantages and disadvantages of reusable and disposable drapes and gowns.

Table 9.3 Advantages and disadvantages of reusable and disposable drapes and gowns

Reusable drapes and gowns	Disposable drapes and gowns
Advantages	
Cheaper	Insurance of sterility
Conform better to the patient	Reduction in contamination
Long-term use	More water-resistant (not some papers)
Comfortable to wear	Less laundry
	Always in first-class condition
	Labour saving
Disadvantages	
Contamination greater as very porous	Expensive
Pore size increase with each wash therefore reducing aseptic barrier	Need space to store the stock
Time consuming (washing, drying, sterilising)	Delivery problems
Threads can become loose, contaminating the surgical site	May be less conforming
May fray, 'bobble' or develop holes in time	

Folding a gown

The technique for folding a gown is shown in Figure 9.2.

• Lie the gown face up on a table.
• Fold the one edge into the middle, ensuring that all ties are kept inside and that the arm holes are straight.
• Fold the other side right over to the opposite side, ensuring that all ties are kept inside and that the arm holes are straight.
• Concertina the gown lengthways (from the bottom to the collar).
• Pack in material, peel-and-seal pouches, drums, nylon film, or cartons with an indicator.

Folding a drape

The technique for folding a drape is shown in the Figure 9.3.

• Concertina the drape widthways then concertina it lengthways.
• Pack in peel-and-seal pouches, drums, nylon film, or cartons with an indicator.

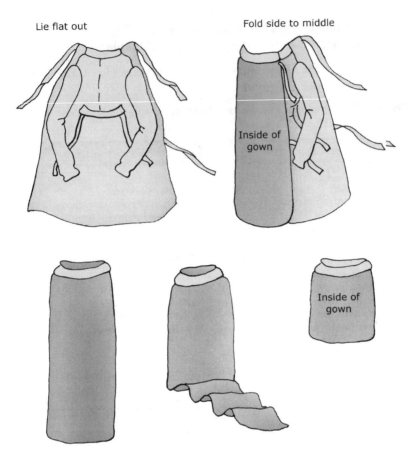

Lie flat out

Fold side to middle

Inside of gown

Inside of gown

Fold over other edge to side   Concertina lengthways   Pick up by inside of gown after autoclaving

Figure 9.2 How to fold a gown.

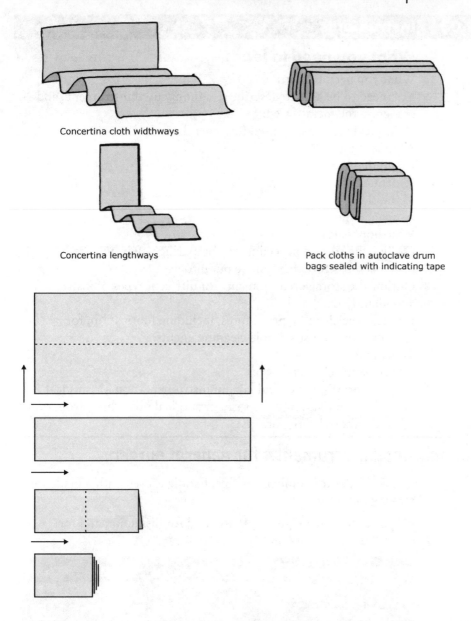

Concertina cloth widthways

Concertina lengthways

Pack cloths in autoclave drum
bags sealed with indicating tape

Figure 9.3 How to fold a drape.

What you need to learn

❧ What you need to learn

❧ You need to be able to describe commonly used instruments and recognise the metals used:
   ❧ surgical instruments used for general surgical
   ❧ abdominal
   ❧ ophthalmic
   ❧ dental
   ❧ thoracic
   ❧ uro-genital
   ❧ orthopaedics.

❧ Outline the correct procedure for preparing newly acquired instruments before they can be put into use.

❧ Outline the storage requirements for different types of instruments and identify their faults.

❧ Describe the cleaning procedures, including lubrication, for instruments and list suitable cleaning agents:
   ❧ manual
   ❧ ultra sonic cleaner.

❧ Describe how to select and lay out instrumentation for surgical procedures maintaining asepsis. For surgical procedures from range (gloved hands/cheatle forceps).

Commonly used instruments for general surgery

The Bard–Parker number 3 scalpel handle is used with a blade for making incisions.

Mayo scissors (see Figure 9.4) are used for dissection and for extending surgical wounds.

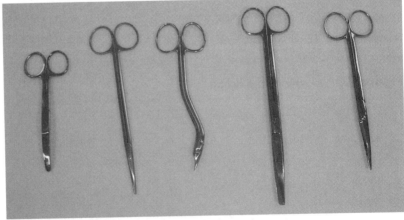

Figure 9.4 Scissors: dressing, Metzenbaum, Heath, Mayo and Mayo fine tipped straight.

Metzenbaum scissors (see Figure 9.5) are used for dissection, for extending surgical wounds and also for more delicate work.

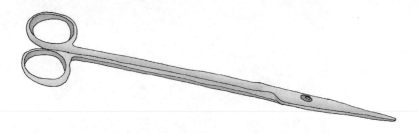

Figure 9.5 Metzenbaum scissors.

Treves rat-tooth forceps (see Figure 9.6) are used for handling tissue. They cause trauma to the held tissue so their use is generally limited to the skin.

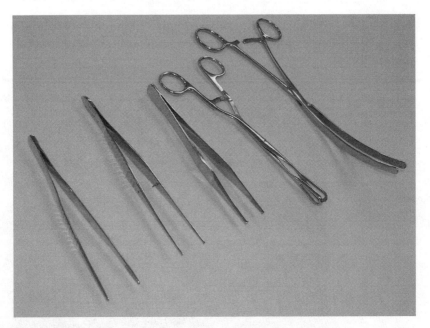

Figure 9.6 Forceps: plain dressing, Treves, Lane, Rampley's sponge-holding forceps and Doyen bowel clamp.

Plain dressing forceps (see Figure 9.6) are used for handling tissue. They are atraumatic so can be used to handle more delicate tissue.

Spencer Wells artery forceps (see Figure 9.7) are used to provide haemostasis.

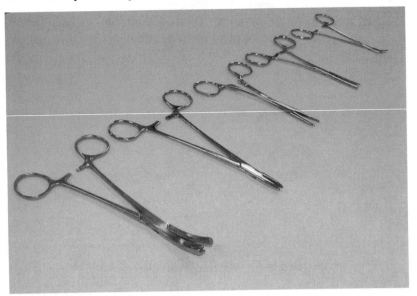

Figure 9.7 Ferguson angiotribes haemostat, Mayo needle holders, Spencer Wells forceps, Kocher and Halstead mosquito.

Allis tissue forceps (see Figure 9.8) are used for holding tissue (they should not be used as retractors or to hold drapes/tubing).

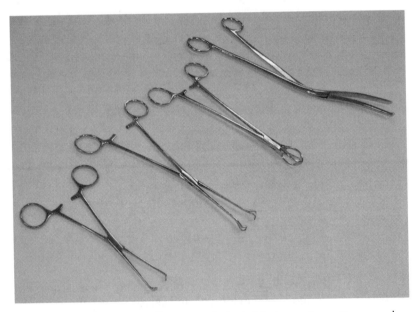

Figure 9.8 Forceps: Allis tissue, Babcock's tissue, Lane tissue and Cheatle forceps.

Gillies needle holders (see Figure 9.9) are used to hold the needle while suturing; they also have a scissor part to cut the suture material.

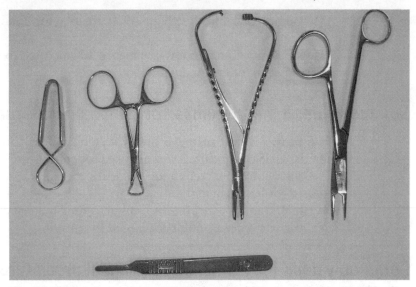

Figure 9.9 Cross-action towel clip, Backhaus towel clip, MacPhail's needle holders, Gilles needle holders and Bard-Parker scalpel handle.

The Backhaus towel clip (see Figure 9.9) is used for attaching drapes to the patient; winged versions are available where tubing, eg suction tubing, may be placed through and secured.

Commonly used instruments for abdominal surgery

Gelpi retractors (see Figure 9.10) are self-retaining retractors that can be used to hold open incisions.

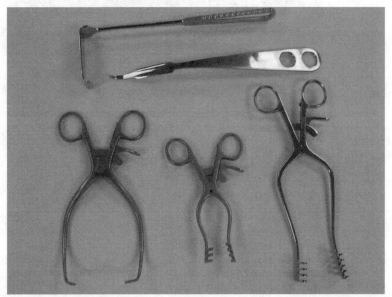

Figure 9.10 Retractors: Lagenbeck, Hohmann, Gelpi, West and Travers.

Doyen bowel clamps (see Figure 9.6) are used for holding intestines.

Halstead mosquito forceps (see Figure 9.7) are used to provided haemostasis for fine or small blood vessels.

Commonly used instruments for ophthalmic surgery

- A Beaver-handle scalpel is used with a blade for making incisions.
- Castroviejo corneal scissors are used for cutting and dissecting.
- Colibri corneal forceps and St Martins corneal forceps can both be used for handling tissue.
- The Barraquer wire eyelid speculum is used to keep the eye open.
- Castroviejo needle holders are used for suturing.

Commonly used instruments for dental procedures

An explorer/measuring probe (see Figure 9.11) is used for examining the enamel and for measuring the subgingival pocket depth.

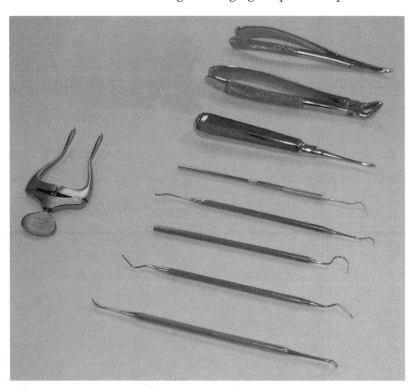

Figure 9.11 Left: rodent mouth gag. Right: dental extraction forceps, root elevator, dental probe, scaler, dental explorer, subgingival curette, double-ended dental scaler.

The subgingival curette is used for removing tartar from the subgingival area (below the gum line). The points on the end of the curette are rounded and blunt.

A supragingival scaler is used when removing tartar rom above the gum line (ie from the crown). The points on the end of the scaler are shaped and pointed.

Luxators can be used for detaching the tooth from the periodontal ligament.

Elevators (see Figure 9.11) are used for elevating the tooth from the socket.

Extraction forceps (see Figure 9.11) are used to remove the tooth.

Commonly used instruments for thoracic surgery

Spencer Wells forceps, Halstead mosquito forceps, rat-tooth and plain dressing forceps and Metzenbaum scissors (described earlier) are all used but for thoracic surgery as they have longer handles.

A Finochetto rib retractor can be used to maintain the opening into the thorax.

A Satinsky clamp is used for haemostasis and is atraumatic.

Commonly used instruments for uro-genital surgery

Spay hooks and angiotribes are commonly used instruments for uro-genital surgery.

Commonly used instruments for orthopaedic surgery

The Hohmann retractors (see Figure 9.10) are used for retracting muscles and for the manipulation of bone fragments and joints.

Twin-pointed fragment forceps are used to hold bone fragments while drilling or screwing.

Kern bone-holding forceps are used when holding long bones.

Liston bone cutters (see Figure 9.12) are used for cutting bone.

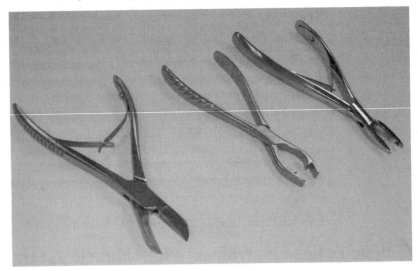

Figure 9.12 Liston bone cutters, Kern bone-holding forceps and Lempert rongeurs.

The Lempert rongeurs are used for 'nibbling' bone.

A chisel (see Figure 9.13) can be used for bone removal. It should be bevelled on one edge only. Chisels are usually used with an orthopaedic mallet.

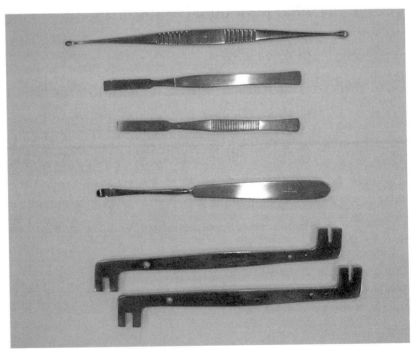

Figure 9.13 Volkman's scoop, chisel, osteotome, periosteal elevator and plate benders.

An osteotome is used for precise cuts into the bone. It is bevelled on both edges and is commonly used with an orthopaedic mallet.

The Volkman scoop (see Figure 9.13) is used for collection of cancellous bone grafts. Jacob's chuck and key (see Figure 9.14) can be used for introducing or removing intramedullary pins.

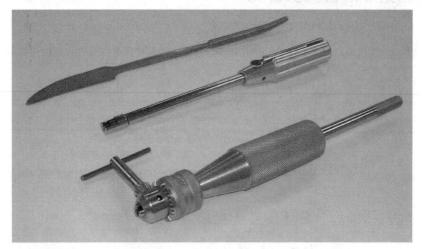

Figure 9.14   Rasp, orthopaedic screwdriver and Jacob's chuck.

Metals used in instrumentation

Instruments can be made of:

- stainless steel – martensitic or austenitic
- chromium-plated carbon
- titanium
- tungsten carbide inserts – used on tips and jaws of needle holders to increase resistance to wear; they can be replaced. These instruments have gold handles.

Newly acquired instruments

Newly acquired instruments should be thoroughly checked to ensure that they are complete and in full working order. The instruments should be washed, either manually or using an ultrasonic cleaner, then dried and lubricated. They should be packed appropriately with an indicator and then sterilised using an appropriate method.

Storage of instruments

Instrument storage should follow these guidelines:

- Store in closed cabinets if possible; if stored on open shelves they will need damp-dusting daily.
- Store evenly; do not place heavy instruments on top of light

instruments.
- Store at room temperature.
- Store away from the floor.
- Store in an area where the instruments cannot easily fall.

Cleaning procedures

Manual cleaning

- Remove visible debris immediately; do not allow it to dry on the instrument.
- The instruments may be soaked in warm (below 60 °C) deionised water containing an instrument-cleaning agent.
- Clean the instruments with a scrubbing brush; ensure all joints, serrations and grooves are fully cleaned.
- Rinse the instruments in deionised water and dry.
- Lubricate all instruments – avoid mineral oils and grease as these leave a film on the instrument that can trap bacterial spores.

Suitable lubricants are Silicon or Teflon®.

Ultrasonic cleaning

- Remove excess debris by rinsing in deionised water.
- Place instruments in the wire basket and half fill the bath with an appropriate instrument cleaner.
- A cycle of approximately 15 minutes is usually sufficient.
- Debris is removed by cavitation (implosion of air bubbles on the instrument's surface). The energy released from cavitation removes the debris.
- After completing the cycle in the ultrasonic cleaner the instruments should be rinsed in deionised water.
- When this method is used lubrication of the instruments must be performed – avoid mineral oils and grease as these leave a film on the instrument that can trap bacterial spores.

Cleaning agents

Chlorohexidine, Rapidex®, or Mediscrub® are suitable cleaning agents.

How to lay out instrumentation for surgical procedures

- Ensure that the instrument trolley was damp-dusted that morning.
- Cover the trolley with a water-resistant drape to prevent strike-through.
- A double layer of sterile cotton drapes should be placed on top; these may be provided by the drapes in which the kit is wrapped. A

scrubbed nurse wearing sterile gloves may place them on or they may be placed using Cheatle forceps (see Figure 9.8)

- If a fully prepared, prepacked kit is not used, then a scrubbed nurse wearing sterile gloves can place the instruments onto the drape, from left to right in the order the surgeon will use them.
- Add extra swabs, instruments, bowls and suture material if required.
- Place a sterile cover over the top until ready for use.

3.9.04   Sutures and needles

What you need to learn

- 🐾 You need to be able to list the different types of suture material and identify the properties:
  - 🐾 absorbable
  - 🐾 non-absorbable.
- 🐾 Outline the different types of suture needles available.
- 🐾 Describe common suture patterns and the indications for their use.
- 🐾 Describe the use of alternatives to suture materials:
  - 🐾 staples
  - 🐾 adhesive tapes
  - 🐾 tissue glue.

Absorbable suture material

- **Polyglactin 910 – Vicryl (Ethicon)**
  - synthetic
  - multifilament
  - coated in calcium stearate
  - retains 50% tensile strength at 14 days and 20% at 21 days
  - absorbed by hydrolysis by 60–90 days
  - can be dyed or undyed
  - low tissue reactivity
  - use in subcutaneous tissue, muscle and hollow viscera.
- **Polyglactin 910 – Vicryl Rapide (Ethicon)**
  - synthetic
  - multifilament
  - coated in calcium stearate
  - retains 50% tensile strength at 5 days, provides wound support for 10 days
  - absorbed by hydrolysis by 42 days
  - very similar to vicryl
  - use in perineum, oral cavity, scalp and skin.
- **Polydioxanone – PDS II (Ethicon)**

- synthetic
- monofilament
- not coated
- retains 70% tensile strength at 14 days and 14% at 50 days
- absorbed by hydrolysis by 90–180 days
- very strong, springy, low tissue reaction
- use in subcutaneous tissue, muscle, tendons, ligaments and infected sites.
- **Poliglecaprone 25 – Monocryl (Ethicon)**
  - synthetic
  - monofilament
  - not coated
  - retains 60% tensile strength at 7 days and 13% at 14 days
  - absorbed by hydrolysis by 90–120 days
  - less springy, low tissue reaction and drag
  - use in subcutaneous tissue, muscle and ligatures.
- **Polyglycolic acid – Dexon (Davis and Geck)**
  - synthetic
  - multifilament
  - can be coated in polasmer
  - retains 20% tensile strength at 14 days
  - absorbed by hydrolysis by 100–120 days
  - similar to Vicryl, some tissue drag
  - use in subcutaneous tissue, muscle, hollow viscera and ligatures.
- **Polyglyconate – Maxon (Davis and Geck)**
  - synthetic
  - monofilament
  - not coated
  - retains 70% tensile strength at 14 days
  - absorbed by hydrolysis by 60 days
  - similar to PDS but easier to handle
  - use in subcutaneous tissue and muscle.
- **Plain catgut**
  - natural
  - multifilament
  - not coated
  - loses tensile strength rapidly, wound support for 21 days
  - absorbed by enzymatic degradation and phagocytosis
  - causes inflammatory response
  - use in subcutaneous tissue, muscle, hollow viscera and ligatures.
- **Chromic catgut**
  - natural
  - multifilament
  - coated in chromic salts (resistant to digestion)
  - retains tensile strength for approximately 28 days

- absorbed by enzymatic degradation and phagocytosis after 90 days
- causes moderate inflammatory response
- use in subcutaneous tissue, muscle, hollow viscera and ligatures.

Non-absorbable suture material

- **Polymide – Nylon (Ethicon)**
  - synthetic
  - monofilament
  - not coated
  - fair knot security
  - little tissue drag
  - minimal tissue reaction
  - use in skin, fascia, nerves and blood vessels.
- **Braided Polymide – Supramid (Nurolon)**
  - synthetic
  - multifilament
  - encased in outer sheath (may break)
  - good knot security
  - non-capillary as wax impregnated
  - better handling than monofilament nylon
  - use in tissues and skin (not buried sutures).
- **Polypropylene – Prolene**
  - synthetic
  - monofilament
  - not coated
  - fair knot security but bulky and untie easily
  - minimal tissue reaction
  - string but springy
  - use in skin, fascia and blood vessels.
- **Silk – Mersilk (Ethicon)**
  - natural
  - multifilament
  - wax coat
  - excellent knot security
  - high tissue reaction
  - good handling, will absorb after approximately two years
  - use in ligatures, skin and ophthalmology. Do not use in infected sites.
- **Stainless steel wire**
  - synthetic
  - monofilament or multifilament
  - not coated
  - excellent knot security

- knots difficult to tie
- highest tensile strength of all suture materials
- strong, non-elastic, can cut tissues
- use in bone, tendon and in sternum closure.

Suture needles

The suture needle can be fully curved, half curved, or straight. Its point can be round-bodied, tapercut, reverse cutting, or blunt.

Shape of needle

Fully curved	Entire length of needle is curved into an arc Various degrees are available half circle is most common
Curved on straight/half curved	Sharp end of needle is curved but eye end is straight
Straight	Entire needle is straight

Figure 9.15 Shapes of suture needles.

Design of point and shaft

		Features	Suggested uses
Cutting		Point and sides of needle are sharp Triangular cross section with apex on inside of curve	Skin (other dense tissues)
Reverse cutting		Point and sides of needle are sharp Triangular in cross section with apex on outside of curve design used with small needles	Skin (other dense tissues)
Round bodied		Needle is round in cross section with no sharp edges	Delicate tissues e.g. fat; thin walled viscera
Taper out		Needle is similar to cutting needle at tip As needle widens, becomes round bodied in design	dense tissues other than skin e.g. fascia; thick walled viscera; mucous membranes

Figure 9.16 Design of suture needles' point and shaft.

Suture patterns

Sutures can be interrupted or continuous.
Interrupted suture patterns include:

- Simple interrupted suture – see Figure 9.17(a). This is a standard pattern with good opposition. It can be used for skin closure, and midline and visceral sutures.

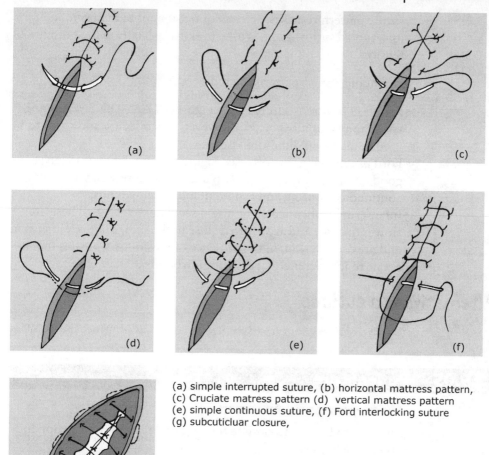

(a) simple interrupted suture, (b) horizontal mattress pattern,
(c) Cruciate matress pattern (d) vertical mattress pattern
(e) simple continuous suture, (f) Ford interlocking suture
(g) subcuticluar closure,

Figure 9.17   Suture patterns.

- Vertical mattress suture – see Figure 9.17(d). This suture involves some eversion. It interferes with the blood supply less than horizontal mattress sutures and is used in skin, especially in the presence of tension.
- Horizontal mattress suture – see Figure 9.17(b). This suture involves some eversion. Excess tension can lead to skin necrosis. It is used in skin especially in the presence of tension.
- Cruciate mattress suture – see Figure 9.17(c). The strands of this suture cross over the wound. There is less eversion than in horizontal mattress sutures and they are quicker to place. This

suture pattern resists the effects of tension more than simple interrupted suturing and is used in skin especially in the presence of tension.

Continuous suture patterns include:

- Simple continuous sutures – see Figure 9.17(e). This is a running stitch and is rapidly placed. However, it is insecure and tends to be used in fascia, midline and viscera.
- Ford interlocking sutures – see Figure 9.17(f). This suture gives good opposition and is rapidly placed. It is more secure than simple continuous suturing and is used in long skin wounds.
- Interdermal/subcuticular sutures – see Figure 9.17(g). These are slower to place and are sutured close to the skin. They resist tension and are used in skin, in the presence of tension and in sites that are prone to interference, eg castration wounds.

Alternatives to sutures

Staples, adhesive tapes, or tissue glue can be used instead of sutures.

3.9.05　Patient care

What you need to learn

- You need to be able to outline the required patient preparation for surgery, including:
  - withholding of food
  - diet
  - hygiene
  - defecation
  - urination
  - medication.
- Outline the preferred order of priority for aseptic surgical procedures:
  - Sterile/clean/clean-contaminated/contaminated/dirty.
- Describe the preparation of an animal for surgical procedures. To include:
  - position of animal
  - surgical site
  - surgical drapes
  - pre-medication
  - restraint and handling
  - clippers
  - razors
  - scissors
  - skin disinfectants/antiseptics.

Patient preparation for surgery

- **Withholding food** – Food should be withheld for 12 hours; water may be offered until the morning of surgery.
- **Diet** – The patient's normal diet should be offered unless otherwise indicated by the veterinary surgeon, eg low-fibre diet before large bowel radiography/surgery.
- **Hygiene** – Ideally each patient should be bathed and dried before surgery to decrease contamination.
- **Defaecation and urination** – All owners should be advised to allow their pet to urinate and defaecate before attending the practice. The patient should also be offered a further opportunity once in hospital. For some procedures, eg large bowel radiography/surgery, an enema may be required.
- **Medication** – The patient should receive any prescribed medication as advised by the veterinary surgeon. Further drugs may be given, eg sedatives and analgesia (pre-medication), antibiotics.

Priority of aseptic surgical procedures

Theatre procedure lists should be organised to follow this order:

- clean/sterile procedures, eg orthopaedics
- clean/contaminated procedures, eg gastrointestinal surgery with no break into the gastrointestinal tract
- contaminated procedures, eg pyometra, bowel resection surgery which involves a break into infected organs.
- dirty procedures, eg abscesses.

Preparation of an animal for surgical procedures

- **Position of the animal** – The patient should be positioned in the most appropriate manner for the procedure being undertaken; remember to be careful and to take precautions with any wounds, fractures, dressings, or external fixation work. Check the final position with the veterinary surgeon as it is not ideal to change a patient's position midway through a procedure.
- **Surgical site** – The surgical site must be identified correctly, eg ensure if it is the right or left side; the site should then be prepared as described earlier (see 3.9.02).
- **Surgical drapes** – Arrange plain surgical drapes in the following manner:
  - The first drape is placed between the surgeon and the patient, the other three are then placed in a methodical order, see Figure 9.18.
  - For fenestrated drapes only one drape is used with an

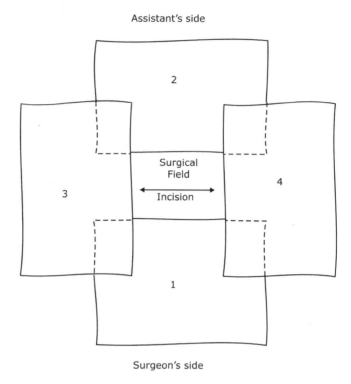

Assistant's side

Surgeon's side

Figure 9.18 Surgical drapes.

appropriately sized hole/window for the procedure. The drape is placed over the patient with the window over the surgical site.

- **Pre-medication** – This will be decided by the veterinary surgeon, if indeed the patient receives any. Pre-medication is usually administered 30 minutes before induction of anaesthesia.
- **Restraint and handling** – The patient should be restrained and handled with care; the method may need adapting if the patient is injured. Always maintain your own safety first.
- **Electric clippers** – These are used in preparing the patient. Clip along the grain of the hair then against it. Keep the blade at the same angle as the skin to prevent clipper rash and cuts. Ensure the teeth on the blade are all present and sharp.
- **Razors** – These should not be used as they create small nicks/grazed areas which then habour bacteria.
- **Scissors** – These can be used to clip hair from the leg for induction, or to identify the surgical area, eg clipping part of the hair over a lump to be removed.
- **Skin disinfectants/antiseptics** – see 3.9.02.

3.9.06   Intra-operative care

What you need to learn

* You need to be able to recognise how to assist the veterinary surgeon during surgical procedures:
    * commonly carried out procedures (see range).
* Outline methods of controlling haemorrhage:
    * swabs
    * instruments
    * ligatures.
* Describe correct swabbing technique.
* Describe methods of preventing heat loss from the patient during surgical procedures:
    * monitoring temperature
    * insulation
    * additional sources of heat
    * species and procedures from range.
* Identify and report hazards that may occur in the theatre.

How to assist during surgical procedures

Prepare yourself for surgery scrubbing, gloving and gowning as needed. The duties of a sterile assistant include passing instruments to the surgeon; holding instruments and tissues for the surgeon as directed; removing soiled or used material from the surgical field; counting swabs and providing fluids for lavage, and suction as required.

Methods of controlling haemorrhage

Haemorrhage can be controlled using swabs, instruments, eg Spencer Wells or Halstead Mosquito artery forceps, ligatures, or diathermy.

Swabbing technique

When using swabs the procedure outlined below should be followed.
* Count the total number of swabs before surgery.
* Use one swab at a time.
* Blot the haemorrhaging area as opposed to wiping it as the latter disrupts the clotting actions.
* Count all swabs again at the end of surgery.

Preventing heat loss

* Monitor temperature, both core and peripheral.

- Insulate the patient – wrap the patient in bubble-wrap, or light-weight blankets.
- Place heat pads or warm water beds underneath the patient.
- Wrap the patient's extremities in foil.
- Maintain theatre temperature between 21 and 23 °C.
- Use heat/moisture exchanges within the anaesthetic circuit.
- Use rebreathing circuits where appropriate.
- Warm all intravenous and lavage fluid.
- Avoid clipping large areas and soaking with preparation agents.

Hazards in the operating theatre

The operating theatre contains many hazards, among them:

- pollution from anaesthetic gases
- equipment – ensure all equipment receives regular maintenance checks and electrical safety tests
- disposal of sharps
- clinical waste.

3.9.07　Post-operative care

What you need to learn

- You need to be able to describe the immediate post-operative care for surgical cases:
  - all commonly carried out procedures (see range).
- Describe the procedures to be undertaken before removing the animal from the operating table:
  - all commonly carried out procedures (see range).
- Outline the importance of intubation, its advantages and disadvantages.
- Describe the procedure for endotracheal intubation:
  - dogs
  - cats.
- Identify when to remove the endotracheal tube:
  - all species from range.
- Describe post-operative emergencies and first aid procedures:
  - haemorrhage
  - laryngospasm
  - shock
  - hypothermia
  - vomiting.
- Describe nursing principles for specific surgical cases post-operatively:
  - all commonly carried out procedures (see range).
- Identify the analgesics commonly used intra- and post-operatively.

☙ Describe signs of common long-term post-operative complications, and associated nursing:
  ☙ shock
  ☙ coughing
  ☙ decubitus ulcers
  ☙ hypostatic pneumonia.

Immediate post-operative care

The airway must be maintained. The animal should be attended at all times in the immediate post-operative period until in sternal recumbency. Any wounds should be observed for haemorrhage. Body temperature should be monitored and maintained. Heart rate and pulse should also be monitored.

Procedures before removing the patient from the operating table

The ET tube should be removed at the appropriate time. All monitoring equipment should be detached. Dressings should be placed before the patient enters recovery. Swabs and purse-string sutures should be removed. Prepare the recovery environment before moving the animal.

Intubation

Intubation has its **advantages**.

• It provides a secure airway.
• It protects the airway from saliva, secretions, or other fluids, such as water during dental procedures.
• It allows positive pressure ventilation (IPPV).
• It reduces anatomical dead space.
• It allows maintenance of anaesthesia or provides a means to supply oxygen.
• It reduces pollution from waste anaesthetic gases.

However, there are also **disadvantages**.

• The tube may kink during positioning.
• Over-inflation of cuffs can occlude the tube and can cause damage to the trachea.
• It can increase resistance to breathing if the diameter of the tube is too small.
• It can cause traumatic laryngitis; this can be a problem particularly in cats due to poor technique, over-sized tubes, or the lack of local anaesthetic used before intubation.

- Chemical tracheitis can occur as a result of contamination with cleaning fluids.
- Endobronchial intubation can be a problem.

How to intubate a dog

- Position the patient in right or left lateral recumbency.
- An assistant holds the head up, supporting the base of the head with the left hand and holding the maxilla and nose upwards with the right hand (keeping fingers out of the mouth).
- Extend the tongue forward out of the mouth, pulling down slightly to lower the mandible – this enables the larynx to be viewed.
- Lubricate a correctly sized tube, insert into the mouth towards the soft palate (you may need to push this dorsally away from the epiglottis.
- Insert the tube over the epiglottis (pushed down by the tip of the tube) and between the vocal folds.

How to intubate a cat

- Position the patient in right or left lateral recumbency.
- An assistant holds the head up, supporting the base of the head with the left hand and holding the maxilla and nose upwards with the right hand (keeping fingers out of the mouth).
- Extend the tongue forward out of the mouth pulling down slightly to lower the mandible – this enables the larynx to be viewed.
- If using a laryngoscope place the tongue between the thumb and forefinger and hold the laryngoscope with the same hand.
- Use the blade of the laryngoscope to push the tongue down, not the epiglottis, as this enables the larynx to be viewed.
- Spray the larynx with local anaesthetic to desensitise it; wait 60-90 seconds.
- Lubricate a correctly sized tube and insert it into the mouth and between the laryngeal folds during inspiration. The laryngeal folds can be seen moving in and out as the cat breathes.

When to remove an endotracheal tube

In dogs the tube should be removed once the gag reflex has returned. In cats it should be removed before the gag reflex returns.

Leave the cuff inflated until removal; some procedures may require you to remove the tube with the cuff still inflated, eg oral surgery. Remove the tube in a smooth downward motion to avoid damage to the trachea and larynx.

Post-operative emergencies

Haemorrhage

- Control external haemorrhage with digital pressure or with pressure bandages.
- Internal haemorrhage is more complicated. Usually the patient will be re-anaesthised, the wound will be incised and the haemorrhage can then be controlled with instruments or ligatures.
- Prepare intravenous fluids.

Laryngospasm

- Keep the endotracheal tube in place if it has not been removed and begin steroidal treatment if necessary. A tracheotomy can be performed if needed.

Shock

- Monitor all vital parameters – heart rate, pulse, mucous membrane colour, capillary refill time, and respiration rate and pattern.
- Prepare intravenous fluids.
- Keep the patient warm with light-weight blankets or bubble-wrap; do not apply direct heat using heat pads.
- Prepare any antidotes to anaesthetic agents used.

Hypothermia

- Prepare any antidotes to anaesthetic agents used.
- Keep the patient warm using blankets, foil, bubble-wrap, or heat pads.
- Keep all windows and doors shut.
- Maintain the temperature of the room between 21 and 23 °C.
- Monitor rectal temperature every 10 minutes.
- Warm any intravenous fluids.

Vomiting

- Stay with the patient at all times.
- Hold the head and neck down or hang over the side of the table. The body may also be raised so the head and neck are in a downward direction.
- Maintain the position of the head and neck until the animal is fully conscious.
- Prepare any anti-emetic drugs the veterinary surgeon has requested.
- Keep the patient and its bedding clean and dry.

Analgesics used intra- and post-operatively

Also see 3.10.03.

The following drugs can be used:

- carprofen
- meloxicam
- morphine
- buprenorphine
- pethidine
- fentanyl
- butorphanol.

Long-term post-operative complications

Shock

Signs of shock include:

- tachycardia
- a weak rapid pulse
- pale or cyanotic mucous membranes
- slow capillary refill time
- cold extremities
- shallow breathing
- tachypnoea.

Nursing for shock requires the following procedures.

- Monitor all vital parameters – heart rate, pulse, mucous membrane colour, capillary refill time, and respiration rate and pattern every five minutes.
- Prepare warm intravenous fluids.
- Keep the patient warm with light-weight blankets or bubble-wrap; do not apply direct heat using heat pads.
- Prepare any antidotes to the anaesthetic agents used.

Coughing

Signs of coughing can be:

- harsh coughing
- grunting noises
- wheezing
- the patient becomes restless and agitated
- the patient refuses to eat when offered food.

Nursing a patient with coughing requires the following procedures.

- Differentiate the problem from kennel cough.
- Examine the throat and mouth – check for ulcers or inflammation and ensure they are clean and patent.

- Prepare any drugs requested by the veterinary surgeon.
- Feed mushy soft food (by hand if required) when appropriate.
- Remember tender loving care (TLC).

Decubitus ulcers

The signs of decubitus ulcers are:

- red sores on bony prominences
- possible ulceration or bleeding
- patient may demonstrate signs of pain or restlessness.

Nursing a patient with decubitus ulcers requires:

- Clean and dry the area with a suitable skin antiseptic.
- Apply extra padding or bedding.
- Turn the patient frequently.
- Remember TLC.

Hypostatic pneumonia

The signs of hypostatic pneumonia include:

- shallow rapid respiration
- signs of restlessness or discomfort
- pale or cyanotic mucous membranes
- slow capillary refill time.

Nursing a patient with hypostatic pneumonia requires:

- Supply oxygen if required.
- Monitor all vital parameters – heart rate, pulse, mucous membrane colour, capillary refill time, and respiration rate and pattern every five minutes.
- Turn the patient every two hours.
- Position the patient in sternal recumbency using foam pads or bedding.
- Remember TLC.

Multiple choice questions

1. Asepsis is defined as
   - ☐ A The removal of micro-organisms but not always bacterial spores.
   - ☐ B The presence of pathogens in the blood of the patient
   - ☐ C Freedom from all micro-organisms including bacterial spores.
   - ☐ D Prevention of sepsis by inhibiting or destroying micro-organisms.

2. The sterilising time for an autoclave at 126 °C and pressure of 20 psi is
   - ☐ A 5 minutes
   - ☐ B 10 minutes
   - ☐ C 15 minutes
   - ☐ D 20 minutes

3. Hot air ovens cannot be used to sterilise
   - ☐ A rubber
   - ☐ B glass
   - ☐ C cutting instruments
   - ☐ D drill bits

4. The **most** accurate sterility monitoring method which can be used in an autoclave is
   - ☐ A Bowie–Dick tape
   - ☐ B TST strips
   - ☐ C Browne's tubes
   - ☐ D Spore tests.

5. Items sterilised by ethylene oxide must be left to allow the gas to dissipate for
   - ☐ A 12 hours
   - ☐ B 24 hours
   - ☐ C 36 hours
   - ☐ D 48 hours.

6. A sterile gown should initially be picked up by the
   - ☐ A outside of the gown at the cuffs
   - ☐ B inside of the gown by the waist
   - ☐ C inside of the gown at the shoulder seams
   - ☐ D outside of the gown at the shoulder seams.

7. It is recommended that unused sterile packs should be repacked and resterilised after
   - ☐ A 2 weeks
   - ☐ B 4–6 weeks
   - ☐ C 6–8 weeks
   - ☐ D 8–10 weeks.

8. When draping a patient using the 'four drape' technique the first drape should be placed
   - ☐ A furthest away from the surgeon on the opposite side of the patient
   - ☐ B between the surgeon and the nearest side of the table
   - ☐ C covering the extremities
   - ☐ D covering the cranial aspect of the patient.

9. To help reduce hypothermia in the patient the ambient temperature of an operating theatre should be maintained between
   - ☐ A 12–15°C
   - ☐ B 15–20°C
   - ☐ C 20–25°C
   - ☐ D 25–30°C.

10. Which of the following is not a self-retaining retractor?
   - ☐ A West
   - ☐ B Travers
   - ☐ C Gelpi
   - ☐ D Hohmann.

11. The forceps used to aseptically lay out an instrument trolley are
   - ☐ A Allis
   - ☐ B Cheatle
   - ☐ C Spencer Wells
   - ☐ D Treves.

12. The instrument depicted in the diagram is
   - ☐ A Gillies needle holders
   - ☐ B Macphails needle holders
   - ☐ C Metzenbaum scissors
   - ☐ D Heath scissors.

13. The instrument most likely to have the following serrations at their tips is
   - ☐ A Spencer Wells artery forceps
   - ☐ B Allis tissue forceps
   - ☐ C Doyen bowel clamps
   - ☐ D Lane forceps.

14. The suture material which is absorbed by enzymatid degradation and phagocytosis is
    ☐ A Polyglactin 910
    ☐ B Polydioxanone
    ☐ C Chromic catgut
    ☐ D Polymide.

15. An example of a synthetic, monofilament absorbable suture material is
    ☐ A polyglactin 910
    ☐ B polydioxanone
    ☐ C polyglycolic acid
    ☐ D polymide.

16. The skin suture pattern illustrated in the diagram is
    ☐ A vertical mattress
    ☐ B horizontal mattress
    ☐ C cruciate mattress
    ☐ D simple continuous.

17. An incision made into the abdomen to remove a foreign body from the small intestine would be classified as
    ☐ A clean
    ☐ B clean-contaminated
    ☐ C contaminated
    ☐ D dirty.

18. The correct time to remove an endotracheal tube from a cat following anaesthesia is
    ☐ A once the gag reflex has returned
    ☐ B before the gag reflex returns
    ☐ C cats should only be given anaesthetic via a mask
    ☐ D as soon as the anaesthetic agents are turned off

19. Which of the following patients is least likely to be susceptible to hypothermia:
    ☐ A   a neonatal puppy
    ☐ B   a rabbit spay
    ☐ C   a geriatric dog
    ☐ D   a cat spay.

20. On a busy day's operating schedule the procedure which should be performed first is
    ☐ A   cat dental
    ☐ B   perineal hernia repair
    ☐ C   anterior cruciate repair
    ☐ D   dog castration.

Anaesthesia

3.10.01 Physiology of anaesthesia

What you need to learn

* You need to be able to identify the types of anaesthesia, and know their advantages and disadvantages:
  * general
  * spinal
  * regional
  * local
  * topical.
* Outline the reasons for anaesthesia.
* Outline the central nervous control of respiration and the effects of anaesthesia on the respiratory system:
  * changes of respiratory rate and character.
* Explain normal and abnormal breathing patterns:
  * bradypnoea
  * tachypnoea
  * dyspnoea
  * apnoea.
* Outline the central control of heart rate and blood pressure, and understand associated terms:
  * tachycardia
  * bradycardia
  * arrhythmia
  * dysrhythmia
  * hypertension
  * hypotension.
* Outline the effects of anaesthesia on the heart and circulation:
  * heart rate and pulse characteristics.
* Describe briefly the peripheral control of blood pressure and tissue perfusion.

Types of anaesthesia

General anaesthesia

Advantages of general anaesthesia are that it allows surgical procedures to be performed and it can be controlled.

However, **disadvantages** are that there can be effects of the drugs on organs, more preparation is involved, skill is needed in administering the anaesthetic and equipment such as anaesthetic trolley, circuits and monitoring devices are required.

Spinal anaesthesia (epidural)

Advantages of spinal anaesthesia include the fact that surgical procedures of the lower half of the body can be performed without causing pain, eg Caesarean section, the effects of the drugs are less than those for general anaesthesia and the patient maintains consciousness throughout.

A **disadvantage** with this type of anaesthesia is that experience and skill are required for its administration. There is also the risk of damage to the spinal cord and the introduction of infection.

Analgesia may be given by this route.

Regional anaesthesia

Advantages of regional anaesthesia are that the anaesthetic is administered locally so there are very few effects on the organs from drugs; procedures such as de-horning and Caesarean sections in large animals can be performed; it can be used in the field and no monitoring devices are needed. Little equipment is needed and consciousness is maintained.

Disadvantages can be that time may be limited as the effects of the local anaesthetic diminish, although some types of local anaesthetic can be 'topped up'. This type of anaesthesia is restricted to a certain area and producing regional anaesthesia may be painful.

Local anaesthesia

Advantages of local anaesthesia are many. It can be used on any part of the body and is excellent for short procedures. Consciousness is maintained and there are few effects on the organs from the drugs used. It can be used in the field and requires no monitoring devices and little equipment.

Disadvantages, however, are that its use is restricted to certain areas. Producing the local anaesthesia may be painful and time may be limited as the effects of the local anaesthetic diminish, although some types of local anaesthetic may be 'topped up'.

Topical anaesthesia

Advantages of topical anaesthesia include the fact that it can be applied directly to the skin or mucous membranes. It is useful for providing a certain level of anaesthesia, eg cream can be applied to a limb before introduction of a catheter. It is cheap and can be given to the owner to use at home. There are no effects of the drug on organs. **Disadvantages**, however, are that its use is limited and its effects may be variable.

Reasons for anaesthesia

Anaesthesia is used to:

• perform painless and humane surgery or procedures
• provide analgesia
• provide muscle relaxation.

Respiration

Respiration is controlled by the pons and medulla oblongata in the hindbrain. The medulla oblongata and chemoreceptors control the rate and depth of respiration by monitoring carbon dioxide levels in the cerebrospinal fluid and blood. The effects of anaesthetic drugs (used in general anaesthesia) depress both the respiration rate and depth (character).

The normal breathing pattern is 10 to 30 breaths per minute with adequate depth.

• **Bradypnoea** is a decreased respiration rate.
• **Tachypnoea** is an increased respiration rate.
• **Dyspnoea** describes difficulty in breathing.
• **Apnoea** is the cessation of respiration.

Heart rate and blood pressure

The heart rate is controlled by the autonomic nervous system (sympathetic and parasympathetic). Blood pressure is controlled by baroreceptors (which stretch when blood pressure is high) relaying information to the medulla.

• **Tachycardia** is an increased heart rate.
• **Bradycardia** is a decreased heart rate.
• **Arrhythmia** describes an irregular heart beat.
• **Dysrhythmia** describes an irregular heart beat.
• **Hypertension** is high blood pressure.
• **Hypotension** is low blood pressure.

General anaesthesia depresses the cardiovascular system, producing decreased heart rates, contractility and pulse rates. The character of the pulse may weaken.

Blood pressure and tissue perfusion

Blood pressure is controlled by baroreceptors (which stretch when blood pressure is high) relaying information to the medulla.

If the **blood pressure is high** the medulla will:

- reduce sympathetic activity – lowering the heart rate
- increase parasympathetic activity – causing the heart to slow down
- produce vasodilatation – lowering peripheral blood pressure.

If **blood pressure is low** it works in the opposite direction.

Adequate blood pressure maintains tissue perfusion as sufficient levels of oxygen are delivered and carbon dioxide is removed. If blood pressure is low tissues are in danger of hypoxia which in turn will cause damage to the tissues.

- **General anaesthesia:** (loss of consciousness and memory of the procedure and the ability to be unaware of noxious stimuli).
- **Spinal anaesthesia:** local anaesthetic administered into the epidural space, producing loss of motor function and sensation.
- **Regional anaesthesia:** local anaesthetic administered into a nerve plexus, eg local anaesthetic administered into the brachial plexus produces anaesthesia of the forelimb.
- **Local anaesthesia:** temporary loss of pain, movement and sensation produced by blocking the motor and sensory nerves.
- **Topical anaesthesia:** absorption of local anesthetic through the mucous membranes. As the drug molecules are quite large they are unable to create loss of sensation on the skin.

3.10.02 Pre-operative care

What you need to learn

- ☙ You need to be able to outline the instructions which should be given to clients to enable them to present their animals in a suitable condition for anaesthesia.
- ☙ Describe the patient assessment procedures carried out before anaesthesia and the requirement for recording animal details:
  - ☙ animal weight
  - ☙ laboratory results
  - ☙ animal general health state
  - ☙ TPR.
- ☙ Describe a 'poor risk' patient and identify classes of risk from an animal's physical status.
- ☙ Outline procedures for anaesthetising common exotic species and the associated problems:

❀ small mammals
❀ birds
❀ reptiles.
❀ Identify factors which may determine the choice of anaesthetic drug/agent.

Instructions to clients

The following instructions should be given to the clients before anaesthesia of their animals.

- The patient should not receive food or milk after 8 pm or from the previous evening.
- Water may be available to them until the morning of the procedure.
- Give the patient an opportunity to empty their bladder and bowels.
- Give any medication prescribed by the veterinary surgeon.

Patient assessment

Before anaesthesia patients should be assessed:

- Record the patient's weight.
- Record any laboratory results.
- Record the patient's general health state (assess cardiac function, respiratory function, mucous membrane colour and capillary refill time).
- Take the patient's temperature, pulse, and respiration rate (TPR).
- Ask the owner if the patient has been coughing or sneezing, has demonstrated exercise intolerance, or has had vomiting or diarrhoea.
- Ask the owner if the patient has been starved.

Classes of risks

Anaesthesia carries a certain risk. The level of this risk will vary between patients.

A **poor risk patient** is one with an underlying disease, eg renal, liver, cardiac, making them more susceptible to the effects of the drugs used in general anaesthesia.

The American Society of Anaesthesiologists (ASA) risk assessment is as follows:

- Class I – healthy patients, eg routine bitch spay
- Class II – mild systemic disease, eg grade II/VI heart murmur with no clinical signs
- Class III – severe systemic disease, eg grade IV/VI heart murmur with clinical signs of heart failure

- Class IV – severe systemic disease which is a constant threat to life, eg pyometra
- Class V – patient unlikely to survive 24 hours with or without surgery, eg bleeding splenic haemangiosarcoma.

Anaesthesia in exotics

General anaesthesia in exotic species should be undertaken with caution for a number of reasons.

- Most exotic species (birds, rabbits, guinea-pigs and chinchillas in particular) are very susceptible to stress and can become shocked very easily. Stress during induction can cause respiratory arrest.
- Exotic species are often smaller than cats and dogs and can quickly cool while under general anaesthesia. Great care must be taken to minimise heat loss during the procedure.
- Doses of anaesthetic agents must be calculated very carefully to avoid accidental overdose.
- Prolonged recovery from anaesthesia can result in gastrointestinal disorders.
- Poikilothermic (cold-blooded) species such as reptiles will take much longer to recover from general anaesthesia if their temperature falls.
- Small rodents and birds have a very high metabolic rate. Care should be taken to avoid starving these animals to avoid a dangerous drop in blood glucose levels.
- Animals which are being anaesthetised for dental treatment are often in poor condition and may be suffering from concurrent bacterial infections. Rabbits and rodents in particular are often dehydrated and in poor body condition when suffering from dental disease. Many are suffering from respiratory infections such as pasteurellosis. These animals require fluid therapy and nutritional support before, during, and after anaesthesia.

There are a number of methods of general anaesthesia used in exotic species:

Inhalational agents can be administered through a mask or an anaesthetic chamber.

- Halothane and Isofluorane are used commonly. Isofluorane is often favoured as it is short-acting.
- The smell of the anaesthetic gas can cause some animals (rabbits and rodents in particular) to breath hold.
- Gas chambers can be very stressful for an unsedated animal.

A number of **injectable agents** can be used to produce sedation or surgical anaesthesia.

- Agents used include Alphaxolone/Alphadolone, Ketamine, Medetomidine, Diazepam, Fentanyl/fluanisone, Midazolam and propofol.
- Doxapram is an injectable respiratory stimulant which can be used during anaesthesia (**NB** high doses can cause seizures).
- Many of the injectable anaesthetic agents cause respiratory depression. Oxygen should be supplemented for animal where respiratory depression is noted during anaesthesia.

Factors determining the choice of drug

There are many factors that determine the choice of anaesthetic drug to be used:

- age of the patient
- health status of the patient
- pregnancy
- previous reactions to drugs
- emergency situation, eg unstarved patient
- temperament of the patient
- skill of the veterinary surgeon
- the nature and duration of the procedure.

3.10.03 Pre-medication

What you need to learn

- You need to be able to describe pre-medication and state and understand the reasons for this procedure including associated terms:
  - sedative
  - hypnotic
  - neuroleptic
  - ataractic.
- Outline the main pre-medicants in use and the physical forms in which they can be used.
- Calculate and prepare pre-medicants in correct form and dose for use in a clinical situation.
- Outline the main pharmacological properties of each of the commonly used premedicant drugs, and recognise their differences:
  - acepromazime
  - diazepam
  - medetomidine
  - opiate
  - analgesics.
- Describe the effect that the route of administration will have on the clinical performance of pre-medicants

🐾 intravenous

🐾 intramuscular

🐾 subcutaneous.

🐾 Identify which pre-medicants are controlled drugs.

Pre-medication will:

• calm and control the patient
• reduce stress
• minimise pain
• produce muscle relaxation
• decrease the amount of anaesthetic drug required
• produce safe, uncomplicated induction, maintenance and recovery.

Various forms of pre-medication are available.

• **sedative** – a drug that calms and causes drowsiness
• **hypnotic** – a drug that induces sleep but the patient can be aroused
• **neuroleptic** – a combination of a sedative drug and an opioid drug
• **ataractic/tranquilliser** – a drug that calms and relieves anxiety but does not cause drowsiness.

Pre-medicant drugs available include:

• phenothiazines, eg acepromazine (ACP), available as tablets or injectable
• benzodiazepines, eg diazepam, available as tablets and injectable
• alpha 2 adrenoceptor agonists, eg medetomidine, available as injectable
• opioids, eg morphine, available as injectable
• non-steroidal anti-inflammatory drugs (NSAID), eg carprofen, available as tablets or injectable
• anticholinergics, eg atropine, available as injectable.

Calculating doses

General calculation of dose is:

weight of patient (in kg) × mg of dose rate of the drug, divided by the mg/ml of the drug

Example:

A 20 kg dog is to be administered ACP 2 mg/ml, used at a dose rate of 0.05 mg/kg. Weight × dose rate will give 20 (kg) × 0.05 (mg/kg) = 1. This is then divided by 2 mg/ml to give 0.5 ml.

The correct dose for a 20 kg dog is therefore 0.5 ml.

Phenothiazine – ACP

• ACP is available as 2 mg/ml and 10 mg/ml injection and 10 mg and

25 mg tablets.
* It causes sedation and tranquillisation.
* It can cause hypotension and bradycardia.
* Increasing the dose does not give increased sedation, only increased side-effects.
* Use with caution in boxers.

Benzodiazepine – Diazepam

* Diazepam is available as 10 mg/2 ml injectable and 10 mg tablets.
* It causes tranquillisation.
* It can be used as an anti-epileptic and as an appetite stimulant.

Alpha 2 adrenoceptor agonist – medetomidine

* Medetomidine effects can be reversed by administration of the alpha 2 adrenoceptor antagonist, atipamezole.
* It causes sedation.
* It may cause vomiting or nausea.
* It causes hypotension and bradycardia.
* It markedly reduces the amount of anaesthetic agent required.
* It is available as injectables.

Opiates/Opioids

* Opiates are available as full agonists, eg morphine, or partial agonists, eg buprenorphine.
* Opioids produce analgesia.
* They can cause euphoria.
* They may cause vomiting or nausea.
* They are available as injectables.
* They can cause constipation.
* They cause respiratory depression and depression of the cough reflex.

Analgesics

* Opiates, NSAID, or local anaesthetics can be used.
* NSAID are available as drops, tablets or injectables.

Routes of administration

Routes available for administration of pre-medication are:

* intravenous (iv) – rapid uptake
* intramuscular (im) – moderate uptake
* subcutaneous (sc) – slow uptake.

Always refer to the manufacturer's instructions for each drug to check the administration method. Not all drugs can be given by all the described routes.

Controlled drugs

The following are controlled drugs for use in pre-medication.

- morphine
- pethidine
- methadone
- omnipon
- fentanyl
- fentanyl/fluanisone
- etorphine hydrochloride/methotrimeprazine.

3.10.04 Analgesia

What you need to learn

- You need to be able to describe the difference between analgesia and anaesthesia.
- Explain the importance and benefits of analgesia in:
  - dogs
  - cats
  - small mammals.
- Recognise the use of analgesics in different species and the possibility of them not being licensed for use in that species:
  - small mammals
  - birds
  - reptiles.
- Outline the main pharmacological properties of each of the commonly used analgesic agents:
  - effects of analgesics by various routes.

Analgesia differs from anaesthesia. **Analgesia** produces pain relief while **anaesthesia** produces a state where a procedure can be performed without causing pain, with or without consciousness.

There are several benefits of analgesia.

- Analgesia controls both acute and chronic pain.
- It provides balanced anaesthesia – reducing the amount of anaesthetic drugs required in a procedure.
- It assists in the handling of patients when used as pre-medication.

Agents for use in analgesia

Morphine is an opiate and is a full agonist. It has the following characteristics:

- produces analgesia
- can cause euphoria
- may cause vomiting or nausea
- is available as injectables
- can cause constipation
- causes respiratory depression
- causes depression of the cough reflex
- has a duration of action of four hours
- is contraindicated in head trauma
- can cause pain on injection
- can be administered sc, im, or iv.

Pethidine is an opiate and a full agonist. It has the following characteristics:

- it is the only full agonist licensed for use in cats and dogs
- is less potent than morphine
- has a rapid onset of action
- does not cause vomiting
- has a duration of action of 40–60 minutes
- can be administered im or sc.

Buprenorphine is an opiate and is a partial agonist. It has the following characteristics:

- has a slow onset of action
- has a duration of action of 4–6 hours
- increased doses can reduce analgesia
- can be administered sc or im.

Carprofen is an NSAID. It has the following characteristics:

- diminishes certain components of the inflammatory response
- should be used with caution in patients with renal disease
- should not be used if the patient is in shock
- can be administered orally, sc, or iv.

Meloxicam is also an NSAID. It has the following characteristics.

- diminishes certain components of the inflammatory response
- should be used with caution in patients with renal disease
- should not be used if the patient is in shock
- can be administered either orally or sc.

Analgesia in exotic species

Analgesia is often overlooked in exotic species but is an extremely important tool in the treatment of these animals. Analgesia hastens anaesthetic recovery and reduces the likelihood of post-operative shock.

Various analgesic agents are commonly used in exotic species. They include opiate agents, such as morphine and buprenorphine, and NSAIDS, such as meloxicam, carprofen and ketoprofen.

Very few analgesic agents are licensed for use in exotic species. However, data is available regarding the use of these agents in exotic species (particularly laboratory species). Unlicensed products may be used when there is not a licensed alternative and when the product is recognised for use in that species.

3.10.05 Care and maintenance of apparatus and anaesthetic equipment

What you need to learn

* You need to be able to describe the principal and working parts of an anaesthetic machine.
* Describe the use of the anaesthetic machine and equipment.
* Describe how to clean, care for, maintain and store all equipment.
* Outline commonly occurring faults of equipment.
* Describe the colour coding of gas cylinders and the sizes available.
* Describe how to evaluate the amount of gas in a cylinder.

Anaesthetic machine and equipment

The following are the components of the equipment required for anaesthesia:

* trolley unit – has four wheels and shelves, provides storage space but takes up space itself, or a trolley stand – has three/four wheels, no store for nitrous oxide, limited storage, take up less space
* attachments for gas cylinders
* reducing valve – placed between cylinder and flowmeter, allows control of the gas flow
* pressure gauge – indicates gas levels
* flowmeters – control gas flow to the patient, gas-specific
* vaporiser – allows a volatile agent to be used
* alarm – driven either by oxygen or nitrous oxide, is usually audible but some are visual
* oxygen flush valve – delivers high flow of oxygen only
* reservoir bag – supplies a gas reservoir and is essential for intermittent positive pressure ventilation (IPPV)
* corrugated tubing – conducts gas
* expiratory valve – allows gas to escape in semi-closed systems
* soda lime canister – allows re-breathing of gas
* face masks – placed around the face to deliver gas
* scavenging systems – conduct waste gases

• endotracheal tubes – rubber or silicone, allow delivery of gas

Cleaning and maintenance of equipment

It is important that the anaesthetic equipment is maintained in good working order.

• Turn off all cylinder valves, flowmeters and vaporisers.
• Dispose of soda lime if exhausted.
• Most machines require little maintenance.
• Vaporisers require annual servicing.
• All rubber equipment should be washed thoroughly in antiseptic solution and rinsed with water. Allow to drain and dry. Replace any worn parts, eg cuffs on endotracheal tubes. When washing endotracheal tubes close the cuff so water does not enter the cuff.
• Any circuit valves showing a tendency to stick should be dismantled, washed, dried and reassembled.
• Wash all circuits with antiseptic solution and allow to dry.

Faults of equipment

Equipment can have the following faults.

• Vaporisers may stick.
• There may be leaks in the tubing of circuits.
• The cuffs of the endotracheal tubes may not inflate because of a tear or leak.
• The bobbins of the flowmeters may not be spinning – indicating a fault with the flowmeter.
• The Bodock washer may be missing on the cylinder connections, causing hissing of gas.

Colour coding of cylinders

• **Oxygen** cylinders are black with white shoulders/neck, available in sizes AA–J, filled to a pressure of 132 atmospheres.
• **Nitrous oxide** cylinders are blue, available in sizes AA–J, filled to a pressure of 51 atmospheres.
• **Carbon dioxide** are grey.
• **Cycloproprane** are orange.

Evaluating contents of a gas cylinder

Checking the pressure gauges will allow the amount of gas in the cylinder to be ascertained.

Weighing the cylinder, then deducting that weight from the weight printed on the cylinder is the only accurate method with which to evaluate nitrous oxide.

3.10.06　Signs of anaesthesia

What you need to learn

☙ You need to be able to describe signs of light anaesthesia:
  ☙ voluntary/involuntary excitement stage.
☙ Describe and know the importance of the signs of medium and deep anaesthesia:
  ☙ respiration character
  ☙ eye movement/position
  ☙ palpebral reflexes
  ☙ degree of muscle relaxation.
☙ Describe the signs of anaesthetic overdose.

Signs of **light anaesthesia** can be divided into voluntary and involuntary.

Voluntary signs are:

• increased respiration
• increased heart rate
• eye position – the eye rotates back to the centre
• reflexes become more marked.

Involuntary excitement is seen when insufficient induction agent is used; the patient becomes excited and panicky.

Signs of **medium anaesthesia** are:

• regular smooth respiration
• eye position – rotated medially and ventrally
• diminished palpebral reflex
• good muscle relaxation
• pulse – regular and strong.

Signs of **deep anaesthesia** are:

• variable and shallow respiration
• eye position – centrally fixed
• absent palpebral reflex
• greatly reduced muscle relaxation
• pulse – weak as the blood pressure drops.

Signs of an **anaesthetic overdose** are:

• irregular, shallow respiration
• decreased heart rate, blood pressure and capillary refill time
• cool skin
• eye position – centrally fixed
• pupil – dilated and unresponsive to light

• all reflexes are absent
• muscle tone is flaccid.

3.10.07 Monitoring of anaesthesia

What you need to learn

❧ You need to be able to explain the importance of patient monitoring and recording during anaesthesia and describe the methods used:
  ❧ respiration
  ❧ heart rate
  ❧ pulse
  ❧ mucous membranes
  ❧ capillary refill time
  ❧ reflexes
  ❧ body temperature.
❧ Describe different types of monitoring equipment:
  ❧ oesophageal stethoscope
  ❧ electrocardiogram
  ❧ respiratory monitors
  ❧ pulse oximeters
  ❧ capnograph.
❧ Outline the limitations of mechanical monitoring devices.

It is important to monitor and record anaesthesia so that the depth of anaesthesia and dose of anaesthetic agents can be adjusted accordingly. A written record provides better visualisation of the anaesthetic and is also proof of the anaesthetic if anything goes wrong.

The following should be monitored:

• respiration
• heart rate
• pulse
• mucous membrane colour
• capillary refill time
• all reflexes – pedal, palpebral, jaw tone, corneal
• body temperature – core and peripheral
• eye position.

Monitoring equipment

An **oesophageal stethoscope** – a tube placed down the oesophagus – allows heart and lung sounds to be heard.

An **electrocardiogram** (ECG) indicates the electrical activity of the heart; most display the heart rate.

Respiratory monitors – such as Wright's respiratory monitor – measure tidal and minute volumes.

Pulse oximeters measure the amount of saturated oxygen in the blood.

Capnography measures the amount of carbon dioxide in expired air.

Blood gas analysis measures arterial levels of oxygen and carbon dioxide.

Mechanical monitoring devices are there as an aid to monitoring. They are not a replacement for the veterinary nurse and manual monitoring must be performed alongside these devices.

3.10.08 Intravenous anaesthesia

What you need to learn

- You need to be able to describe the induction of anaesthesia and outline the common intravenous agents in clinical use.
- Outline how intravenous agents are distributed in the body after administration and describe how they are eliminated from the body.
- Describe the preparation of intravenous anaesthetics and understand calculations to obtain a solution of a specific percentage concentration.
- Describe the correct placement of an intravenous catheter and the alternative sites for intravenous injection with particular importance to cleansing the site for injection.
- Identify the hazards of misuse of anaesthetic agents and describe the safe storage of anaesthetic drugs.
- Describe the alternative routes by which injectable anaesthetic agents may be administered.
- List the drugs commonly used by these alternative routes.
- Outline the licensed drugs and those not licensed for anaesthesia in animals and have awareness of the possible consequences of using an unlicensed product.
- Explain the hazards in the use of the common intravenous anaesthetic agents.

Induction of anaesthesia

Induction can be performed either intravenously, using an intravenous agent, or by face mask, using a volatile agent (use oxygen first and gradually increase the amount of volatile agent).

Commonly used intravenous agents are:

• propofol

- thiopentone sodium
- alphaxalone/alphadolone
- methohexitone.

Elimination and excretion of intravenous agents

Emergence from sleep depends on the redistribution of the drug from the brain and plasma to the body tissues. After administration the drug is taken from the plasma and redistributed to other well-perfused tissues, such as fat, where it can remain here for up to six hours before it is metabolised.

Thiopentone is unsuitable for sighthounds; as they have little fat the drug remains in the plasma for longer, therefore producing a longer recovery. Propofol is rapidly metabolised, making it a suitable agent for sighthounds, and for patients with renal and hepatic disease. The anaesthetic drug is excreted after hepatic metabolism, and in the case of Propofol may also be metabolised by the lungs. Drugs are then excreted in the urine over several days. Repeated doses of Thiopentone have a cumulative effect.

Preparing intravenous anaesthetics

Preparing Thiopentone sodium:

- Although the percentage of the solution is ultimately up to the veterinary surgeon it is conveniently available in 'ready-to-make' solutions of 1.25%, 2.5% and 5%.
- Remove the covers from both bottles.
- Apply the adapter to the water bottle in a downwards motion without touching its end.
- Apply the other end of the adapter to the bottle containing the powder.
- Turn the bottles around so the water bottle is now on top.
- Allow the water to drain in and mix thoroughly until all the powder has saturated.
- Discard the glass bottle and sharp adapter appropriately.

Calculation of the specific percentage concentration is as follows:

When 1 g is made up with 100 ml of water or another solution it gives a concentration of 1%. Therefore if a solution is 5% the drug content is 5 g.

Placing an intravenous catheter

The procedure for placement of an intravenous catheter is as follows.

- Have all equipment available and to hand.

- The full circumference of the area of the limb should be clipped using electric clippers; scissors are sufficient if the patient will not tolerate clippers.
- Clean the area with a solution of antiseptic and water, eg chlorohexidine, and complete by applying surgical spirit.
- Remove the outer casing of the catheter but do not touch the catheter itself – leave the bung end in as this prevents blood escaping.
- Apply into the vein and wait for flow back of blood (a blade may be required to perform a cut down onto the vein or to make a small skin incision to facilitate placing the catheter).
- Place a piece of tape over the catheter entrance.
- Attach the giving set (which should have previously been run through with the fluid).
- Apply further tape to various points on the catheter and giving set to ensure security.
- Place a bandage over the top to prevent patient interference and accidental damage.

Suitable sites for catheter placement include:

- cephalic
- saphenous
- jugular
- marginal ear vein in rabbits.

Hazards of anaesthetic drug misuse

Misuse includes accidental self-administration with the drug, exposure to anaesthetic gases and addiction to certain anaesthetic drugs.

Storage of anaesthetic drugs

Certain controlled drugs are required by law to be stored in a locked unbreakable cabinet and their purchase and use are recorded. It is wise to store all anaesthetic drugs in a locked cabinet. Some drugs degrade on exposure to light so are stored in amber-coloured bottles, eg halothane.

Alternative routes for injectable anaesthetic agents

Alphaxalone/alphadolone and ketamine can be administered intramuscularly. Ketamine can also be given via the mucous membranes.

Licensed drugs

The following are licensed for use in veterinary practice:

- thiopentone sodium
- propofol
- alphaxalone/alphadolone – for cats
- ketamine (not for sole use in dogs)
- halothane
- isoflurane
- pethidine
- buprenorphine.

Pethidine is the only full agonist opiate licensed for use in cats and dogs.

Hazards of intravenous anaesthetic agents

The following are hazards associated with the use of intravenous anaesthetic agents:

- accidental self-administration of the drug
- peri-vascular injection of thiopentone, causing sloughing of the skin
- addiction to certain anaesthetic drugs
- overdose with the anaesthetic drug.

3.10.09 Muscle relaxants

What you need to learn

- You need to be able to identify the commonly used muscle relaxants and explain the advantages and disadvantages of their use:
  - non-depolarising (eg atracurium)
  - depolarising (eg suxamethonium).
- Describe the requirements for the use of muscle relaxants:
  - intermittent positive pressure ventilation (IPPV).

Muscle relaxants can be either non-depolarising or depolarising. Depolarising agents cause initial twitching and then flaccid paralysis.

Non-depolarising agents include:

- Atacurium
- Vecuronium
- Alcuronium
- Pancuronium.

An example of a depolarising agent is Suxamethonium.

The use of muscle relaxants has **advantages**.

- They produce excellent muscle relaxation, which aids surgical procedures.
- They do not cross the blood-brain barrier or the placenta in

significant amounts.

- They provide better access to the cornea during surgery of the eye.
- Reduction of joint luxations is easier but not fracture reduction.

However, there are **disadvantages**.

- They can produce paralysis of muscles, including the respiratory muscles so IPPV is essential.
- They produce no analgesia or hypnotic effect.
- They cause hypothermia.

3.10.10 Inhalation anaesthesia

What you need to learn

- You need to be able to identify the properties of oxygen, nitrous oxide and outline their uses in anaesthesia.
- Define inhalation anaesthesia.
- Describe the properties and use of the common volatile anaesthetic agents.
- Identify the hazards encountered in the use and storage of the common volatile anaesthetic agents and outline the health and safety risks associated with anaesthesia.
- Describe how the risk of explosions and fires caused by specific anaesthetic agents may be minimised.
- Describe equipment and its maintenance, designed to minimise health and safety risks associated with anaesthesia.
- Describe the various types of scavenging systems and their benefits:
  - absorption
  - passive
  - active.

Oxygen can be used as 100% oxygen. It supports combustion but can be delivered to the patient at a controlled level, which is essential to maintain adequate perfusion of tissues and to keep the patient alive.

Nitrous oxide produces good analgesia but is a weak anaesthetic. It has a wide safety margin and its use reduces the amount of volatile agent and oxygen needed for the procedure. Nitrous oxide diffuses into gas-filled areas/air pockets and should be turned off 10 minutes before the procedure finishing to prevent diffusion hypoxia.

Inhalation anaesthesia can be defined as producing unconsciousness/hypnosis by delivering a volatile agent (gas).

Volatile anaesthetic agents

Halothane

Halothane has a minimal alveolar concentration (MAC) of 0.8%. It has the following characteristics:

- dose-dependent depression of myocardial activity inducing hypotension
- dose-dependent respiratory depression which depresses the minute volume
- cardiac arrhythmias are more common as the myocardium is sensitised to circulating catecholamines
- excreted by the lungs; one-third is excreted by the liver
- shivering and tremors can be seen in recovery
- non-irritant
- non-flammable
- produces no analgesia and poor muscle relaxation
- compatible with soda lime.

Isoflurane

Isoflurane has a MAC of 1.5%. Its solubility is low so rapid inductions and recoveries are seen. It has the following characteristics:

- dose-dependent respiratory depression which depresses the minute volume
- affects myocardial contractility less than halothane
- does not sensitise the myocardium to circulating catecholamines
- blood pressure is reduced
- excreted almost entirely by the lungs
- non-irritant
- compatible with dampened soda lime.

Sevoflurane

Sevoflurane has a MAC of between 1.7% and 2.3%. It has the following characteristics:

- lower solubility than isoflurane
- metabolised and unstable with soda lime
- excitement can be provoked in recovery.

Ether

Ether is rarely used, very safe and produces excessive salivation and secretions, so pre-medicate with atropine. The effects on the cardiovascular and respiratory systems are relative to the depth of anaesthesia. Ether can be explosive.

Methoxyflurane

This is rarely used, has a high solubility (not suitable as an induction agent). It is excreted mainly by the lungs, some is metabolised and excreted in the urine. There is a decreased respiration rate and blood pressure during deep levels of anaesthesia. It does possess good analgesic properties.

Hazards of using volatile agents

Volatile agents have a key port filling system, which prevents the wrong anaesthetic agent being administered into the wrong vaporiser and from a health and safety issue, prevents spillage of the contents. The following are precautions that should be taken with volatile agents.

- Volatile agents should be stored in the original bottles; these are amber because the agent degrades on exposure to light.
- Thymol (a preservative used in halothane) can cause the vaporiser to stick.
- A scavenging system should be used with these agents to maintain health and safety.
- Personnel monitors should be used to monitor exposure to volatile agents and nitrous oxide.
- Endotracheal tubes should be used to deliver the anaesthetic gas rather than masks to reduce personnel exposure.
- Vaporisers should be refilled at the end of the day.

The risk of **explosions and fires** can be reduced by following these rules.

- Do not use flammable agents such as ether near heat, eg diathermy equipment.
- Do not use naked flames around inflammable agents or oxygen cylinders.
- Do not use carbon- or petroleum-based lubricants on parts of equipment using oxygen.
- Store gas cylinders safely.

Maintaining equipment

- Service vaporisers annually.
- Check for leaks in anaesthetic equipment daily.
- Ensure scavenging systems are working effectively – they need to be checked every 14 months (health and safety requirement).

• Check that the endotracheal tubes used to deliver the anaesthetic gases are not damaged or leaking.

Scavenging systems

These systems remove waste gas from the expiratory limb of the anaesthetic circuit.

Absorption system

This is a passive system. Gases are transported through a piece of corrugated tubing to an activated charcoal system where the gas is absorbed (these systems do not absorb nitrous oxide). Absorption systems are easy to use. They need weighing after each use and disposing of when they reach a certain weight, as they exhaust quickly.

Passive systems

Passive systems comprise a piece of tubing attached to the expiratory valve on the circuit, the other end of which is then placed through a hole in the wall to the outside atmosphere. They are cheap and easy to use.

Active systems

Active systems comprise a piece of tubing attached to the expiratory valve on the circuit, the other end of which is then attached to further tubing, to an extractor fan and then finally to the outside atmosphere. The extractor fan generates negative pressure which enables the gas to move along the tubing. An air brake receiver is incorporated to prevent excessive negative pressure being enforced on the patient and prevents a build-up of excess pressure if the system fails. They are more expensive than passive systems but several anaesthetic systems can be scavenged using the same system.

3.10.11 Anaesthetic equipment and circuits

What you need to learn

- You need to be able to outline the main methods of administering inhalation agents.
- Describe the advantages and disadvantages of administering volatile anaesthetic agents via an endotracheal tube or face mask.
- Outline the limitations of this method of induction.
- Outline the advantages of an accurately calibrated vaporiser and their use to maintain anaesthesia.

- Describe the method of calculating respiratory minute volume and its importance when selecting anaesthetic circuits and the correct gas flow rates.
- Describe open and closed circuits and explain their differences.
  - circle
  - Humphrey ADE.
- Describe rebreathing and non-rebreathing circuits and outline their advantages/disadvantages.
- Identify different non-rebreathing circuits in common use:
  - Magill
  - Lack
  - Ayre's T Piece
  - Bain.
- Recognise the purpose of the Jackson-Rees modified T piece and its use in the maintenance of anaesthesia.
- Identify a closed circuit system and indicate the direction of gas flow:
  - The To and Fro (Water's canister)
  - Circle systems.
- Outline which gases are unsuitable for use in closed circuits and those which are unsuitable for use with soda lime.
- Describe which chemicals are used in this apparatus and identify the colour changes that occur as carbon dioxide is absorbed.
- Describe a suitable circuit for the anaesthesia of small mammals and birds:
  - small animal anaesthetic chamber.

Administering inhalation agents

Inhalation agents can be delivered to the patient by:

- endotracheal tubes
- masks
- tracheostomy tubes.

Using endotracheal tubes and their limitations

There are **advantages** to the use of endotracheal tubes.

- They provide more efficient delivery of anaesthetic gases.
- They provide safer delivery of anaesthetic gas with regard to personnel exposure.
- They maintain a patent airway.
- They allow direct delivery of oxygen.
- They allow the use of NMBD (neuromuscular blocking drugs).
- They allow IPPV.
- Inflated cuffs reduce the risk of inhaled, saliva, vomit, or blood.

However, there are **disadvantages**.

- Skill is needed to place the tube, especially in bracycaephalic patients.
- The larynx, pharynx and soft palate may be damaged if the tube is placed using force.
- If the tube is too long it may be inserted into a bronchus so that only one lung is receiving the gas.
- Damage to the trachea can be caused if the cuff is overinflated.
- They can kink or occlude with secretions.
- They may cause irritation, with a cough seen for a few days following removal.

Using face masks and their limitations

The use of face masks has **advantages**.

- Little skill is needed for their use.
- They are useful to deliver oxygen to conscious patients.
- There is no damage to the trachea, larynx, pharynx, or soft palate.
- There is no irritation.

However, there are also **disadvantages**.

- On induction, their stress levels can increase, therefore increasing circulating catecholamines.
- There is a risk of personnel exposure to the inhalational agent used.
- There is no patent airway.
- IPPV cannot be performed using a face mask.
- They are less efficient at delivering anaesthetic gas.
- They provide no protection from secretions.

Calibrated vaporisers

There are advantages to the use of accurately calibrated vaporisers.

- They deliver the exact concentration of anaesthetic agent selected.
- Percentages are graduated on the vaporisers, which increases accuracy and control.
- They are temperature-compensated, ie the temperature of the room does not affect the amount of anaesthetic gas vaporised.
- They are flow-compensated, ie the amount of anaesthetic vaporised is not affected by the amount of gas flowing over the anaesthetic liquid (apart from at high flow rates of >10 l/min or at low flow rates <500 ml/min.
- They are back pressure-compensated, ie the amount of anaesthetic vaporised is not affected by anaesthetic gas being delivered under pressure, eg when 'bagging'.

Calculating the minute volume

Minute volume = Volume of inspired air / Volume of expired air in one breath (ie tidal volume) × Respiratory rate

The tidal volume is between 10 and 15 ml/kg body weight [eg for a 20 kg dog its minute volume would be (10 ml × 20 breaths per minute) = 200 ml minute volume.

The minute volume determines the amount of gas the patient will require when using anaesthetic circuits. In addition, there is usually a circuit factor by which the minute volume needs to be multiplied.

Flow rates

To calculate the amount of gas needed to support a patient when using anaesthetic circuits the minute volume should be multiplied by the circuit factor. The following are the circuit factors for various systems.

- Jackson-Rees modified Ayre T-piece – circuit factor is 2.5–3 or 400 ml/kg/min.
- Magill – circuit factor is equal to the minute volume or 200 ml/kg/min.
- Bain – circuit factor is 2.5–3 or 400 ml/kg/min.
- Lack – circuit factor is equal to the minute volume or 200 ml/kg/min.
- To-and-fro – circuit factor is 0.5–2 or 50 ml/kg/min if using the system semi-closed or 15 ml/kg/min if using the system closed
- Circle – circuit factor is 0.5–2 or 50 ml/kg/min if using the system semi-closed or 15 ml/kg/min if using the system closed.

Open and closed circuits

When using the circle or to-and-fro circuits, the valve on the respiratory bag can be 'open' so re-breathing of the gases does not occur and higher flow rates are needed.

If semi-open, the pop-off valve is semi-closed, allowing some re-breathing of gas and lower flow rates. If closed, the pop-off valve is fully closed, allowing all gas to be re-breathed and very low flow rates can be used.

Humphrey's ADE system aims to assist the transition from a Mapleson D or E configuration during controlled ventilation to a Mapleson A mode for spontaneous ventilation.

Re-breathing circuits

These circuits allow the gas expired in each breath to be re-used. The expired gas is transported to a canister containing soda lime which removes any carbon dioxide; the remaining gas is then transported back into the anaesthetic system and re-breathed.

Advantages of these circuits are that:

• they are more economical because of the low flow rates used
• they reduce the risk of hypothermia because the gases are warm.

Disadvantages of the system, however, are:

• The circuits are more complex to use.
• The anaesthetic agent level cannot be adjusted quickly.
• Irritant from soda lime dust can be a potential problem.
• Concentration of anaesthetic gas is not as accurate as with non-re-breathing circuits.
• Dead space increases as the soda lime becomes exhausted.
• Nitrous oxide cannot be used unless there is adequate respiratory monitoring, eg blood gas analysis, capnography.

Non-re-breathing circuits

In these circuits all the expired gases are transported away by a scavenging system so no gas is re-breathed.

Advantages of these circuits are that:

• they provide accurate delivery of gases
• the anaesthetic agent level can be adjusted quickly
• nitrous oxide can be used safely
• they are not as cumbersome to handle as the re-breathing systems.

However, **disadvantages** are:

• they require higher flow rates to prevent re-breathing
• they are less economical because of the high flow rates
• the inspired gases are cold, increasing the risk of hypothermia
• the respiratory tract may become dry during long procedures.

The Magill circuit is shown in Figure 10.1.

An Ayres T-piece circuit (with Jackson-Rees modification) is show in Figure 10.2.

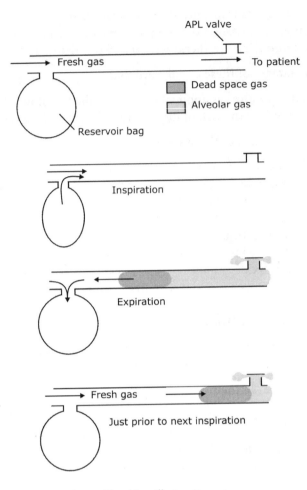

Figure 10.1 The Magill circuit.

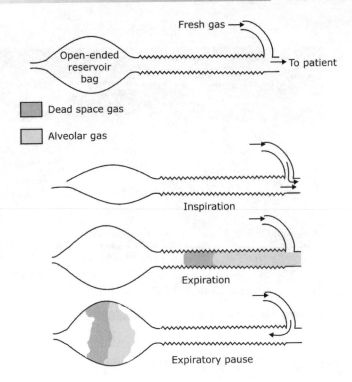

Fresh gas →

Open-ended reservoir bag

→ To patient

Dead space gas

Alveolar gas

Inspiration

Expiration

Expiratory pause

Figure 10.2 An Ayres T-piece circuit. (See Jackson-Rees modification.)

The Bain circuit is shown in Figure 10.3.

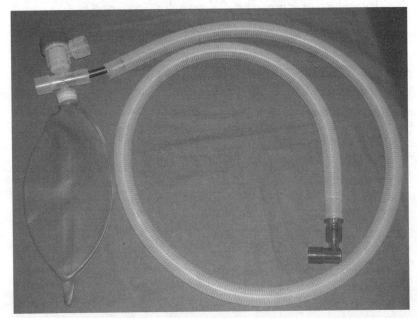

Figure 10.3 The Bain circuit.

A Lack circuit is shown in Figure 10.4.

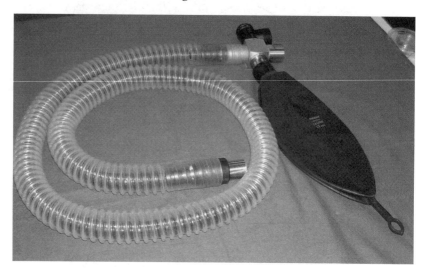

Figure 10.4 A Lack circuit (Co-axial).

Jackson-Rees modification

The Jackson-Rees modification has an open-ended bag that is incorporated onto the original Ayres T-piece (a length of corrugated tubing with no bag or valves). The modification of the bag facilitates IPPV.

Re-breathing circuits (closed systems)

A closed system is where all the expired gas is re-breathed. A To-and-fro circuit is shown in Figure 10.5.

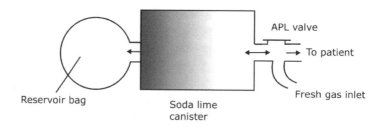

Figure 10.5 To-and-fro circuit.

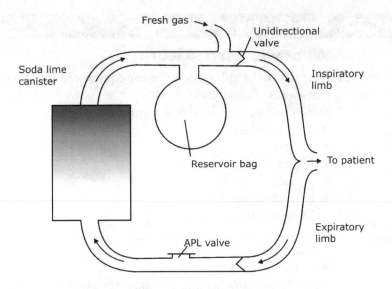

Figure 10.6 Circle circuit.

The canister containing the soda lime is called a Water's canister.

Gases unsuitable for use with to and fro and circle circuits

Nitrous oxide cannot be used with closed circuits unless there is adequate respiratory monitoring, eg blood gas analysis, capnography. Isoflurane cannot be used with soda lime unless it is dampened soda lime.

Absorbing carbon dioxide

Chemicals used for absorbing the carbon dioxide include soda lime and barium hydroxide lime.

It is the calcium hydroxide part of both of these chemicals that absorbs the carbon dioxide.

There are two different colour changes (depending on the manufacturer) as carbon dioxide is used and the chemical is becoming exhausted: pink to white and white to purple.

For anaesthesia of small mammals and birds the following may be used:

• Small animal anaesthetic chamber – like a Tupperware® with inspiratory and expiratory limbs

An Ayres T-piece circuit is secured by tape to the nose or face.

What you need to learn

❧ You need to be able to describe the equipment and drugs required for emergency resuscitation.

❧ Describe the clinical signs of respiratory obstruction and understand its associated terms:

- ❧ anoxia
- ❧ hypoxia
- ❧ apnoea
- ❧ hypoventilation
- ❧ hyperventilation
- ❧ dead space
- ❧ tidal volume
- ❧ minute volume.

❧ Describe the circumstances when respiratory obstruction is most likely to occur.

❧ Outline the principles of emergency procedures carried out in the management of a patient with respiratory obstruction.

❧ Identify how to reduce the likelihood of respiratory obstruction occurring.

❧ Describe the clinical signs of apnoea and recognise the need to carry out IPPV.

❧ Outline the procedure and relevant circuits used for performing IPPV.

❧ Describe the clinical signs of cardiac arrest and carry out external cardiac massage (simulated or actual).

❧ Describe the circumstances under which cardiac arrest may occur

❧ Describe the signs of a return of effective circulation.

❧ Outline the problems and injuries that may be caused by misuse of anaesthetic equipment:

- ❧ eg excessive inflation of endotracheal cuff.

Equipment

- Stethoscope
- Intravenous catheters – various sizes
- Needles – various sizes
- Syringes – various sizes
- Blades
- Endotracheal tubes – various sizes
- Tracheotomy tubes
- Scissors
- Artery forceps
- Portex dog urinary catheters – can be applied down the centre of an

ET tube for administering drugs
• Pen torch

Drugs

• Adrenaline
• Dopram
• Atropine
• Dexamethosome
• Dobutamine

Respiratory obstruction

• Clinical signs

• Dyspnoea
  • No movement of the reservoir bag
  • Cyanotic mucous membranes

• Anoxia – failure of oxygen to the brain

• Hypoxia – tissues deficient in oxygen

• Apnoea – cessation of breathing

• Hypoventilation – decreased ventilation

• Hyperventilation – increased ventilation

• Dead space – an area where gases exchange cannot happen, divided into anatomic dead space and mechanical (apparatus dead space)

• Tidal volume – the amount of inspired and expired air in one normal breath

• Minute volume – tidal volume × respiratory rate

Respiratory obstruction can occur in:
• Oral or nasal surgery due to blood, saliva
• The endotracheal has become occluded or kinked
• From foreign bodies

Emergency procedure
• Clear the airway, remove any foreign bodies
• Intubate if not already and administer oxygen only
• Prepare to perform a tracheotomy if attempts to intubate have failed

Prevention of a respiratory obstruction
• Ensure the ET tube is kept straight at all times
• Place a pack with a visible piece of tape at the back of the mouth to prevent blood, saliva or secretions blocking the airway
• Suction could be used during oral or nasal surgery

Clinical signs of apnoea
• No respiratory movement, pale or cyanotic mucous membranes
• If a patient shows signs of apnoea for longer than 30 seconds, turn any anaesthetic agent off and deliver oxygen only by IPPV

Performing IPPV
• Use 100% oxygen
• Squeeze the reservoir bag 10–30 times a minute to mimic their own respiratory rate. The valve may need to be closed to re fill the bag and then opened to allow delivery of the oxygen to the patient
• All circuits can be used for IPPV apart from the Magill and Lack circuit as re-breathing of the gases would occur.

Cardiac arrest
Signs of cardiac arrest:
• May be some respiratory movement but quiet often there is none
• Cyanotic mucous membranes
• Dilated pupils
• No pulse
• No heart beat

External cardiac massage (cardio pulmonary resuscitation – CPR)
• Intubate if not already intubated
• Ensure the airway is patent
• Turn any anaesthetic agents off
• Perform IPPV at 10–30 breaths a minute with oxygen only
• Perform cardiac massage in right lateral recumbency at 60–80 compressions a minute
• Keep checking for pulses
• Administer drugs as directed by the veterinary surgeon; these can administered intravenously, intracardiac, intratracheal, or via the endotracheal tube

Remember if you are becoming good at CPR you are doing something wrong.

Cardiac arrest may occur due to:
• Overdose of anaesthetic agents
• Systemic illness eg cardiac disease

Return of an effective circulation
• Pulses become palpable
• Heart beat becomes audible and palpable
• Mucous membranes return to a pink colour
• Respiration returns to normal
• Pupils start to constrict

Misuse of anaesthetic equipment
• Over-inflation of cuffs on ET tubes causes pressure necrosis on the

trachea
- Forcing an ET tube will cause damage to the larynx, pharynx and soft palate, especially in cats
- Leaving or forgetting to turn down vaporiser settings leads to overdose of anaesthetic agents
- Turning nitrous oxide on only – results in hypoxia and navy blue mucous membranes – always turn the oxygen on first before any anaesthetic gas.

3.10.13 Local anaesthesia

What you need to learn

- You need to be able to describe types of local anaesthesia:
  - topical application
  - intradermal
  - regional anaesthesia.
- Describe types of regional anaesthesia:
  - perineural
  - intravenous
  - spinal block.
- Outline the various techniques by which local anaesthetics are introduced to their site of action.
- Describe the main pharmacological properties and the commonly used local anaesthetic agents.
- Outline the factors which influence their speed of action and duration of their effects.
- Explain how epidural block, peri-neural block and intravenous local anaesthesia are produced.
- Outline the common clinical indications for local anaesthesia in practice.

Topical anaesthesia

Topical anaesthesia can be applied directly to the skin or mucous membranes. It is useful for providing a certain level of anaesthesia, eg cream applied to a limb before introducing a catheter. The drug has no effects on the organs but there are limitations in its use. Its effects may be variable as the drug molecules are unable to reach the dermis where the peripheral nerves are found.

Intradermal (infiltration)

Intradermal anaesthesia is infiltrated into tissues close to the nerves. It can also be infiltrated subcutaneously and in between muscles. The area must be clipped and prepared aseptically. The drug can be applied as a nerve block or a line block. There are little or no effects of the drugs on organs.

Regional anaesthesia

For regional anaesthesia a local anaesthetic is injected into a nerve plexus blood vessel, or close to the spinal cord. This method can be used to anaesthetise large areas, eg a limb, and there are few if any effects of the drugs on organs. The area must be clipped and prepared aseptically.

Types of regional anaesthesia

Regional anaesthesia can be described as:

• intravenous
• spinal block
• epidural
• brachial plexus.

Introduction of local anaesthetic

Local anaesthetics can be administered using:

• syringe and needle
• intravenous catheters
• spinal needles
• intravenous infusion

Lignocaine

• Lignocaine is available in concentrations between 0.5% and 35%.
• It provides good surface anaesthesia and spreads well throughout the tissues.
• It has a rapid onset of action, within 3–5 minutes.
• The duration of action is 1.5 hours.
• It has low toxicity.
• The toxic effects include drowsiness, sedation, twitching, convulsions, coma and death.
• There is an anti-arrhythmic action on the heart.
• Lignocaine is available with or without adrenaline.

Bupivicaine

• Bupivicaine is longer acting than lignocaine.
• It is available in concentrations of 0.25%, 0.5% and 0.75%.
• Onset of action is slow, 20 minutes or more.
• It is more potent than lignocaine.
• Contains adrenaline.

Procaine

Procaine is available in concentrations between 1 and 5%. It provides good local anaesthesia and its duration of action is approximately 1 hour. Procaine is weak at penetrating tissues but toxicity is rare. It is available with or without adrenaline.

Speed of action

The speed and duration of action of an anaesthetic agent are reduced by:

- scar tissue
- fat
- oedema
- haemorrhage
- inflammation – inactivates the drug.

An **epidural block** is produced by administering a local anaesthetic into the epidural space (between the dura mater and vertebrae). The site is between lumbar vertebra 7 and the sacrum.

A **perineural block** (spinal block) is produced by introducing a local anaesthetic into the cerebrospinal fluid by penetrating the dura mater and the arachnoid mater.

Intravenous local anaesthesia is produced by administering a local anaesthetic into a vein of a limb with a tourniquet tied around the proximal limb.

Indications for local anaesthesia

- Local anaesthesia can be used for short surgical procedures, eg skin tag removal, scraping of the cornea.
- It can be used in systemically ill patients.
- It is useful in large animal work, eg cow caesareans; as it is not feasible to perform general anaesthesia on these patients, local anaesthesia must be used.
- Local anaesthesia is used to treat cardiac arrhythmias.
- Local anaesthesia is used to provide analgesia.

Multiple choice questions

1. Decreased respiratory rate is termed
   - ☐ A   dyspnoea
   - ☐ B   tachypnoea
   - ☐ C   bradypnoea
   - ☐ D   apnoea

2. An example of an Alpha 2 adrenoceptor agonist is
   - ☐ A   pethidine
   - ☐ B   carprophen
   - ☐ C   acepromazine
   - ☐ D   buprenorphine

3. An example of an anticholinergic drug is
   - ☐ A   atipamazole
   - ☐ B   atropine
   - ☐ C   acepromazine
   - ☐ D   buprenorphine

4. An example of a non-steroidal, non-barbiturate intravenous induction agent is
   - ☐ A   propofol
   - ☐ B   thiopentone
   - ☐ C   saffan
   - ☐ D   halothane

5. The volume of propofol required to anaesthetise a 20 kg collie cross if the dose rate is 10 mg/kg and the solution contains 25 mg/ml is
   - ☐ A   0.8 ml
   - ☐ B   6 ml
   - ☐ C   8 ml
   - ☐ D   10 ml

6. The volume of morphine required to provide analgesia to a 5 kg Westie if the dosage rate is 0.1 mg/kg and the solution contains 5 mg/ml is
   - ☐ A   0.1 ml
   - ☐ B   1 ml
   - ☐ C   10 ml
   - ☐ D   100 ml

7. The colour of an oxygen cylinder is
   - ☐ A   black
   - ☐ B   black with white shoulders
   - ☐ C   blue
   - ☐ D   grey

8. Acepromazine is not recommended for use in
   - ☐ A Scottish Terriers
   - ☐ B Dalmations
   - ☐ C Basenjis
   - ☐ D Boxers

9. An example of a depolarising muscle relaxant is
   - ☐ A atacurium
   - ☐ B pancuronium
   - ☐ C suxomethonium
   - ☐ D vercuronium

10. A 2.5% solution of thiopentone contains / ml
    - ☐ A 0.25 mg
    - ☐ B 2.5 mg
    - ☐ C 25 mg
    - ☐ D 50 mg

11. Tidal volume is defined as the volume of air
    - ☐ A exchanged each breath
    - ☐ B exchanged each minute
    - ☐ C exhaled in a maximal expiration following a maximal inspiration
    - ☐ D remaining in the lungs following a maximal expiration

12. The minute volume of a 5 kg cat if its tidal volume factor is 15 ml/kg and its respiratory rate is 20 breaths a minute would be
    - ☐ A 75 ml
    - ☐ B 150 ml
    - ☐ C 300 ml
    - ☐ D 1500 ml

13. The most suitable circuit to maintain a 4 kg cat under general anaesthetic is a/an
    - ☐ A Lack
    - ☐ B Baines
    - ☐ C Ayres T Piece
    - ☐ D Magill

14. The circuit in the diagram is a/an
   - ☐ A Magill
   - ☐ B Lack
   - ☐ C Ayres T Piece
   - ☐ D Baines

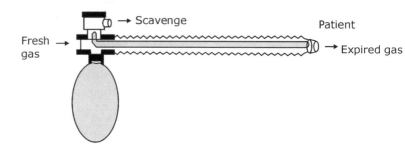

15. The circuit factor of the anaesthetic circuit in the diagram is equal to
   - ☐ A tidal volume
   - ☐ B minute volume
   - ☐ C 2.5–3 times tidal volume
   - ☐ D 2.5–3 times minute volume

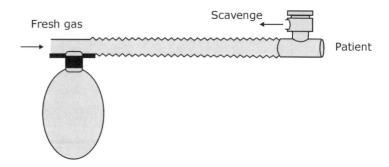

16. An example of a closed circuit is a
   - ☐ A Lack
   - ☐ B Magill
   - ☐ C To and fro
   - ☐ D Waters

17. Capnography measures the
   - ☐ A electrical activity of the heart
   - ☐ B tidal volume
   - ☐ C amount of saturated oxygen
   - ☐ D amount of CO_2

18. If injected perivascularly the induction agent which will cause tissue sloughing is
    ☐ A propofol
    ☐ B thiopentone
    ☐ C alphaxalone/alphadolone
    ☐ D methohoxitone

19. The flow rate that should be delivered through a Lack circuit to a 20 kg Labrador if its respiratory rate is 15 bpm and its tidal volume factor is 10 ml/kg is
    ☐ A 1 litre/min
    ☐ B 2 litres/min
    ☐ C 3 litres/min
    ☐ D 4 litres/min

20. An example of a non steroidal anti-inflammatory drug is
    ☐ A atropine
    ☐ B diazepam
    ☐ C morphine
    ☐ D carprofen

Level 3: Unit 11

Other species – exotics and wildlife

3.11.01 Definitions

What you need to learn

- You need to be able to identify the animals and birds commonly known as exotic or 'other' species and the advantages/disadvantages as common pets:
  - mammals – cavies, chinchillas, chipmunks, ferrets, lagomorphs, gerbils, mice and rats degus, jirds
  - birds – budgerigars, canaries, finches, parrots, etc, also fowl kept as pets and raptors
  - others – fish tropical freshwater, coldwater and marine, amphibian-salamanders, frogs
  - reptiles – snakes such as pythons, colubrids, garter snakes, and lizards such as green iguana, bearded dragon, leopard gecko, bosc monitor lizard, veiled chameleon
  - chelonian – Mediterranean tortoises, red-eared terrapins.
- Basic knowledge of biology and requirements of those animals normally kept as pets:
  - heat
  - light
  - humidity
  - type of enclosure.
- Identify special requirements for food and care of those special animals normally kept as pets, recognise common problems and advise owners accordingly:
  - knowledge to include vitamin supplementation in the diet, calcium deficiency in lizards, chelonians and birds, thiamine deficiency in garter snakes, hypovitaminosis A
  - food types for different species eg iguanas are vegetarian other lizards can be insectivorous species or carnivores
  - correct balanced diet for birds
  - low humidity problems in reptiles causing dysecdysis and in birds causing feather problems, retained spectacles in snakes
  - lack of 'chewing material' causing overgrown teeth in rodents and overgrown beaks in birds.
- Identify the requirements for caring and nursing wild animals

normally presented as casualties:

* ❧ barrier nursing, risk of zoonoses, aggressiveness of wildlife casualties, need for isolation from people/domestic pets, need for warm, quiet environment with minimal contact.
* ❧ Recognise specific species behaviour and normal habitat:
  * ❧ coprophagia, cannibalism in some reptiles (particularly kingsnakes and milksnakes.)
  * ❧ habitats for arboreal, ground, desert, tropical species.
* ❧ Outline common clinical parameters:
  * ❧ common mammals, birds and reptiles, rabbit, guinea pig, rat, Burmese python, cornsnake, green iguana, Mediterranean tortoise, red-eared terrapin.

In recent years there has been a great increase in the number of 'exotic animals' which are being kept as pets in the UK. For most purposes the term 'exotic' is used to describe a pet animal other than a cat or a dog. The most commonly encountered exotic species are described now.

Birds

There are many orders of bird. Those commonly encountered in veterinary medicine include:

* ducks, geese and swans (Anseriformes)
* birds of prey (Falconiformes)
* grouse, pheasants, domestic fowl (Galliformes)
* pigeons and doves (Columbiformes)
* parrots (Psittaciformes; this order includes the parakeets such as cockatiels and budgerigars)
* perching birds such as finches and canaries (Passeriformes).

Birds are generally more difficult animals to keep properly in captivity. They are very intelligent animals and can become bored and depressed if sufficient attention is not paid to enriching their environment. Many pet birds suffer from chronic malnutrition and poor husbandry.

Birds can become very distressed when handled but tame birds may sit unrestrained on their owner's hands, head, or shoulders.

The easiest birds to keep are the small parakeets such as budgerigars and cockatiels, and the small finches and canaries. Larger birds such as parrots and birds of prey should only be kept by experienced bird owners who are willing to dedicate a great deal of time and effort to their pet.

Birds are adept at disguising symptoms of ill health. For this reason they are often presented at the veterinary surgery in an advanced disease state.

Some birds can be quite noisy which may not suit some owners. All birds will bite if they feel threatened. Parakeets can break human skin with their beaks. Some of the larger parrots and birds of prey are able to remove a human finger tip. Birds of prey are also armed with powerful talons which can cause injury to their owner.

Mammals

Rodents

Rodents include rats, mice, gerbils, guinea-pigs, chipmunks, degus, jirds and hamsters.

Their axial and appendicular skeleton resembles those of cats and dogs in many ways.

Rodents have continuously erupting teeth which are specialised for gnawing.

Rodents are very popular pets. They are generally easy to look after and are fairly clean and odour-free. They can be tamed easily and can be easy to handle. Some rodents are more nervous than others. Chinchillas in particular are very sensitive and easily frightened. They should be handled by more experienced pet owners as rough handling can cause the coat to be shed (fur slip). See plate section.

Rodents are able to administer a nasty bite with their strong teeth. Even smaller rodents such as hamsters can break the skin. Dwarf hamsters can be short-tempered and care should be taken when young children handle these animals. Chipmunks generally do not like being handled.

Some rodents are able to shed their tails when handled roughly. Gerbils and their close relatives the degus and jirds are able to do this and should therefore never be handled by the tail.

Many rodents tend to be nocturnal (hamsters and gerbils in particular). These animals are therefore sleeping during the day when an owner may want to interact with their pet.

Guinea-pigs are generally friendly and make very good pets for children but can be timid if they are not used to regular handling.

Rats and mice also make very good pets for children. They can become very tame and can generally be easily handled.

Table 11.1 Common Clinical Parameters

Species	Adult weight	Temperature (°C)	Life-span (years)	Heart rate (per minute)	Reproduction
Rabbit	1–8 kg	37–39	8–12	180–250	Altricial young born after 30 day pregnancy
Guinea-pig	0.6–1.0 kg	37–39	5–8	150–200	Precocious young born after 63 day pregnancy.
Rat	0.4–0.8 kg	38	2–3	250–400	Altricial young born after 21 day pregnancy
Budgerigar	35–80 g		10–15	250–350	4–6 eggs laid, hatch after 16–18 days.
African Grey Parrot	320–550 g		25–30	150–200	3–4 eggs laid, hatch after 26–28 days
Burmese Python	5–10 kg	Not applicable as cold blooded	20–25	*	Eggs laid
Cornsnake	300–800g	N/A	5–10	*	Eggs laid
Green Iguana	5–15 kg	N/A	15–25	*	Eggs laid
Mediterranean Tortoise	1.5–3.0 kg	N/A	70–100	*	Eggs laid, hatch after about 60 days.
Red-eared Terrapin	1–2 kg	N/A	15–25	*	Eggs laid

* Heart rate in reptiles varies with temperature but is generally much slower than in mammals.

Lagomorphs

Lagomorphs are the rabbits and hares. They are similar to rodents except that they have a third pair of incisors on the upper jaw – the peg teeth.

Rabbits are very popular pets in the UK. However, they suffer from a variety of health problems related to poor husbandry as many owners are poorly informed about proper care of their pet.

Rabbits are generally docile but often do not enjoy handling. Occasionally rabbits can be aggressive. Large rabbits can bite and kick and are able to inflict injury on their owner. Children should therefore be supervised when handling rabbits.

Ferrets

Ferrets are intelligent animals which can be tamed. Nervous ferrets can be unpredictable and are able to administer a nasty bite similar to a cat bite. Entire male ferrets in particular can smell very pungent which can be off-putting for owners.

Reptiles

Reptiles are cold-blooded and include four orders:

• chelonians
• snakes and lizards
• crocodilians
• tuatara.

Chelonians

The chelonians (tortoises, turtles and terrapins) are difficult animals to keep properly in captivity. They are expensive to buy, and the correct equipment for keeping them is also expensive.

Chelonians suffer from health problems related to poor husbandry and malnutrition.

Although tortoises are generally amiable some terrapins and turtles can administer nasty bites and should be handled with great care. Chelonia can be a source of infection with zoonotic diseases such as *Salmonella*.

Commonly kept tortoises include the Mediterranean tortoises (Greek spur-thighed tortoise and Herman's tortoise), Horsfield's tortoise and leopard tortoises. Red-eared terrapins are the most commonly seen terrapin species.

Snakes and lizards

The snakes and lizards form the biggest group of reptiles. They are difficult animals to keep properly in captivity. They are expensive to buy and the correct equipment for keeping snakes and lizards can also be expensive.

Snakes and lizards suffer from health problems related to poor husbandry and malnutrition.

Snakes and lizards can be a source of infection with zoonotic diseases such as *Salmonella*.

Commonly kept snakes are the pythons and boas, the colubrids, and garter snakes. Some snakes are poisonous and should only be kept by specialist herpetologists with the correct licences. Large constrictor snakes, such as reticulated pythons, rock pythons and anacondas should be handled by more than one person as they are easily capable of killing a human being. These animals should also only be kept by specialist herpetologists.

Commonly kept lizards are green iguanas, bearded dragons, water dragons, leopard geckos, Bosc monitor lizards and veiled chameleons. Leopard geckos are nocturnal. Chameleons are particularly difficult to keep properly in captivity.

Many species of lizard are capable of losing their tail when handled roughly (**autotomy**). Lizards will bite if threatened and can use their sharp claws to inflict injury to their handler. Large lizards, such as green iguanas and Bosc monitors, can cause serious injury.

Crocodilians

The crocodilians (crocodiles, alligators, gharials, etc) are potentially dangerous animals and should only be kept by specialist herpetologists.

Tuatara

The Tuatara is an order containing a single species, similar to a lizard, that lives in New Zealand. These are not available as pets.

Amphibians

Amphibians are cold blooded and most live in a semi-aquatic environment. They include frogs and toads, newts, salamanders and axolotls. Amphibians are less commonly kept as pets in the UK.

Correct housing and good water quality are essential for keeping healthy amphibians. Any owner interested in keeping amphibians as pets should be advised to research thoroughly the species they intend to keep.

Amphibians generally do not tolerate handling and their delicate skin can easily be injured by handling using dry human hands. Hands should be wet but not washed with any chemicals before handling.

Commonly kept amphibians include salamanders, axolotls (the immature form of the Mexican salamander), tree frogs, clawed toads and cane toads. Cane toads and many tree frogs are poisonous and should only be kept by specialists.

Fish

Fish are cold blooded. Nearly all fish are completely aquatic. The fish are divided into the bony fish which have an ossified skeleton (such as cod, goldfish, trout); and the cartilaginous fish which have a cartilaginous skeleton (such as the sharks and rays).

Cold-water fish are popular pets. Goldfish, Koi carp and orfe are commonly kept as pets.

Tropical fish are also kept in large numbers in the UK. Many species are kept but those encountered commonly include tetras, mollies, guppies, Siamese fighting fish, cichlids, angelfish and a variety of loaches and catfish.

Brackish water and salt-water fish are more difficult to keep and are seen less frequently. To keep fish in good condition an owner must invest in good quality tanks and equipment such as pumps, lighting heaters and filters.

The water quality in the fish tank should be monitored and the temperature should not be allowed to fluctuate.

Fish food is readily available commercially but care must be taken not to overfeed fish because this results in spoilage of the water.

Fish welfare can easily be overlooked but poor husbandry can cause the fish considerable distress.

Exotic animal accommodation

See Level 2, 2.4.03.

Feeding exotics

See Level 2, 2.4.03.

Rabbits

Note that it is normal for rabbits to practice **coprophagia**. The first time food passes through the digestive system it is only partially digested and it emerges from the anus as a **caecotroph**. This is eaten immediately and is completely digested during its second pass through the digestive system. Rabbits which are unable to eat the caecotrophs (due to injury, obesity or dental disease) may suffer from weight loss and digestive disorders.

Reptiles

Red-eared terrapins are predominantly carnivorous and should be fed on a fish-based diet, eg herring, sardines, pilchards and other small whole fish. Appropriate calcium and phosphorus supplementation should be provided. As many terrapins prefer to eat in the water care should be taken that any uneaten food is removed to prevent spoiling of the water.

Wildlife patients

See Level 2, 2.4.26.

Remember that the aim of treating wildlife casualties is a return to the wild. Few species (with the exception of hedgehogs, rabbits and some bird species such as crows) will adapt to living in captivity. If an animal is too badly injured euthanasia should be considered.

It is illegal to release non-indigenous (non-native) species into the wild in the UK. Non-indigenous species include grey squirrels, rabbits and some species of deer (muntjac, Chinese water deer).

Similar safety principles apply for restraint and transport of wildlife casualties.

- Injured birds can cause themselves further injury by flapping their wings in panic. The wings should be held to the bird's side. This can be achieved by wrapping the bird lightly in material. Do not obstruct the bird's airway. Special carrying bags are available for the safe transport of large birds such as geese and swans.
- Large exotic birds such as parrots have strong beaks which can easily remove a human finger.
- Birds of prey have extremely sharp, strong beaks and claws.
- If an animal is caught in netting or has fishing line in its beak the excess material should be cut away but do not try to remove material which is wrapped tightly unless respiration is being obstructed. This material should be removed under control at the surgery.
- Fish should obviously be transported in water. If possible they should be transported in the water in which they were living rather than tap water.
- Amphibians should be transported in a moist container (eg a plastic container lined with moist kitchen paper). They should not normally be transported in water because of the risk of drowning in very weakened animals.
- Potentially dangerous exotic animals such as snakes and spiders should not be handled directly. A blanket can be thrown over them and the animal moved with the blanket into a container. Snakes can be carried in a cloth bag.

Never handle bats without wearing gloves. Bats can transmit a virus which is similar to rabies.

Wild animals panic less if they are transported in the dark. A blanket should be thrown over the carrying box. Deer should have a blindfold placed gently over the eyes to prevent panic.

3.11.02 Anatomy and physiology

What you need to learn

🐾 You need to be able to describe anatomical landmarks in mammals, birds, reptiles and chelonia:

* 🐾 birds – types of feathers. How to clip feathers correctly, beak, position of air sacs, cloaca
* 🐾 rodents – lagomorphs
* 🐾 reptiles – cloaca, Jacobson's organ in snakes, 'third eye' in iguanas, hemipenes in reptiles, lack of diaphragm in some reptiles and birds, tail spectacle scale in snakes, the position of the ventral midline vein in lizards, dorsal tail vein in snakes and chelonians
* 🐾 chelonians – structure of shell, carapace and plastron, hinge, the names of the scutes of the shell (eg vertebral, pleural, marginal and cervical scutes), jugular vein and dorsal tail vein.

🐾 Recognise normal digit number:

* 🐾 birds – parrots, canaries, finches, raptors (parrots have a different digit number), rodents, lagomorphs, green iguana (state reasons lizards may lose digits).

🐾 Describe dentition of various species and identify abnormalities:

* 🐾 rodents and lagomorphs – overgrown incisors, hooked molars, malocclusion.

🐾 Identify obvious anatomical differences in skeletal structure:

* 🐾 birds, rodents, lagomorphs, reptiles, amphibians, and fish.

🐾 Describe features of digestive system:

* 🐾 carnivores, omnivores, herbivores, reptiles (snakes, lizards, chelonia) and fish.

🐾 Describe optimal environment for each species:

* 🐾 reptiles – Burmese python, com snake, bearded dragon, leopard gecko, veiled chameleon
* 🐾 Birds – budgie, parrot, finch, Harris hawk, duck
* 🐾 Chelonia – Mediterranean tortoise, red-eared terrapin.

🐾 Describe normal urinary deposits in various species:

* 🐾 birds, rodents, lagomorphs and reptiles.

🐾 Identify normal feeding requirements and feeding patterns for each species:

* 🐾 birds, finches, parrots, raptors, fowl, rodents Vit C in guinea pigs, lagomorphs and reptiles – snakes, insectivorous lizards, carnivorous lizards, vegetarian lizards, Mediterranean tortoises, red-eared terrapins.

Birds

For the skeletal system, see Level 2, 2.3.04.

Feathers are unique to birds and are vital for providing insulation and the ability to fly (in most species). Feathers vary greatly in their structure and function. The **primary feathers** provide the forward thrust during flight. The **secondary feathers** provide the lift which keeps the bird in the air.

To prevent flight some owners request that their bird's flight feathers are clipped. Usually the feathers of just one wing should be clipped so that the bird is less aerodynamic. The primary feathers should be clipped one at a time to the level of the covert feathers so that the feather stump is not visible. The last few primaries should be left to retain the contour and appearance of the wing. It should be remembered that many birds with clipped wings are still able to glide and should not be left unattended.

The **air sacs** extend from the lungs through the body cavity and into some hollow bones. Gas exchange does not occur in these air sacs.

Birds do not possess a diaphragm. The combined thoracic and abdominal cavities are instead called the coelomic cavity. Respiratory movement is mainly provided by the abdominal muscles. Care must therefore be taken not to restrict this movement when handling birds.

In birds the gastrointestinal tract terminates in the **cloaca** which receives the excreted products of the urinary and digestive tracts.

Reptiles

The gastrointestinal tract terminates in the **cloaca** which receives the excreted products of the urinary and digestive tracts. Most reptiles do not possess a diaphragm. The combined thoracic and abdominal cavities are instead called the coelomic cavity.

In chelonia the action of moving the forelimbs allows air to move in and out of the lungs, as the ribs are fused and rigid in these animals.

Blood samples can be taken from the jugular vein or the dorsal tail vein in most reptile species. The ventral midline vein can also be used in lizards.

Snakes possess a sensory organ called the **Jacobson's Organ** (or vomeronasal organ) which contributes to their keen sense of smell. The Jacobson's organ is a pit in the roof of the mouth which picks up scent particles which have been picked up from the snake's tongue.

In snakes the eye is covered by a transparent scale called the **spectacle**.

Many lizards possess a photoreceptive 'third eye'. This is actually the pineal gland which is situated beneath a transparent scale on the dorsal surface of the head. It is thought to play a role in thermoregulatory behaviour and possibly reproduction.

The copulatory organs in male snakes and lizards are the paired **hemipenes**. These normally lie internally at the base of the tail.

During mating they are extruded and semen runs along a groove on the outer surface.

The appendicular skeleton

See Level 2, 2.3.10.

Teeth

See Level 2, 2.3.61.

Birds

Birds possess a horny beak rather than teeth. In birds the shape and function of the beak depends on the lifestyle and diet of the species.

Reptiles

Chelonians posses a horny beak rather than teeth.

Some carnivorous reptiles such as crocodilians possess teeth which are used for slicing prey. In snakes the teeth are often modified to inject venom into prey and can sometimes be retracted.

The digestive system

See Level 2, 2.3.35.

Urinary sediments seen in exotic species

Birds and reptiles excrete the majority of nitrogenous waste as **uric acid** and **urates** (compared with most mammals which excrete nitrogenous waste as urea). These urates form the normal white crystals which are seen in the urine of birds and reptiles.

There is great variation in the colour of normal rabbit urine. The variation in colour is caused by a variety of pigments which come from plant material and can range from white through to dark red. Rabbits excrete excess calcium via the urine as calcium carbonate. This results in creamy urine. Struvite crystals can also be found in small amounts in normal rabbit urine.

Other herbivorous rodents such as guinea-pigs can show a similar range of colour for normal urine.

Feeding requirements

See Level 2, 2.4.21.

Red-eared terrapins are predominantly carnivorous, and should be fed on a fish-based diet such as herring, sardines, pilchards and other small whole fish. Appropriate calcium and phosphorous supplementation should be provided. As many terrapins prefer to eat in the water care should be taken that any uneaten food is removed to prevent spoiling of the water.

3.11.03 Housing

What you need to learn

- You need to be able to explain the optimum and acceptable housing requirements of any individual species based upon a knowledge of the animal's biology and basic requirements:
  - heat, lighting and guarding of heating and lighting to prevent injury of animal, humidity, substrate, cage furniture, type of enclosure for different species, perch types for birds, cage toys, cage locks, outdoor runs/aviaries, cage security to prevent escape.

See Level 2, 2.4.03.

Rabbits and rodents

Numerous cages are available commercially for rabbits and rodents. Small rodents should be provided with escape-proof accommodation which cannot easily be damaged through gnawing. The cage should allow the animal as much room as possible.

The environment should be enriched to allow the animal to express normal behaviour. This can be achieved by providing objects of interest to the animal.

3.11.04 Management and nutrition

What you need to learn

- You need to be able to outline the management, nutrition and general husbandry including basic breeding of species variation:
  - gestation period and breeding for cornsnake, live bearing snakes (boas, garter snake) egg incubation in snakes, lizards, chelonia and birds.
  - gestation periods for rat, rabbit, chinchilla, guinea pig
  - importance of Ca and Vit D3 in the diet of reptiles and importance of Vit C in guinea pig diet
  - humidity levels for birds and reptiles
  - food container placement for birds, reptiles and chelonians
  - importance of feeding individually and recording food intake
  - importance of record keeping, particularly daily temperature, humidity, feeding records and shedding records.

❧ State the common foods and feeding methods of the common animals and birds kept as pets including common foods and feeding methods:
  ❧ insectivores
  ❧ vegetarians
  ❧ omnivores
  ❧ carnivores
  ❧ lizards
  ❧ snakes
  ❧ chelonia
  ❧ birds
  ❧ rodents.
❧ Describe safe handling methods for common species including wildlife:
  ❧ snake hooks
  ❧ gloves
  ❧ identification of venomous species
  ❧ safe handling of birds
  ❧ aggressiveness of wild animals.
❧ Describe the use of assisted feeding and oral therapy in some species and the correct method for placing a nasogastric tube:
  ❧ stomach tube placement in chelonia to facilitate tube feeding
  ❧ types of food stuffs that can be used for tube feeding
  ❧ calorific values.
❧ Outline the accessible intravenous sites in common species:
  ❧ ventral tail vein in lizards and snakes
  ❧ jugular vein in chelonia
  ❧ dorsal tail vein in lizards and chelonia
  ❧ jugular vein
  ❧ femoral vein and ventral wing vein in birds
  ❧ cephalic vein and marginal ear vein in rabbits
  ❧ cephalic, jugular and dorsal tail vein in rodents.
❧ Identify the intramuscular and subcutaneous injection sites in common species:
  ❧ injection site should be in the top third of the body in snakes
  ❧ front leg injection site in chelonia
  ❧ IM injection into the pectoral breast muscle of birds
  ❧ the scruff in rodents.
❧ Describe common diseases/conditions:
  ❧ nutritional diseases
  ❧ disease caused by poor husbandry
  ❧ dysecdysis in reptiles
  ❧ shell rot in chelonia
  ❧ retained spectacle in snakes
  ❧ feather picking/plucking in birds

* thiamine deficiency in garter snakes
* feather cysts in birds
* malocclusion in rodents and birds.

Breeding

Owners who are intending to breed their animals should be fully informed about the management of the pregnant animal. They should be aware of gestation periods so that any problem can be quickly identified. The young of some animals are born at a fairly immature stage. They are often blind, hairless and helpless. These offspring are called **altricial** neonates.

The young of other species are born at a more mature stage. They are able to see, have full coats and are generally more mobile. These are called **precocious** neonates.

Table 11.2

Species	Usual gestation period (days)	Type of young
Rat	20–22	Altricial
Mouse	19–21	Altricial
Rabbit	30–33	Altricial
Chinchilla	111	Precocious
Guinea-pig	59–72	Precocious
Chipmunks	31–32	Altricial
Gerbils	24–26	Altricial
Hamsters	15–18	Altricial

Reptiles

Most reptiles (including crocodilians, chelonia, most lizards, and many snakes) lay eggs (they are **oviparous**).

The oviparous snakes include corn snakes. Corn snakes lay their eggs 5–14 days after mating. The eggs are incubated at 80–83 °F in a substrate such as vermiculite. The incubation chamber should be kept at a humidity of 100% and the eggs should not be handled once they are in the chamber. Corn snake eggs hatch 58–66 days after they are laid.

Some snakes and lizards give birth to live young (without an egg). These are called **viviparous** species. Examples include boas and garter snakes. Garter snakes give birth to the young approximately 3–4 months after mating. There are usually 10–20 young. The young should be removed from the vivarium as the parents will eat the offspring if given the opportunity.

Ovo-viviparous species retain the eggs within the body until they are ready to hatch.

Chelonia are all oviparous. The eggs are incubated in a similar way to that described above for corn snake eggs. The sex of the hatchlings depends on the temperature at which the eggs are incubated. For example, for Mediterranean tortoises the clutch will all hatch as males if the incubation temperature is kept below 30°C. Above 30°C the hatchlings will all be female. If the temperature varies during incubation there will be a mixture of sexes in the clutch.

Birds

Birds are also all oviparous. The owner should familiarise themselves with the breeding cycle of their species. Birds incubate their own eggs under normal circumstances. The incubation period varies between species. It is 18 days in budgerigars, 21 days in cockatiels and approximately four weeks in larger birds such as macaws, African Grey parrots and Amazon parrots.

Safe handling methods for common exotic and wildlife species

See Level 2, 2.4.02.

Assisted feeding in exotics and wildlife

See Level 2, 2.4.16.

Intravenous sites in exotic species

Birds

The following are suitable sites in birds:

- **Jugular vein** – The bird should normally be anaesthetised unless it is large and very easily handled. The feathers are parted on the **right** side of the neck and the area over the vein is swabbed with surgical spirit. The vein is raised using gentle pressure on the distal portion of the vein. There is no need to remove any feathers. Care must be taken to apply pressure after venepuncture as haematomas commonly develop at this site.
- **Brachial vein** (ventral wing vein) – The wing is extended and the vein can be seen passing over the distal part of the elbow. The vein is raised using gentle pressure on the distal portion of the vein. Care must be taken to apply pressure after venepuncture as haematomas commonly develop at this site.
- **Medial metatarsal vein** – This vein can be used easily in large birds such as geese and swans. It passes over the medial aspect of the

proximal metatarsus. Haematomas do not form as easily as for the other veins.

Mammals

The following are suitable sites in mammals.

- **Cephalic vein** – This can be easily accessed in larger rodents and rabbits. The technique is the same as for cats and dogs.
- **Jugular vein** – This vein is in the same position as it is in dogs and cats. Smaller rodents need to be anaesthetised for the venepuncture as they are very difficult to restrain when conscious. Female rabbits often have a large dewlap which obscures the vein and makes this technique difficult.
- **Marginal ear vein** (rabbits) – This is the easiest method of venepuncture in most rabbits. The hair should be clipped over the outside of the lateral edge of the pinna. The vein passes along the edge of the pinna. An assistant raises the vein by applying gentle pressure at the base of the vein. Haematoma formation is avoided by applying gentle pressure for a few minutes after the needle is withdrawn.
- **Dorsal and lateral tail veins** (small rodents) – This procedure is easier if the veins are made more prominent by warming the tail first. The skin is cleaned to make the vein more visible. A very small needle such as an insulin needle is usually necessary to gain access to these veins.

Reptiles: Chelonia

The following are suitable sites in Chelonians.

- **Jugular vein** – The head is extended while the patient is restrained by an assistant. The jugular vein can often be seen passing from just caudal to the tympanic membrane caudally down the neck. The vein is more dorsal in chelonia than it is in mammals.
- **Dorsal tail vein** – The vein courses up the tail in the dorsal midline. It is often more difficult to use for venepuncture as it is smaller and is covered by thicker skin than the jugular vein.

Reptiles: Snakes and lizards

The following are suitable sites in snakes and lizards.

- **Ventral tail vein** – This vein passes up the ventral midline of the tail. It can easily be accessed in larger lizards and snakes.
- **Dorsal tail vein** – This is smaller and more difficult to use for blood sampling than the ventral tail vein.
- **Cardiac sampling** – This can be performed in anaesthetised snakes

without harm to the patient. It should only be performed by veterinary surgeons experienced in this technique.

Intramuscular and subcutaneous injection sites

Birds

Intramuscular injections should be given into the pectoral (breast) muscles.

Subcutaneous injections should be given under the loose skin around the neck, taking care to withdraw the plunger before injecting to ensure the needle is not in an airway or vessel.

Mammals

Intramuscular injections should be given into the quadriceps muscles or the hypaxial muscles over the rump.

Subcutaneous injections should be given under the loose skin over the scruff of the neck or thorax.

Reptiles

In reptiles injections should always be given in the cranial half of the body. This is because some reptiles possess a renal portal blood supply which bypasses the rest of the circulation. This means that unusually high doses of medication will enter the kidney because they have not been altered by other organs (particularly the liver). Many drugs are potentially nephrotoxic.

In chelonia the muscles of the forelimb can be used for intramuscular injection. In snakes and lizards the longissimus muscles (on either side of the spine) are suitable for intramuscular injection.

Subcutaneous injections can be given under the looser skin in the neck area of most reptiles, taking care to withdraw the plunger before injecting to ensure the needle is not in an airway or vessel.

Common diseases and conditions in exotic species

Most of the diseases encountered in exotic species are as a direct result of poor husbandry and nutrition.

Dental disease

Dental disease is common in rodents, particularly the rabbit.

Nutritional disorders

Great care should be taken that the diet of reptiles contains sufficient calcium and phosphorus to prevent **metabolic bone disease**. This condition is caused by improper diet containing incorrect proportions of calcium and phosphorus, as well as inadequate access to natural sunlight leading to a deficiency of vitamin D3. A number of feed and natural light supplements are available and should always be used in conjunction with a balanced diet.

Some snakes are fish-eaters (eg garter snakes). Care should be taken when feeding them white fish as it contains an enzyme which causes **thiamine deficiency**. Freezing the fish increases thiaminase activity. Symptoms of thiamine deficiency are neurological disorders such as lack of co-ordination, convulsions and eventually death.

Disorders as a result of poor husbandry

Snakes should normally shed their skin in one or more large pieces. Piecemeal shedding is abnormal and is called **dysecdysis**. It is usually due to the humidity in the environment being too low or lack of provision of a bath for the animal to soak in. Scars can also cause difficulty in shedding.

Retained spectacles can be a consequence of dysecdysis in snakes. The spectacle scale covering the eye is retained. This can happen over a number of skin sheds so that a thick layer of spectacle builds up. These should be removed with great care and can take a few days of soaking with tear-replacement solutions.

Feather plucking in birds can be the result of infections or parasites but is often a sign of psychological disorders because of poor husbandry. If the bird is plucking its own feathers the feathers on the head will remain untouched as the bird cannot reach these with its beak. Treatment involves preventing the plucking using an Elizabethan collar; improving the nutrition; providing the bird with more attention and enriching the environment with toys, distractions and increased exercise. Birds also benefit from regular spraying with water. This prevents them from getting too dusty and then over-grooming.

Other diseases

Feather cysts are occasionally seen in birds. They are swellings at the base of the feathers which are sometimes mistaken for tumours.

Shell rot in chelonia is usually caused by a fungal infection. It may be a result of poor water quality in aquatic chelonia. The lesions can be treated using topical anti-fungal agents.

3.11.05 Pain assessment and welfare considerations

What you need to learn

❧ You need to be able to recognise signs of pain or distress exhibited by the various species:
  - ❧ normal/abnormal behaviour 'hunching' in rabbits, rodents
  - ❧ mouth gaping in lizards, snakes
  - ❧ recognise normal/abnormal breathing patterns.
❧ Outline pain assessments based on subjectivity, clinical indications and responses:
  - ❧ normal reflexes
  - ❧ normal vocalisations.
❧ Consider euthanasia as an alternative.
❧ Demonstrate knowledge of the current legislation and policies, both nationally and locally with regard to the keeping and handling of exotics and wildlife:
  - ❧ Dangerous Wild Animals Act, Local council licensing, release of wildlife.

Many exotic species and wild animals are prey animals so avoid showing signs of pain, as any weakness could be detected by a predator. This often results in illness being overlooked by the owner until it is advanced and can no longer be disguised by the animal.

Care must be taken to observe an animal for subtle changes in behaviour which could suggest that the animal is unwell or in pain.

A report from an owner that an exotic animal is 'not himself' should therefore always be taken seriously and investigated.

Signs of pain include the following.

- Sick rabbits and rodents will be less mobile and often have a hunched stance.
- Tooth grinding (**bruxism**) is often a sign of pain.
- Elevated respiratory rate and effort can be a sign of pain or respiratory distress.
- Elevated heart rate can also be a sign of pain or distress.
- A sick animal or one in pain may show signs of aggression.
- Different vocalisations may be noted in painful or distressed animals. Rodents and rabbits may squeak when in distress. Birds vocalise when they are frightened or in pain.
- Refusal to eat and weight loss are usually a sign of ill health in exotics.
- Sick birds often have a hunched stance with ruffled feathers.
- Animals which are not normally easy to handle can become more

docile and do not resist handling as much when they are weakened by illness.

- The skin of brightly coloured reptiles may become dull when the animal is poorly.
- Reptiles may exhibit open-mouth breathing when in respiratory compromise.

Many exotic species and wild animals are presented for veterinary attention when they are in an advanced state of disease. If the animal is in intractable pain or is unlikely to recover to an acceptable level euthanasia should be considered as a humane alternative.

A number of laws and policies apply to exotic animals and wildlife. These must be followed by owners and the veterinary practice while these animals are being treated.

The **Dangerous Wild Animals Act** ensures that all potentially dangerous animals, such as poisonous reptiles, insects and spiders; primates (except marmosets); and wild cats, can only be kept by people with the appropriate licences. Licences are granted once housing, welfare and safety criteria have been met by the owner.

Dangerous animals such as those listed above must be reported to the local council and a licence must be granted to allow the owner to keep the animals on their premises.

A number of laws apply to wildlife. In particular it is illegal to release any animal into the wild which is not a native species. Non-native species include grey squirrels, rabbits and certain deer species. It is illegal to keep a wild animal in captivity unless it is in temporary captivity while an injury or illness is being treated.

3.11.06 Sexing

What you need to learn

- You need to be able to describe how sex of exotics is determined and knowledge of sexing sexually dimorphic avian species:
  - small mammals
  - budgerigars
  - tortoises
  - snakes and reptiles
  - sexing of cockatoos, cockatiels and eclectus parrots can be 'by sight'
  - endoscopic sexing of bird species which do not show sexual dimorphism
  - DNA sexing of birds.
- Knowledge of methods of sexing snakes, reptiles and birds:
  - hemipenal probing of snakes and large lizards

❧ presence of enlarged femoral pores and enlarged hemipenal bulges in large species of lizards
❧ endoscopic sexing of lizards.

Birds

See Level 2, 2.3.61.

3.11.07 Transport

What you need to learn

❧ You need to be able to outline the most acceptable method of transporting exotics:
  ❧ use of wire transport carriers
  ❧ reptile bags
  ❧ security of transport vessel
  ❧ importance of maintaining temperature during the transport of reptiles
  ❧ importance of maintaining a stress-free environment when transporting birds (covered container with perch included)
  ❧ transporting rodents in an indestructible container.
❧ Value of subdued light with diurnal birds and mammals:
  ❧ for rest, breeding, stress factors.

Transportation of exotic and wild animals should be undertaken only when absolutely necessary and should be performed in a manner which causes the animal as little stress as possible.

Most mammals, reptiles and birds can be transported safely in a carrier constructed from wire. This is a strong material and prevents escape by larger animals.

Small mammals may need to be transported in a narrow-mesh wire cage to prevent them from escaping between the bars. If given enough time rodents are able to gnaw through plastic, wooden, or cardboard containers so these should only be used if the journey is short and supervised and if there is no better alternative.

Cloth bags or pillow cases can be used to transport snakes and large lizards. The top of the bag should be carefully sealed to prevent escape. The bag should be handled with care to protect the animal's body from injury.

The vehicle being used to transport the animal should also be secure, particularly if it is being left unattended even for a brief period.

Animals which escape from their cages must not be able to escape from the vehicle.

When transporting reptiles, fish, or amphibians, care must be taken to keep the animal's environment as similar to the home environment as possible. This usually involves controlling the temperature and the water quality and oxygenation where applicable.

Birds and some rodents (such as chinchillas and rabbits) are particularly sensitive to stress during transportation. These animals should always be covered during transportation as this makes them feel less vulnerable to predators.

Birds should be provided with a perch for transportation to make the journey as comfortable as possible. Most birds will be unaccustomed to standing on a flat surface.

Noise should be kept to a minimum when transporting any animal.

Lighting

Care should be given to the lighting when any diurnal exotic species is being kept.

In most households there will be light for up to 18 hours of the day. This is not a natural situation and can cause health problems.

Larger birds such as parrots and macaws will become over-tired if they are not allowed sufficient sleep. These birds should be allowed a natural day length and then should be covered and kept away from noise. This encourages them to sleep.

Some species such as cockatiels will lay eggs persistently if the day length is too long. Again the photoperiod should be reduced in these animals.

Multiple choice questions

1. Pigeons are classified into which of the following orders of birds:
   - ☐ A Falconiformes
   - ☐ B Passeriformes
   - ☐ C Galliformes
   - ☐ D Columbiformes

2. Axolotls are
   - ☐ A chelonians
   - ☐ B amphibians
   - ☐ C lizards
   - ☐ D crocodilians

3. Geckos are
   - ☐ A herbivorous
   - ☐ B carnivorous
   - ☐ C insectivorous
   - ☐ D omnivorous

4. Following recovery which of the following wildlife casualty species would you not return to the wild:
   - ☐ A Sparrow
   - ☐ B Hedgehog
   - ☐ C Fox
   - ☐ D Grey squirrel

5. Considering birds, which of the following is NOT true:
   - ☐ A the coelomic cavity encloses the air sacs
   - ☐ B gas exchange occurs in the air sacs
   - ☐ C the keel is an enlarged sternum
   - ☐ D the pelvic bones are hollow and fused

6. Which of the following species has the dental formula $\frac{1003}{1003}$: (Refer back to Level 2).
   - ☐ A Guinea pig
   - ☐ B Lagomorph
   - ☐ C Ferret
   - ☐ D Rat

7. Some species of snakes and lizards reproduce without producing eggs. They are known as
   - ☐ A viviparous
   - ☐ B oviparous
   - ☐ C altricial
   - ☐ D precocious

8. The most accessible vein for venipuncture in a rabbit would be the
   - ☐ A brachial
   - ☐ B jugular
   - ☐ C cephalic
   - ☐ D marginal ear

9. Abnormal skin shedding in captive snakes is known as
   - ☐ A dacryocystitis
   - ☐ B dysecdysis
   - ☐ C autotomy
   - ☐ D demodicosis

Level 3: Unit 12

Managing resources

3.12.01 Ordering and receiving supplies

What you need to learn

- You need to be able to describe methods to identify supplies of veterinary material required to maintain working stock levels:
  - manual
  - electronic
  - stock rotation.
- Describe working procedures for placing an order for veterinary supplies:
  - telephone
  - post
  - electronic.
- Outline handling problems involved in maintaining the condition of different veterinary materials upon delivery:
  - vaccines
  - sterile supplies
  - controlled drugs, etc.
- Identify, upon delivery, stock condition (ie damaged) and discrepancies and understand the reporting and returning procedures for:
  - drugs
  - sterile supplies
  - consumables
  - stationery.
- Describe the format of delivery documentation and the importance of checking received stock against delivery note accurately.
- Outline correct handling of packaging materials and their disposal.

Identifying stock levels

This can be done either:

- manually – by physically counting stock content or
- electronic – computer systems record the stock level then delete the amount of stock as items are sold or used.

Stock must be rotated – newly purchased items should be placed at the rear of the stock, any items with short sell-by-dates or soon-to-expire dates should be placed at the front and veterinary surgeons should be informed.

Placing an order

This can be done:

- over the telephone
- by post – certain controlled drugs require original prescriptions to be sent in the post
- electronically – the computer deletes stock items as they are used or sold, it will automatically add these items to the order which is then transmitted by modem.

Maintaining conditions of materials upon delivery

Vaccines need to be signed for as a fridge item and then placed in the fridge immediately. The expiry date should also be checked.

Sterile supplies will be delivered pre-sterilised. Check that there is no damage to the outer packaging and store the supplies in the appropriate cupboards. The expiry date should also be checked.

Some **controlled drugs** require a signature from the veterinary surgeon which is then posted back to the supplier. All controlled drug items should then be entered as purchases in the controlled drug register (within 24 hours) and placed in the controlled drug cabinet.

Receiving stock

All stock delivered should be checked for the following.

- Expiry date – Drugs should have a long shelf life.
- Damage – Both the packaging and the item itself should be checked.
- Strength of drug – Is the strength correct?
- Amount – Has the correct amount been sent?
- Food – Is it the correct diet amount and pack-size?

These checks apply to:

- drugs
- sterile supplies
- consumables
- stationery
- food.

Delivery documentation

All deliveries will come with an invoice stating the contents and the amount of the contents within the order. The items in the order should be checked against those listed on the invoice for, amount, strength, correct item name and size. Once checked, tick the item on the invoice so that it is visible that examination of the order has been carried out. This invoice should then be compared with the order placed by the practice to ensure that the items ordered are the items that have been received.

Correct handling and disposal of packaging

It may be necessary to wear gloves when handling packaging. All packaging should be handled carefully and without mess. Dispose of packaging such as paper or cellophane wrapping in the office waste or paper-waste bin. Glass should be disposed of in a dedicated glass bin.

3.12.02 Maintaining stock quality

What you need to learn

* You need to be able to describe suitable methods for ensuring stock is kept at its optimum condition:
  * stock rotation
  * monitoring of storage areas eg fridge temperatures, expiry dates.
* Outline correct disposal of surplus and outdated waste veterinary materials with the knowledge of health and safety guidelines and medicine legislation:
  * Legislation: Health and Safety at Work Act 1974
  * Control of Substances Hazardous to Health (COSHH) Regulations 1999
  * Misuse of Drugs Act 1971, Misuse of Drugs Regulations 1985.

Stock levels

It is important that stock is maintained at its optimum condition. This can be done by following the guidelines below.

* **Stock rotation** – Place newly acquired stock at the back of old stock. Use old stock first.
* **Monitoring storage areas** – Areas such as the fridge containing vaccines and some drugs should be checked daily for correct temperature (2–8 °C), that they are working correctly and that they are not leaking.
* **Expiry dates** – All items should have their expiry dates checked

weekly. This prevents stock going out of date; out-of-date stock cannot be sold. Rotate stock accordingly.

- **Drugs** – Unless otherwise stated on the drug data, all drugs should be stored at room temperature.

Disposal of surplus and out of date stock

The disposal of stock is governed by some important Acts and Regulations:

- Health and Safety at Work Act 1974
- Control of Substances Hazardous to Health (COSHH) Regulations 1999
- Misuse of Drugs Act 1971
- Misuse of Drugs Regulations 1985.

Drugs

Drugs that are not controlled drugs are disposed of in special pharmaceutical bins; any containers contaminated with drugs, eg empty injection bottles or vaccines bottles, should also be disposed of in this bin. A written record of the drug name and quantity disposed of should be kept (the practice can be fined if this written record is not performed).

Controlled drugs

Disposal of these agents needs to be supervised by a member of the Home Office or a policeman. The name of the disposed drug and the amount disposed should then be entered in the controlled-drug register.

3.12.03 Veterinary practice equipment

What you need to learn

- You need to be able to outline different equipment commonly used in veterinary practice:
  - surgical (powered/manual)
  - diagnostic
  - laboratory
  - imaging
  - anaesthetic.
- Identify where equipment and equipment parts may be obtained if replacements or repairs are required.
- Describe possible faults for commonly used equipment in veterinary practice.

♣ Outline practice protocol for ensuring equipment is maintained and faults identified and responded to.

♣ Outline the principles of record keeping with regard to equipment maintenance.

Commonly used equipment

A wide variety of equipment is used in veterinary practice.

- **Surgical powered**
  - drills
  - diathermy equipment
  - suction equipment
  - cryosurgery equipment
  - steriliser
  - electric clippers
  - operating lights.
- **Surgical manual**
  - instruments
  - kidney dishes and bowls
  - nail clippers.
- **Diagnostic imaging**
  - X-ray machine
  - ultrasound machine
  - endoscopes.
- **Laboratory**
  - wet or dry chemistry analyses
  - haematology reading equipment
  - centrifuge
  - microscope.
- **Imaging** – see Diagnostic imaging.
- **Anaesthetic equipment**
  - anaesthetic machine
  - circuits
  - endotracheal tubes
  - pulse oximeters
  - capnograph
  - blood pressure reading machine
  - oesophageal stethoscope
  - electrocardiogram (ECG).

If new equipment or parts for equipment are required, either to replace or repair the existing equipment, contact the supplier of the equipment or the manufacturer.

Common faults

Surgical equipment can suffer from the following faults:

• electrical faults, eg blown fuse, blown light bulbs, loose wires
• faults with heating elements, eg in diathermy equipment, steriliser
• broken, damaged or blunt instruments/clipper blades.

Diagnostic imaging equipment can have the following faults:

• X-ray machine continuing to expose after the radiograph has been taken
• failure of the X-ray machine to turn on
• anode not spinning
• damage to transducers on ultrasound machines
• dirty, scratched or broken lenses on endoscopes
• electrical faults, eg blown fuse.

In the **laboratory** the equipment can suffer from:

• blockage of dry analyses
• electrical faults, eg blown fuse or light bulbs
• abnormal readings of biochemistry and haematology machines
• dirty, scratched or broken lenses on the microscope.

Anaesthetic equipment can have the following problems:

• vaporisers may stick
• leaks in the tubing of circuits
• cuffs of endotracheal tubes may not inflate because of a tear or leak
• bobbins of flowmeters not spinning – fault with flowmeter
• Bodock washers may be missing on cylinder connections – causes hissing of gas
• electrical faults, eg blown fuse
• abnormal readings on monitoring equipment.

Equipment should be checked daily for any faults. Faults identified should be reported immediately to the head nurse or to the practice manager. In the case of faults with the X-ray machine the report should be to the radiation protection supervisor.

Any equipment repairs or maintenance carried out by professional engineers should be noted in a record book or file specific to that piece of equipment. Any maintenance reports, contracts, or repair work carried out will have a report issued by the engineer. This should be filed in a file specific to that piece of equipment.

Level 3

Multiple choice answers

Unit 5: Diagnostic aids

1. Answer: C.
   (A) RIDDOR: These regulations describe the procedures which must take place if death, serious injury or work-related diseases occur in the workplace.
   (B) Health and Safety at Work Act: This is designed to maintain and improve health and safety standards at work.
   (D) Collection and Disposal of Waste Regulations describes the safe handling and disposal of products including clinical waste and chemicals.

2. Answer: B.
   The total magnification of a specimen under a microscope is the power of the objective lens times the power of the eye-piece. The total magnification with the × 10 objective if the eye-piece magnification was also 10 would be $10 \times 10 = 100$. The object would therefore be magnified 100 times.

3. Answer: D.
   Pink is the answer because of the presence of the haemoglobin released from the damaged red blood cells.
   (A) milky: Presence of lipids resulting in lipaemia. Normal post feeding therefore the need to starve animals before taking a blood sample.
   (B) yellow: Presence of bilirubin indicative of liver damage.
   (C) clear: Normal canine and feline plasma is a clear pale straw coloured liquid.

4. Answer: A.
   The normal range in the dog is 37–55%.

5. Answer: B.
   Routine haematology includes total red and white red blood cell counts, differential white blood cell counts and PCVs.
   (A) Heparin: Biochemistry.
   (C) Sodium citrate: Clotting defects and prothrombin levels.
   (D) Fluoride oxalate: Glucose estimation.

6. Answer: D

7. Answer: B
   (B) Neutrophils are approximately 65%.
   (C) Lymphocytes are the next most common at 25% with monocytes and eosinophils making up a much lower %.

8. Answer: C.
   (A) Calcium: Hypercalcaemia.
   (B) Sodium: Hyperneutraemia.
   (D) Phosphate: Hyperphosphataemia.
   Hypo would be reduced levels.

9. Answer: B.
   (A) AST: Muscle and liver.
   (C) ALKP: Present in many body tissues.
   (D) Amylase: Digestive enzyme which comes mainly from the pancreas, liver and small intestine.

10. Answer: D.
    (A) ACTH stimulation test assesses cortisol levels.
    (B) TSH Stimulation test distinguishes hypothyroid animals from those with falsely low T4 levels.
    (C) Low Dose Dexamethasone test is used to diagnose Cushings.

11. Answer: B.
    Answer C is the normal range of specific gravity in the cat.

12. Answer: D.
    Triple phosphate.

13. Answer: C.
    (A) Felicola subrostratus: Biting louse of the cat.
    (B) Trichodectes canis: Biting louse of the dog.
    (C) Trixacarus caviae: Mite similar to sarcoptes found on guinea pigs rats and mice.

14. Answer: C
    The flea acts as the intermediate host in the lifecycle of Dipylidium caninum, the commonest tapeworm of the dog and cat.

15. Answer: B.
    The scolex (pleural scolices) is the head of the tapeworm from which the segments (proglottids) develop. The rostellum is the anterior part of the head often with hooks to facilitate the attachment of the parasite to the intestinal wall. Onchospheres are the tapeworm eggs.

16. Answer: C
    Man becomes the intermediate host.

17. Answer: B.
    Streptococci.

18. Answer: C
    An example of a facultative anaerobe is E coli.
    (A) Obligate anaerobes must have an air-free environment to grow.
    (B) Microaerophiles require a lower amount of oxygen than normal but cannot survive without oxygen.
    (D) Obligate aerobes must have oxygen to grow.

19. Answer: A
    Selective for Salmonella.
    (B) and (C) are enriched media which encourage the growth of more fastidious bateria.
    (D) is a simple media.

20. Answer: B.
    (A) Methylated spirit causes excessive shrinkage of the sample.
    (C) Potassium hydroxide is used to clear skin samples to enable the parasites to be seen.
    (D) Boric acid is used as a urinary preservative especially if bacteriological examination is required.

Unit 6: Medical nursing

1. Answer D.
   Option (A) is distemper virus, (B) is a spiral shaped flexible virus responsible for Leptospirosis or Lyme disease and (C) rabies is caused by a rhabdovirus.

2. Answer A.
   Lyme disease is one example of a disease spread by tick bites. Fomites are inanimate objects which may transmit the disease. Kennel cough is transmitted by inhalation.

3. Answer D.
   Peritonitis results in pyrexia and anorexia, chlamydiosis causes an ocular discharge and rhinitis and calici virus is upper respiratory tract disease.

4. Answer A.
   Viruses contain either DNA or RNA, not both.

5. Answer B.
   This is an accidental host. There is development in intermediate and biological hosts, while the definitive is the final host

6. Answer A.
   Convalescent carriers have recovered but continue to shed. Closed carriers do not release the organism.

7. Answer C.
   This is hypervitaminosis A.

8. Answer C.
   BER = 60 × 3 kg X disease factor for burns (2)

9. Answer C.
   A cation is positively charged.

10. Answer A.

11. Answer D.
    There would be high levels of PCV and plasma proteins and micturition would be less than normal.

12. Answer D.
    Maintenance = 50 ml/kg/day
    $$= 50 \times 10 \times 2 = 1000 \text{ ml}$$
    Surgery = 5-10 ml kg/hour = 100 ml
    Total = 1100 ml

13. Answer D.

14. Answer C.
    Required per hour = 2000 ÷ 12 =166.66
    Prequired per minute = 166.66 ÷ 60 = 2.77ml
    Giving set drip rate = 55.4 drops per minute

15. Answer A.
    The administration of nutrition by injection would be quicker and easier via the jugular vein.

16. Answer B.
    Store at 5 °C. Blood transfused into a syringe with EDTA should be used within 48 hours, with citrate phosphate dextrose as the anticoagulant the blood can be stored for four weeks, and plasma can be frozen for three months.

17. Answer D.
    Options (A) and (B) are symptoms of overinfusion of a fluid. Muscular tremors may be evident but not bradycardia.

18. Answer D.
    TPR would be most likely to indicate unusual reactions.

19. Answer C.
    A prion is also an infectious agent.

20. Answer C.
    Antibodies are produced by the animal in response to the antigen in the vaccine.

21. Answer B.
    These are antibodies which are specific to the foreign antigen.

22. Answer A.
    Adjuvants are used in killed vaccines to enhance the normally short acting immune response.

23. Answer D.

24. Answer B.
    This poison is released when rancid fat is overheated, as in chip pan fires.

25. Answer C.
    An allergic skin condition known as atopic dermatitis. Usually results from allergens such as house dust mites, fungi and pollens.

26. Answer A.
    Chylothorax is the term which describes rupture of the thoracic duct, resulting in a thick, creamy white exudate in the pleural cavity.

27. Answer C.
    Inflammation of the naso-lacrimal duct. Epistaxis is also a possibility but dasolacrimal problems are most frequent.

28. Answer C.
    Gradual acquired thickening of the left atrio-ventricular valve results in endocardiosis and eventually left sided congestive heart failure.

29. Answer B.
    PDA allows blood to bypass the lungs in the foetus but should normally close off at birth.

30. Answer A.
    A regenerative anaemia describes a response by the bone marrow to a decrease in circulating erythrocytes.
    Haemobartonella felis damages red blood cells and is known as Feline Infectious Anaemia.

31. Answer D.
    Fresh blood in the faeces originates from the distal part of the alimentary tract. It may cause difficulty in passing faeces (dyschezia).

32. Answer D.
    A reduced flow of bile to the gut would most likely result in bilirubinuria which is apparent as orange urine.

33. Answer C.
    Increased amounts of urine would be unlikely unless the FLUTD was concurrent with renal disease.

34. Answer C.
    The clinical diet should support kidney function and should contain adequate amounts of high quality protein, low phosphorus and low sodium.

35. Answer A.
    The patient should not be touched and other external stimuli should be reduced until the veterinary surgeon can be informed. Anticonvulsant drugs may then be administered under the direction/ supervision of the Veterinary Surgeon.

36. Answer B.
    This disease is a deficiency in ADH or failure of the kidneys to respond to it. As a result the kidneys produce large amounts of dilute urine (low specific gravity).

37. Answer B.
    Muscle weakness and exercise intolerance is common. Thyroxine controls metabolism (BMR).

38. Answer D.
    Also known as metaphyseal osteopathy, this disease has an unknown origin, unlike nutritional hyperparathyroidism which is caused by feeding a diet low in calcium to growing large breeds.

39. Answer A.
    Inflammation of the uveal tract.

40. Answer D.
    Ear mite which is host specific to rabbits.

Unit 7: Diagnostic imaging

1. Answer A.
   More scatter is produced when a high Kv is employed, particularly over 70Kv.

2. Answer A.
   The remaining options all relate to the duties of the Radiation Protection Supervisor (RPS).

3. Answer C.
   Protective clothing is designed to protect only against scatter and should never be folded or mal-treated otherwise cracks may appear. Check for cracks by X-raying annually.

4. Answer C.
   The other options relate to the atom.

5. Answer B.
   The step down transformer supplies the mA to result in the thermionic emission.

6. Answer A.
   The focal spot is the target on the anode.

7. Answer B.
   Tungsten has a melting point of 3370°C.

8. Answer A.
   All of the other options would not absorb the radiation and so the resultant image would be black.

9. Answer B.
   Contrast is controlled by the amount of penetration, the kV.

10. Answer B.

11. Answer D.
    Slow film requires a long exposure but gives good detail because of the large amount of small fine phosphorescent crystals.

12. Answer C.
    The most suitable storage conditions are vertical storage in a cool, dark, low humidity area away from radiation.

13. Answer C.
    represents the amount by which the exposure should be increased to compensate for the amount (mAs) of the primary beam absorbed by the lead strips. The number of lines per cm and the grid ratio are an indication of the quality of the grid.

14. Answer B.
    The remaining options all relate to the developing solution.

15. Answer D.
    Exposure to white light before processing was complete would result in blackening of all parts of the emulsion.

16. Answer D.
    Ionic iodine preparations are relatively opaque and they exert a
    high osmotic pressure which makes them unsafe for
    myelography. Ionic media such as barium sulphate should
    ideally be used for alimentary studies but may result in adhesions
    if perforations are present.

17. Answer C.
    Cisternal puncture consists of injection of non ionic media into
    the cranial end of the subarachnoid space at the cisterna magna,
    just behind the skull.

18. Answer B.
    This is the most commonly used B mode, where the brightness of
    the dot represents the strength of the echo and movement can be
    seen.

19. Answer B.
    Fluid appears black, therefore a full bladder will give a better
    image, due to the increased contrast.

20. Answer D.
    Computed tomography is cross sectional radiographic scanning
    of a patient's tissues. The tube head moves around the moving
    table top during the exposure to image a different cross sectional
    slice of the tissue.

Unit 8: General Surgical Nursing

1. Answer C.
   The area would be erythematous (red) this together with the heat
   and swelling are all associated with an increase in blood flow to
   the inflammation site. The pain is caused by a combination of the
   irritating effect of toxic products and the swelling of the site
   which results in increased pressure on nerve endings.

2. Answer B.
   (A) An incised wound is produced by a sharp object eg glass
   and the damage is parallel to the skin.
   (B) A lacerated wound involves the tearing away of skin often
   known as a degloving injury.
   (C) A puncture wound is produced by a sharp object eg a tooth.
   They are usually perpendicular to the skin with only an entry
   wound but no evidence of an exit wound.

3. Answer D.
   (A) Organisation is the replacement of damaged tissue by scar tissue(connective tissue).
   (B) Re-epithelialisation is the re-growth of the epithelium it is the covering stage of wound healing.
   (C) Resolution is the situation when the tissue returns to its original state prior to the inflammatory damage.

4. Answer C.
   This could be caused by infection, decreased blood supply, seroma formation, poor surgical technique or post operative care.
   (A) ulceration.
   (B) cellulitis.
   (D) herniation.

5. Answer C.

6. Answer A.
   (B), (C) and (D) are passive drains which rely on gravity, capillary action and overflow from the wound.

7. Answer D.
   An example is a rectovaginal fistula.
   (A) a tear in the lining of a body cavity through which organs may protrude.
   (B) a localised area of pus.
   (C) a blind ending tract lined by granulation tissue.

8. Answer C.
   (A) retain moisture, rehydrate necrotic tissue and encourages sloughing.
   (B) contain significant amounts of water which facilitates rehydration of necrotic tissue. They should always be covered with a secondary dressing to prevent drying out of the area.
   (D) rehydrate necrotic tissue and encourage sloughing.

9. Answer A.
   (B) skin is taken from a separate area on the same patient.
   (C) a type of autogenous graft which is transferred with its blood supply.
   (D) skin taken from another patient but of a different species.

10. Answer A.

11. Answer C.
    An example is an aural haematoma.
    (A) benign tumour of fatty tissue.
    (B) a collection of serum in the tissue spaces.
    (C) benign tumour of fibrous tissue.

12. Answer B.
    (A) anchoring the stomach to the abdominal wall.
    (C) a temporary opening into the stomach.
    (D) removal of a portion of the stomach.

13. Answer C.
    (B) unproductive straining.

14. Answer A.
    Intussusception is telescoping of one section of the bowel into an
    adjoining portion. It is often associated with abnormal intestinal
    motility especially as a complication of diarrhoea.

15. Answer D.

16. Answer C.
    (A) difficulty breathing.
    (B) difficulty passing faeces.
    (D) difficulty passing urine.

17. Answer B.
    (A) there is other serious injury involved.
    (C) a fragment of bone is forced below its normal level. Seen in
    the skull.
    (D) the fracture is across one cortex only. An incomplete
    fracture.

18. Answer A.
    Commonly affects breeds with surplus facial skin folds such as
    Shar-Peis, Chows, Rottweilers and many other breeds.
    (B) eversion of the eyelid seen in St Bernards, Bassett Hounds,
    Bloodhounds and similar breeds.
    (C) overbrimming of tears.
    (D) surgical removal of the globe of the eye.

19. Answer C.

20. Answer B.
    (A) the use of radiation energy to selectively destroy neoplastic
    cells.
    (C) the use of medication to selectively destroy neoplastic cells.
    (D) removal of the bulk of a neoplasm without taking clear
    margins. Often performed on large benign tumours that are
    causing a mechanical problem.

Unit 9: Theatre practice

1. Answer C.
   (A) Disinfection.
   (B) Sepsis.
   (D) Antisepsis.

2. Answer B.

3. Answer A.
   Rubber, plastics and fabrics are damaged by this method of sterilisation.

4. Answer D.
   Most accurate method but delay on the results. Can be used in the autoclave, with ethylene oxide and in hot air ovens.
   (A) – Bowie–Dick tape changes from beige to black/dark brown which indicates it has been exposed to a temperature of 121 °C but gives no indication of exposure time. Can be used in an autoclave and with ethylene oxide changes from beige to green.
   (B) – TST strips (time, steam, temperature) An indicator spot at the end of the strip changes from yellow to purple once it has been exposed to the correct temperature for the correct time. Can be used in an autoclave and with ethylene oxide.
   (C) – Browne's tubes. Changes from red to green. Tubes available which change colour at different temperatures. The colour only indicates that a particular temperature has been reached but gives no indication of the exposure time. Can be used in an autoclave and with ethylene oxide.

5. Answer B.
   Ethylene oxide is toxic, irritant to tissues and highly flammable. COSSH regulations must be followed. Often impractical to use in practice.

6. Answer C.

7. Answer C.
   A sealed pack should remain sterile for a limitless period but it may become contaminated due to moisture, or excessive handling causing damage to the pack.

8. Answer B.
   The first drape should be placed between the surgeon and the patient to reduce the risk of a break in sterility by the surgeon coming into contact with the patient.

9. Answer B.

10. Answer D.
    Hohmann retractors are held by a gowned and gloved assistant in an aseptic manner to retract muscle and manipulate bone fragments and joints in orthopaedic procedures.
    The others are self-retaining retractors used to hold open incisions.

11. Answer B.

12. Answer A.
    Gillies needle holders used to hold the needle during suturing. They also incorporate a scissor part which can be used to cut the suture material.
    (B) Macphails – needle holders

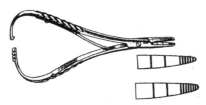

    (C) Metzenbaum scissors. Used for dissection, extending surgical wounds and for more delicate work.

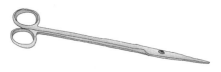

    (D) Heath scissors used for suture removal.

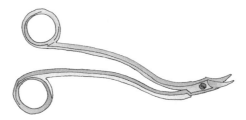

13. Answer C.
    Doyen bowel clamps. Longitudinal serrations are less traumatic to tissue than transverse serrations which tend to be used in haemostats.

14. Answer C.
    (A) and (B) are absorbed by hydrolysis. (D) is non-absorbable.

15. Answer B.
    (A) is multifilament.
    (C) is multifilament.
    (D) is non-absorbable.

16. Answer C.
    Cruciate mattress.

17. Answer C.
    (A) Clean. Where there is no break in asepsis, eg orthopaedic surgery.
    (B) Clean-contaminated. Where a contaminated area is entered but without spillage or spread of contamination.
    (D) Dirty. Where there is pus present or viscus perforation.

18. Answer B.
    Cats are particularly susceptible to laryngeal spasm Therefore the endotracheal tube should be removed before the laryngeal reflex returns. In dogs the endotracheal tube should be removed after the laryngeal reflex returns.

19. Answer D.
    Neonates and small animals are more susceptible to hypothermia because they have a higher surface area to weight ratio which increases heat loss.Geriatric animals are also at greater risk because of their decreased metabolic rate.

20. Answer C.
    This requires the most stringent aseptic technique to prevent the introduction of bacteria into the site with the risk of osteomyelitis developing.

Unit 10: Anaesthesia

1. Answer C.
   (A) Dyspnoea – difficulty breathing.
   (B) Tachypnoea – increased respiratory rate.
   (D) Apnoea – cessation of respiration.

2. Answer D.
   (A) Pethidine – opiate narcotic analgesic.
   (B) Carprofen – NSAID.
   (C) Acetyl promazine – Phenothiazine tranquilliser.

3. Answer B.
   (A) Atipamazole – reversal agent for medetomidine.
   (C) Acetyl promazine – phenothiazine tranquilliser.
   (D) Buprenorphine – opiate narcotic analgesic.

4. Answer A.
   (B) Thiopentone – barbiturate anaesthetic.
   (C) Saffan – steroid anaesthetic.
   (D) Halothane – inhalational anaesthetic.

5. Answer C.
   Dose required = weight of dog × dosage rate
   $$= 20 \times 10 = 200 \text{ mg}$$

   $$\text{Volume required} = \frac{\text{dose required}}{\text{mg/ml of drug}} = \frac{200}{25} = 8 \text{ ml}$$

6. Answer A.
   Dose required = weight of dog × dosage rate
   $$= 5 \times 0.1 = 0.5 \text{ mg}$$

   $$\text{Volume required} = \frac{\text{dose required}}{\text{mg/ml of drug}} = \frac{0.5}{5} = 0.1 \text{ ml}$$

7. Answer B.
   (C) Blue – nitrous oxide.
   (D) Grey – carbon dioxide.

8. Answer D.
   Causes syncope.

9. Answer C.
   The other three are non-depolarising muscle relaxants and need reversing by atropine/neostigmine.

10. Answer C.
    A 1% solution contains 1000 mg/100 ml
    ie 100 ml contains 1000 mg
    $$1 \text{ ml contains } \frac{1000}{100} \times 1 = 10 \text{ mg}$$

    Therefore a 2.5% solution will contain 2.5 times the amount contained in a 1% solution that is 25 mg/ml.

11. Answer A.
    (B) – minute volume.
    (C) – vital capacity.
    (D) – residual volume.

12. Answer D.
    Minute volume = Tidal volume × respiratory rate.
    TV = 5 × 15 = 75 ml
    MV = 75 × 20 = 1500 ml

13. Answer C.

14. Answer B.

15. Answer B.

16. Answer C.
    (A) and (B) are semi-closed circuits.
    A Water's canister is found in a to and fro circuit and contains sodalime which absorbs carbon dioxide.

17. Answer D.
    (A) electrocardiogram.
    (B) respiratory monitor.
    (C) pulse oximeter.

18. Answer B.

19. Answer C.
    TV = 20 × 10 = 200 ml
    MV = 200 × 15 = 3000 ml/min = 3 litres/min
    Circuit factor = equal to minute volume = 3litres/min

20. Answer D.
    (A) Atropine – anticholinergic – antisialogogue.
    (B) Diazapam – benzodiazepine.
    (C) Morphine – narcotic opioid analgesic.

Unit 11: Exotics and wildlife

1. Answer D.
   Includes pigeons and doves.

2. Answer B.
   An axolotl is the immature form of the amphibian salamander.

3. Answer C.
   Should be fed on a mix mealworms, locusts and crickets.

4. Answer D.
   This is a non-indigenous species in the UK and it is therefore illegal to return to the wild.

5. Answer B.
   Gaseous exchange occurs in the lungs. The air sacs suck air in and expel air.

6. Answer D.

7. Answer A.
   Snakes and lizards give birth to live young.

8. Answer D.

9. Answer B.

Level 3

Index